12-Lead
EKG Confidence

Step-by-Step to Mastery

12-Lead EKG Confidence

Step-by-Step to Mastery

Jacqueline M. Green, MS, RN, APN.C
Coordinator,a Center for Congenital Heart Disease
Newark Beth Israel Medical Center
Newark, New Jersey

Anthony J. Chiaramida, MD, FACC
Clinical Associate Professor of Medicine
University of Medicine and Dentistry of New Jersey
Director, Division of Cardiology
Raritan Bay Medical Center
Perth Amboy, New Jersey

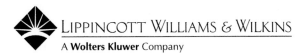
LIPPINCOTT WILLIAMS & WILKINS
A **Wolters Kluwer** Company
Philadelphia • Baltimore • New York • London
Buenos Aires • Hong Kong • Sydney • Tokyo

Acquisitions Editor:
Managing Editor: Joe Morita
Editorial Assistant: Megan Klim
Senior Project Editor: Tom Gibbons
Senior Production Manager: Helen Ewan
Managing Editor / Production: Erika Kors
Design Coordinator: Brett MacNaughton
Cover Designer: Christopher Shea
Interior Designer: Holly Reid McLaughlin
Manufacturing Manager: William Alberti
Indexer:
Compositor: Peirce Graphics
Printer: Quebecor

9 8 7 6 5 4 3 2 1

Library of Congress Cataloging-in-Publication Data

Green, Jackie, M.
   12-lead EKG confidence : step-by-step to mastery / Jackie M. Green, Anthony J. Chiaramida.
      p. ; cm.
   Includes index.
   ISBN 0-7817-3921-7 (pbk.)
   1. Electrocardiography. I. Title: Twelve-lead EKG confidence. II. Chiaramida, Anthony J. III. Title.
   [DNLM: 1. Electrocardiography—methods—Programmed Instruction. WG 18.2 G796 2003]
RC683.5.E5.G685 2003
616.1′207547—dc21

2002043364

Care has been taken to confirm the accuracy of the information presented and to describe generally accepted practices. However, the authors, editors, and publisher are not responsible for errors or omissions or for any consequences from application of the information in this book and make no warranty, express or implied, with respect to the content of the publication.

The authors, editors, and publisher have exerted every effort to ensure that drug selection and dosage set forth in this text are in accordance with the current recommendations and practice at the time of publication. However, in view of ongoing research, changes in government regulations, and the constant flow of information relating to drug therapy and drug reactions, the reader is urged to check the package insert for each drug for any change in indications and dosage and for added warnings and precautions. This is particularly important when the recommended agent is a new or infrequently employed drug.

Some drugs and medical devices presented in this publication have Food and Drug Administration (FDA) clearance for limited use in restricted research settings. It is the responsibility of the health care provider to ascertain the FDA status of each drug or device planned for use in his or her clinical practice.

With love, I dedicate this book to my family who made all this possible, especially my children Caroline and Conor, who were an endless source of encouragement.

Thank you to my Mom, and my Dad, who would have been so proud.

I am forever grateful to Irene Sobolewski who has worked by my side for 11 years, sharing her love and devotion with my family. None of this would have been possible without you.

Thank you to Katherine McGinley for her lifelong love, support and friendship.

A special thank you to my co-author Anthony Chiaramida. You shared with me your dream, your knowledge and your excellence as a cardiologist and teacher. Your belief in me never wavered, and your steadfast loyalty proved to be an inspiration. A simple thank you will never be enough.

- **Jacqueline Green**

To my parents . . . who inspired and taught

my father, Joseph, the doctor I always aspired to be, who taught me that charity and love were the same thing . . .

my mother, Dina, who gave me the notion that I could do anything, and taught me how to find the silver linings along the way . . .

To my children . . . who believed and never stopped

my daughter, Jennifer, the angel of music in so many ways,

my son, Joseph, the open minded, the healer,

my son, Matthew, the wise and knowing.

To my sibs . . . who made such a high standard to follow

my sister Annita ("Teacher of the Year"), whom I have tried to emulate since I was 5 years old

my brother Salvatore ("One of the Best Doctors in NYC," for Pete's sake), who knows everything, and shares it all

To my most difficult student . . .

With whom I tried and failed, always and only . . .

and to you, Jackie . . .

for all that you've endured . . .

who made a dream, that could never be, come true . . .

and who made dreams worth having again . . .

- **Anthony Chiaramida**

Reviewers

Patricia M. Biteman, RN, MSN
Lecturer, Clinical Instructor
Humboldt State University
Arcata, California

Janice M. Judy, RN, MSN
Instructor
University of Nebraska
Scottsbluff, Nebraska

Joan Klemballa, RN, FNP-C, PhD
Professor
Mountain State University
Beckley, West Virginia

Elizabeth M. Long, RN, MSN, CNS, SGNP
Nursing Instructor
Lamar University
Beaumont, Texas

Mary B. Neiheisel, CNS, CFNP, BSN, MSN, EdD
Director, Professor of Nursing
Nursing Graduate Program
University of Louisiana at Lafayette
Lafayette, Louisiana

Nan Smith-Blair, RN, PhD
Assistant Professor
Eleanor Mann School of Nursing
University of Arkansas
Fayetteville, Arkansas

Lisa Wehner, MSN
Associate Professor
State University of New York at Delhi
Delhi, New York

Author's Note

In many ways, teaching is like taking students on a train ride. The goal of a teacher is to get the trainload of students from New York City to California, without losing anyone along the way. The train ride can't take forever, but if it travels too quickly, students "fall off" the train, and the excursion is for naught. The train ride can't have too many side stops or too few. The train should arrive at a destination clear to the student and to the teacher alike. The teacher must have a clear vision and travel a navigable path to that end. **Our goal here is to teach the ability to form an autonomous, useful opinion about any 12-lead EKG.** Many books exist. Some are short, easy rides that do not get to the destination we envision. Others are laborious tomes that serve for reference only.

We believe this book is unique because it uses a step-by-step method, reinforced by practice EKGs. In Chapter 20, the student forms a complete, autonomous opinion about a selection of 12-lead EKGs. We expect the student to be successful because we have used this method for 20 years with a variety of students. It is an achievable goal. We have taken students there many times. The opinion the student forms will be based on comprehension, which always makes memorization simpler. Other EKG books typically rely on EKG interpretation by pattern memorization and never discuss the basis for these patterns.

The first three chapters of the book discuss basic principles of anatomy and physiology and include a review of the heart's electrical system. It is not an exhaustive introduction, and it sacrifices density for clarity. The remaining 16 chapters introduce one concept at a time and build on them with each subsequent chapter.

Each chapter is followed by a practice session of 12-lead EKGs. The sections that should be answered are in bold print. We expect the student to form an opinion only on material covered in the current or previous chapters, and we have grayed out more advanced sections that are covered in subsequent chapters. Upon completion of the book the reader should be able to confidently work through the entire answer sheet, forming an autonomous, useful opinion about a 12-lead EKG.

Each of these EKGs includes an analysis by both authors. Another unique feature of the book is our insistence that each EKG opinion refer back directly to the patient, with diagnostic possibilities. Included in our EKG analysis is useful, pertinent, hands-on clinical information relevant to daily practice. The last chapter of the book is a collection of practice EKGs that includes material covered in all the previous chapters. By the end of the book, the reader should have the knowledge and skills to interpret the entire EKG.

How to Use 12-Lead EKG Confidence

Invest in some colored markers and a good set of calipers. Find a comfortable table and chair to work on. This book is in fact a "workbook," and you should work your way through it.

Begin at the beginning.

Because the book was designed using a "step-by-step" approach, it is important to begin at Chapter 1 and work your way through each section that follows. The first three chapters review basic principles of anatomy and physiology with the intent of providing a foundation for the rest of the book. The remaining 16 chapters are set up to introduce one important concept at a time and build on that concept with each subsequent chapter. The chapters are followed by practice EKGs for the learner to work through.

Each practice EKG provided is accompanied by a specifically designed worksheet that allows you to evaluate only the concepts discussed in that specific chapter or the chapters previous to it. The areas of the worksheet that need to be evaluated are in bold print. These areas of the answer sheet that do not need to be answered are grayed out. Do not attempt to answer these yet. These concepts will be covered, and the questions answered, later in the book.

Each worksheet contains an in-depth interpretation of the EKG by both authors. The interpretation provided contains only the information on the concepts that have been covered. Also included in the interpretation is pertinent hands-on clinical information that would prove useful to the professional caring for the patient.

Once you finish the workbook, you should have the knowledge and skills necessary to form an opinion about the 12-lead EKG. Your knowledge will be based on scientific comprehension, which always makes memorization easier. If you are interested in extra practice, you could go back to Chapter 4 and fully evaluate all the practice EKGs completely.

Acknowledgments

Salvatore Chiaramida, MD

John Middleton, MD

Mark Niemiera, MD

Peter Freis, MD

John Kostis, MD

Cliff Lacy, MD

Dan Shindler, MD

Abel Moreyra, MD

Elizabeth Freis Blom, MS, PA

Rakesh Sahni, MD

Madho Sharma, MD

M., H., and D. Behman, MDs

Rob Wyman, MD

Ira Spiler, MD

Alvin Kravet, MD

Sid Kress, MD

Kong Tan, MD

Fred Stone, MD

Alan Sorkowitz

Michael Porter

Brett MacNaughton

Tom Gibbons

Danielle DiPalma

Carolyn A. Dalton

Carolyn O'Brien

Connie Patten, RN, EdD

Michael Bannon

Brother Stephen Kietzman

Sebastian Palmeri, MD

Harold Paz, MD

Mark Zimmerman, MD

John Morrison, MD

Larry Ong, MD

Robert Schlant, MD

J. Willis Hurst, MD

Nanette K. Wenger, MD

Joel Felner, MD

Gerald Fletcher, MD

Mark Silverman, MD

Eric Holmes, MD

John Stone, MD

Adela Yarcheski, PhD

Virginia Fitzsimmons, PhD

Edward Wyckoff

John Roberts

Evangeline Luna, MD

Rim Al-Bezem, MD

Marie Perrino, RN

Rose Gaven, RN

Linda Marciano

Mary Anne Martyniuk

Nancy Gorka, RN

Paula Perry, RN

Linda Lopazanski, RN

Alexander Pamintuan, RN

The medical, nursing, and technological staffs of
Raritan Bay Medical Center

The medical residents of RBMC over the last 20 years

The USC School of Medicine Class of 1978

The medical students from Robert Wood Johnson and
Ross medical schools

Who's Who

Jackie Green, RN

Anthony J. Chiaramida, MD

Joseph Chiaramida, MD
(Anthony's father)

Dina Chiaramida, MD
(Anthony's mother)

Emily DiBlasi
(Dina's mother)

Anthony DiBlasi
(Dina's father)

Salvatore Chiaramida
(Joseph's father)

Anthony Chiaramida, MD
(as a boy)

Anthony's aunt

Anthony's uncle

Contents

1	Basic Anatomy	1
2	The History and Workings of the Electrocardiogram	14
3	The Electrical System	20
4	Heart Rate	32
5	Intervals	48
6	How to Measure Axis	74
7	The P Wave Axis	136
8	Hemiblock	152
9	Right Bundle Branch Block	174
10	Left Bundle Branch Block	192
11	The T Axis	210
12	ST Segment Depression	238
13	ST Segment Elevation	258
14	Inferior Q Waves (Initial QRS Axis)	280
15	Anterior Q Waves (Initial QRS Axis)	298
16	Atrial Abnormalities	316
17	Left Ventricular Hypertrophy	334
18	Right Ventricular Hypertrophy	354
19	Clinical Conditions Affecting the EKG	372
20	Putting It All Together: Practice EKGs	402

Answers to EKGs 424

Index 429

Some Basic Anatomy

The human heart is a hollow four-chambered muscle that is responsible for pumping blood throughout the body.

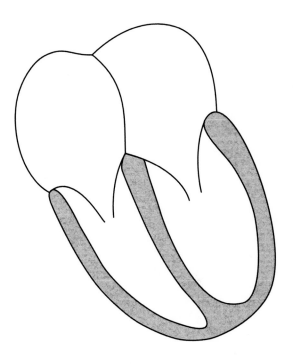

The heart lies in the mediastinum pointing slightly toward the left of the midline.

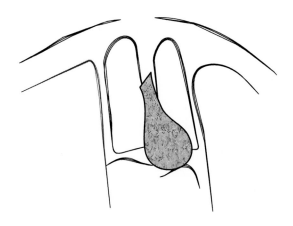

The Pericardium

The heart consists of four main layers: the **pericardium, epicardium, myocardium,** and **endocardium.** The pericardium is a loose-fitting fibroserous sac that covers the heart. Separating the heart muscle from the pericardium is a space called the pericardial space. The space is filled with fluid that acts as a lubricating agent, protecting the heart from injuries caused by friction when it is beating.

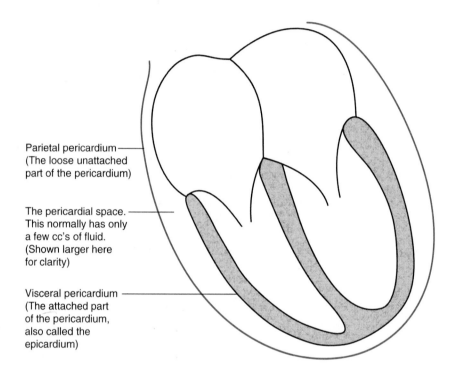

Parietal pericardium (The loose unattached part of the pericardium)

The pericardial space. This normally has only a few cc's of fluid. (Shown larger here for clarity)

Visceral pericardium (The attached part of the pericardium, also called the epicardium)

Layers of the Heart

The epicardium is the outermost layer of the heart and is known as the visceral pericardium. The middle layer of the heart is called the myocardium. The myocardium is the thickest layer of the heart and is responsible for the heart's ability to contract. The innermost layer of the heart is the endocardium. This layer lines the valves and chambers of the heart.

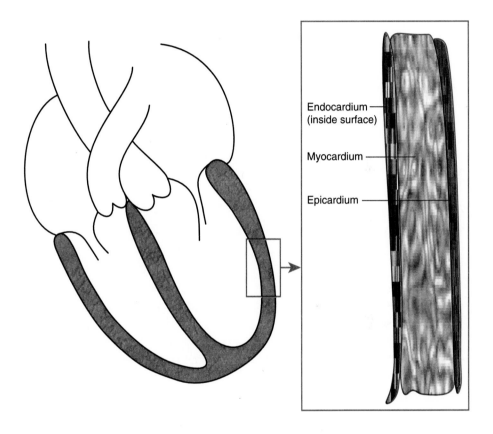

Endocardium — (inside surface)

Myocardium —

Epicardium —

Heart Chambers

The heart is divided into two sides: the right side and the left side. The right side of the heart contains the right atrium and right ventricle. The left side of the heart contains the left atrium and left ventricle. The right and left sides of the heart are anatomically separated by the septum. The two sides of the heart are viewed as two separate pumps and essentially work independently of each other.

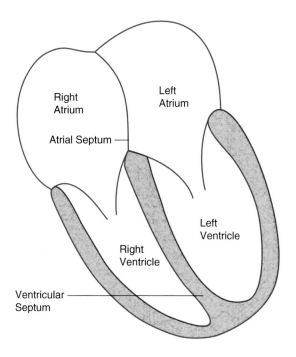

The Circulation

The **right atrium** receives deoxygenated blood from the body via the **superior and inferior vena cavae.** During diastole, the blood is pushed from the **right atrium** into the **right ventricle.** The blood is then forced out of the right ventricle into the pulmonary circulation, where it picks up oxygen. The oxygen-rich blood is transported into the **left atrium** via the **pulmonary veins.** During ventricular diastole, the blood is forced into the **left ventricle.** The left ventricle pumps the oxygen-rich blood to the body.

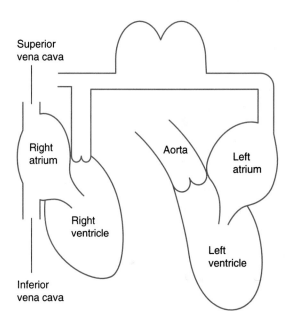

Heart Valves

The heart has four valves that act as tiny doors that keep the blood moving in one direction. The closure of the valves prevents the backward flow of blood. **The right atrium and right ventricle are separated by the tricuspid valve, and the left atrium and left ventricle are separated by the mitral valve.** These valves are known as cuspid valves. The aortic valve and the pulmonic valve are called semilunar valves because of their distinct half-moon appearance. The aortic valve lies between the left ventricle and the aorta, and the pulmonic valve separates the right ventricle from the pulmonary artery.

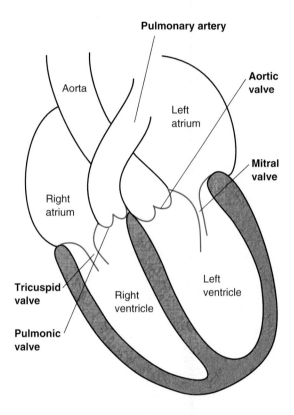

Coronary Circulation

The heart receives oxygen-rich blood via two main vessels: the right coronary artery and the left coronary artery. Both arteries arise from the aortic root and divide into several branches as they travel down the length of the heart.

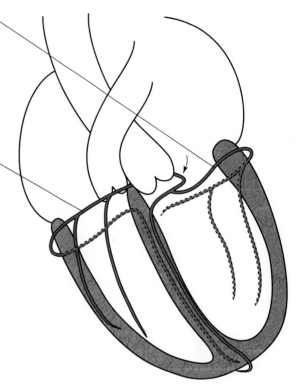

The left coronary artery begins at the aortic root, and splits into the LAD (left anterior descending) and CFX (circumflex) branches. The LAD goes down the front of the septum. The circumflex goes left, around to the back of the ventricle.

The right coronary artery originates at the aortic root, travels around the front of the right ventricle. It loops around to the back of the right ventricle, and then, when it meets the back of the septum, it turns to the apex.

The Right Coronary Artery

The right coronary artery travels along the coronary sulcus, which is the grove between the atria and the ventricles, and continues down the posterior aspect of the septum. It supplies blood to the right ventricle, the atrioventricular (AV) node, part of the septum, and the posterior and inferior walls of the left ventricle.

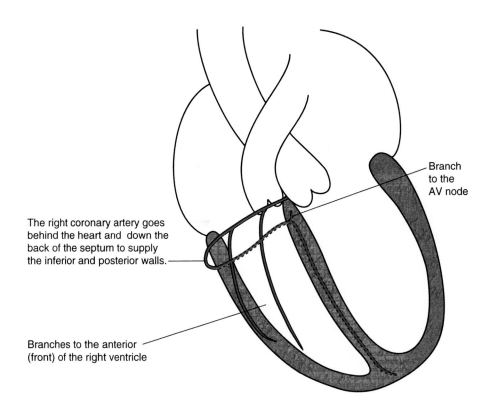

Branch to the AV node

The right coronary artery goes behind the heart and down the back of the septum to supply the inferior and posterior walls.

Branches to the anterior (front) of the right ventricle

The Left Coronary Artery

The left coronary artery consists of two branches: the left anterior descending (LAD) and the circumflex (CFX).

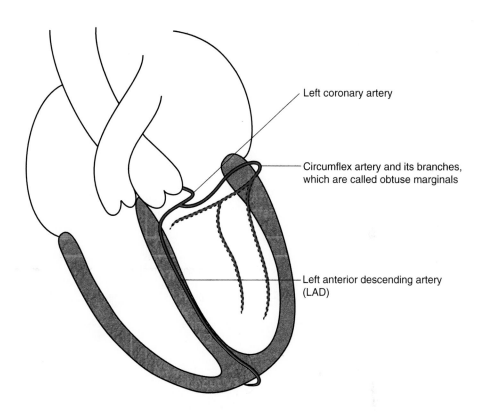

Left coronary artery

Circumflex artery and its branches, which are called obtuse marginals

Left anterior descending artery (LAD)

The Left Anterior Descending Artery

The LAD artery perfuses the anterior wall of the left ventricle, the anterior section of the ventricular septum, and the lateral wall of the left ventricle.

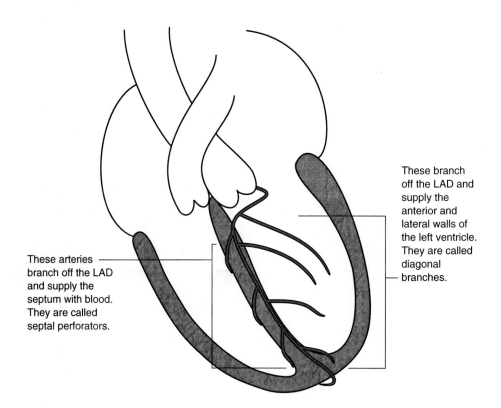

These arteries branch off the LAD and supply the septum with blood. They are called septal perforators.

These branch off the LAD and supply the anterior and lateral walls of the left ventricle. They are called diagonal branches.

The Circumflex Artery

The CFX branch of the left coronary artery supplies blood to the left atrium and the posterior and lateral walls of the left ventricle.

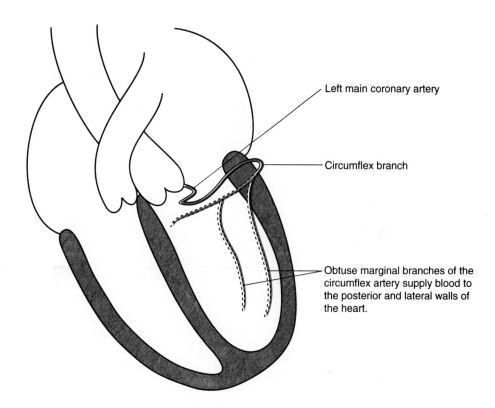

Left main coronary artery

Circumflex branch

Obtuse marginal branches of the circumflex artery supply blood to the posterior and lateral walls of the heart.

Coronary Arteries as End Arteries

The three main branches of the coronary arteries typically do not connect or anastomose with each other at their ends and are therefore called "end arteries." This anatomic feature poses significant problems when atherosclerotic lesions develop in the arteries because there is no alternative route for the blood to travel. This leads to ischemia and necrosis of the myocardial tissue.

Although the main coronary arteries are end arteries and do not connect with each other, the smaller arterial vessels do, in fact, anastomose to some degree, providing what is known as collateral circulation. If collateral circulation develops, it provides a means of supplying blood to the ischemic areas of the heart. Therefore, the factors surrounding the development of collateral circulation are significant in the study and treatment of coronary artery disease.

The end of the right coronary artery at the back of the heart does not connect to the end of the left anterior descending (LAD) artery at the front of the heart.

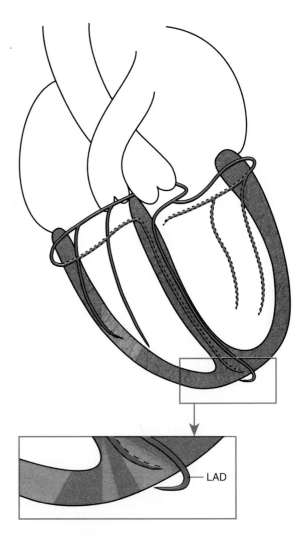

LAD

Blood Supply to the Myocardium

The coronary arteries lie on the outermost layer of the heart, or epicardium, and penetrate in toward the myocardium. The portion of myocardium furthest from the artery lies near the endocardium and is called subendocardial tissue. It has the poorest blood supply of the entire myocardium.

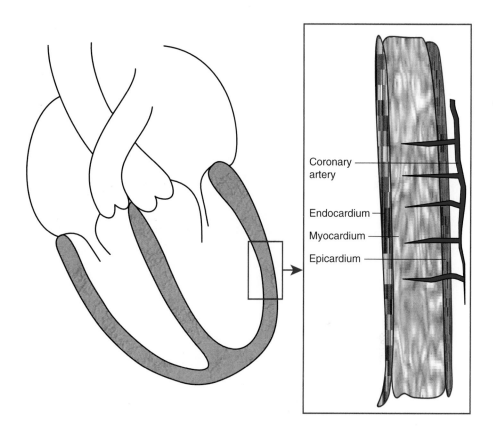

Coronary artery

Endocardium

Myocardium

Epicardium

The History and Workings of the Electrocardiogram

In 1913, Wilhelm Einthoven contributed significantly to the study of the heart by inventing the electrocardiogram (EKG). Einthoven attached wires or electrodes to the right arm, left arm, and left leg. This formed a theoretical triangle. When the electrodes were connected to a galvanometer, they measured the electrical activity, which was eventually recorded on paper and representative of each heart beat.

Modern EKG machines inscribe 12 leads (or views) from differing combinations of the four limb electrodes and six chest electrodes.

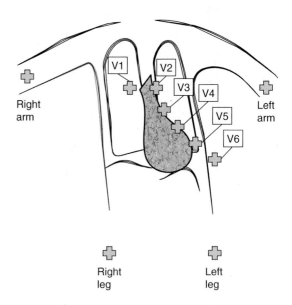

The Twelve EKG Leads

A total of 12 leads or views are represented on the modern EKG. The EKG leads are consistently arranged in a standard pattern. The first six leads represent the frontal plane (or view) of heart. They are called the limb leads and are named I, II, III, AVR, AVL, and AVF. The next six leads represent the horizontal plane (or view) of the heart. They are called precordial (in front of heart) leads and are named V1, V2, V3, V4, V5, and V6.

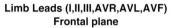

Limb Leads (I,II,III,AVR,AVL,AVF)
Frontal plane

Precordial Leads (V1,V2,V3,V4,V5,V6)
Horizontal plane

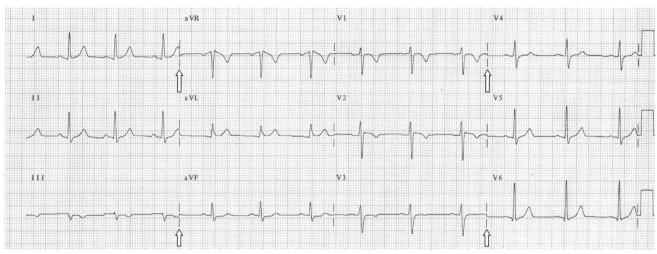

↑ Sometimes an artifact is present where the leads change on the paper. It has no medical meaning.

EKG Paper

The EKG is recorded on special standardized paper that scrolls out of the machine at a specific and controlled speed. Each large box is 5 mm wide and represents 2/10 of a second. Each big box contains 5 smaller 1-mm boxes, each representing 0.04 seconds. Measuring the distance of any wave or interval from left to right determines the duration of that wave in seconds.

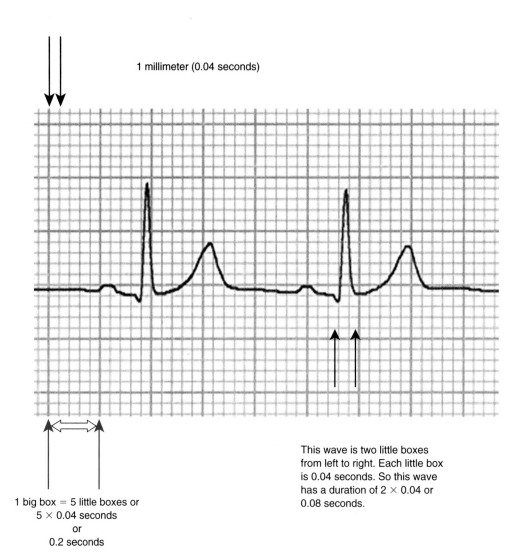

1 millimeter (0.04 seconds)

1 big box = 5 little boxes or
5 × 0.04 seconds
or
0.2 seconds

This wave is two little boxes from left to right. Each little box is 0.04 seconds. So this wave has a duration of 2 × 0.04 or 0.08 seconds.

The Baseline

The baseline on a 12-lead EKG is an imaginary line that connects the end of the T wave to the beginning of the P wave. (See Chapter 3 for more information on P and T waves.) All measurements of other waves are made relative to the baseline.

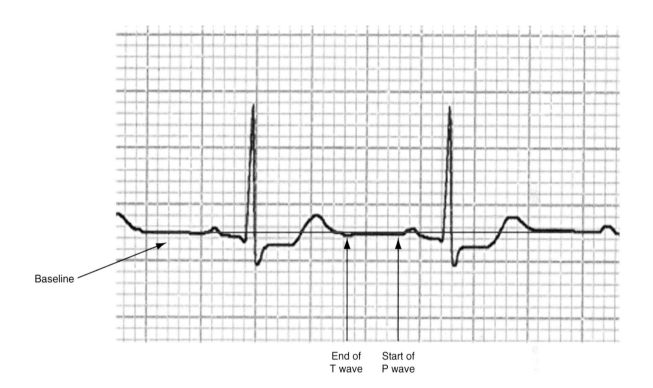

Baseline

End of
T wave

Start of
P wave

Measurements on the EKG

Each little box is 1 mm tall (vertically). A wave that goes upward from the baseline is said to be positive. A wave that goes downward from the baseline is said to be negative. Measuring the distance of any wave above the baseline gives the amplitude (height) of the wave in millimeters. Measuring the distance of any wave below the baseline gives the amplitude (depth) of the wave in millimeters.

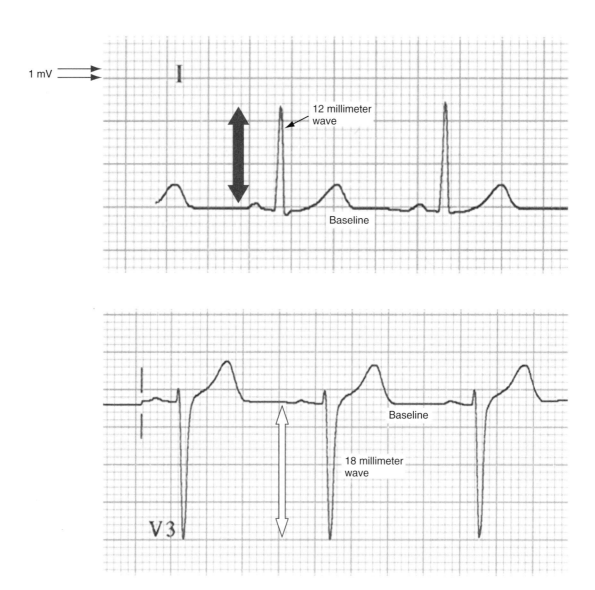

ERRATA

12-Lead EKG Confidence: Step-by-Step to Mastery

Jacqueline M. Green & Anthony J. Chiaramida

The vertical time lines described in the text on page 34, and in the answer sections on pages 275, and 279, are not exactly 3 seconds apart, as indicated. Although 3-second time lines were commonly used on older machines and some current models, computer readings have made the need for the 3-second lines less important. On the strips in this book, these vertical lines serve to separate the leads, not to provide any time information.

To obtain a 6-second sample, take 30 big blocks (each measures 0.2 seconds). This left-to-right measure still gives 6 seconds.

The correct heart rates for these strips are:

Page 34 top: 70
Page 34 bottom: 120
Page 171: 70
Page 275 : 70
Page 279: 70
Page 297: 90
Page 315: 120

Standardization

To ensure that the EKG correctly measures and records the amplitude of waves above and below the baseline, a standardized voltage is inscribed on every EKG, usually on the right side of the EKG. It should measure exactly 10 little boxes in height.

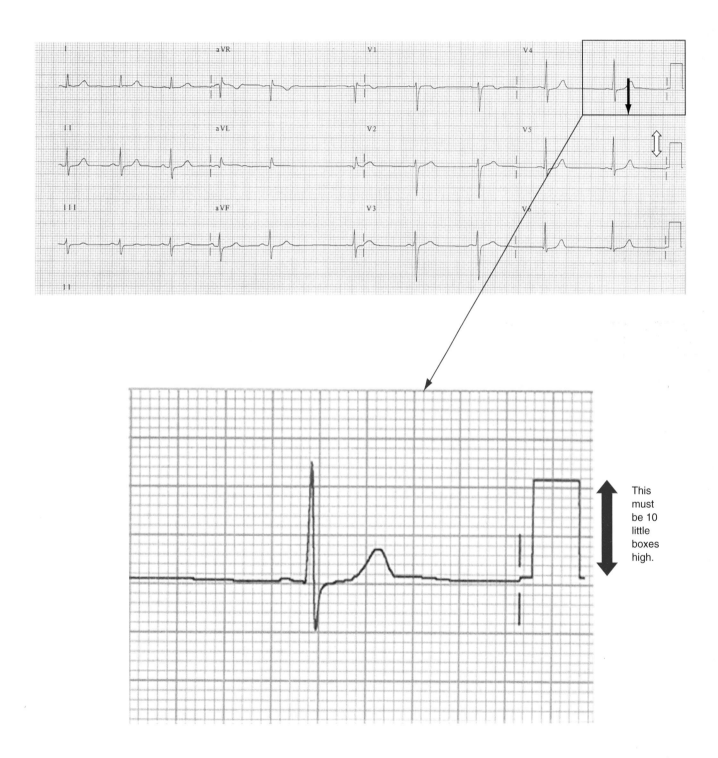

This must be 10 little boxes high.

The Electrical System

The heart has an intricate electrical system that is responsible for generating each heartbeat.

| **Atrial systole** **Ventricular diastole** | **Atrial diastole** **Ventricular systole** |

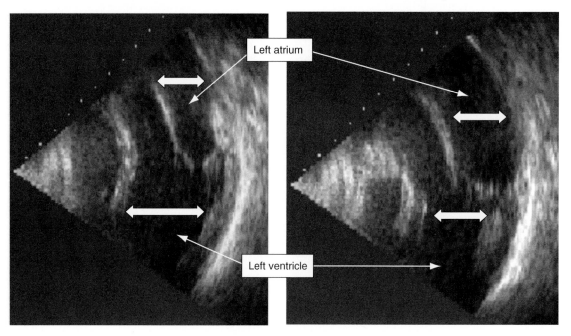

The left ventricle contracts in systole, as the electrical impulse triggers mechanical contraction.

The Electrical Subsystem

The heart has other specialized cells that create and conduct electrical impulses. The heart's electrical system consists of five structures: the sinoatrial (or SA) node, the atrioventricular (or AV) node, the bundle of His, the right and left bundles, and the Purkinje fibers.

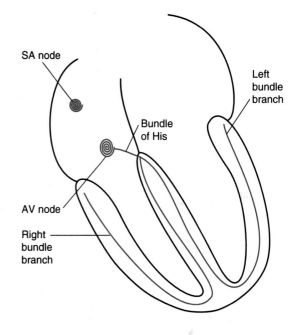

The SA Node

The SA node is known as the heart's natural pacemaker because it initiates each heartbeat and controls the heart's pace. The SA node comprises hundreds of specialized cells and is located in the right atrium.

The *SA node fires electrical impulses* that travel through the atrium, causing them to contract.

The electrical stimulus travels through the atrium via the intra-atrial conduction pathway.

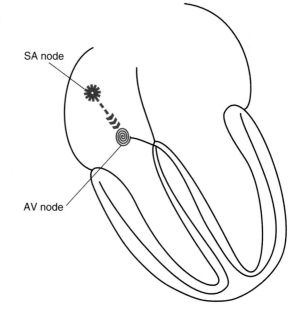

SA node

AV node

The electrical activation (called depolarization) of the atria is represented on the EKG as a P wave. This is normally the first wave or "deflection" on the EKG.

P waves

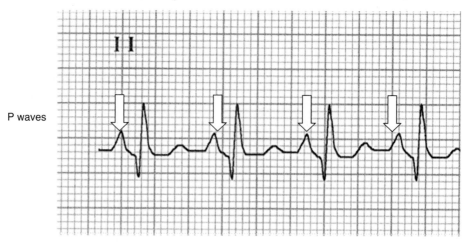

Examples of P Waves

P waves can be positive or negative.

The absence of a P wave is always abnormal.

The P wave amplitude may be small, and it has to be looked for very carefully.

Negative P waves

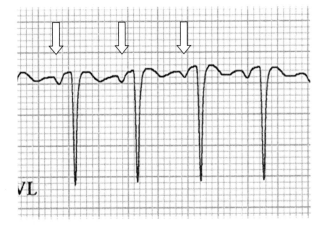

Positive P waves

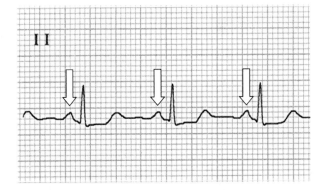

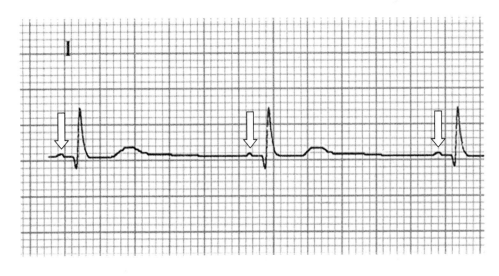

The Atrioventricular Node

The AV node is located in the lower right atrium. The AV node receives the impulse from the SA node and continues transmitting it to the bundle of His.

The bundle of His is found below the AV node and conducts the electrical impulse through to the bundle branches. The bundle branches divide into the right bundle, which leads to the right ventricle, and the left bundle, which leads to the left ventricle. The electrical stimulus travels down the bundle branches to the microscopic Purkinje fibers.

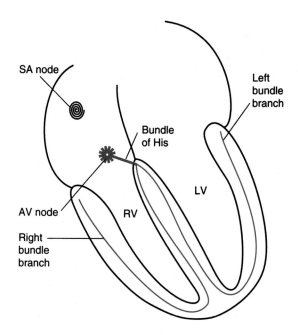

Ventricular Systole

Once the impulse reaches the Purkinje network, it spreads onward across the myocardial cells, causing the ventricles to contract. This is referred to as ventricular depolarization. Ventricular depolarization is represented on the EKG as the QRS complex.

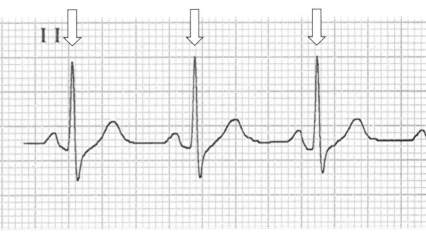

QRS
Complexes

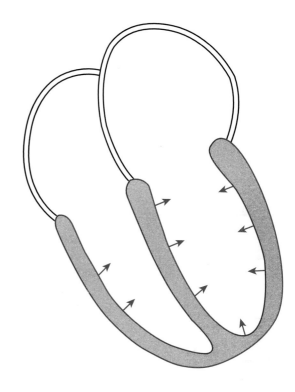

Naming the Parts of the QRS Complex

The QRS complex is the second deflection on the normal EKG. The QRS complex consists of a Q, an R, or an S wave either singly or in any combination. Although the complex is called the QRS complex, it does not always contain a Q wave, an R wave, and an S wave.

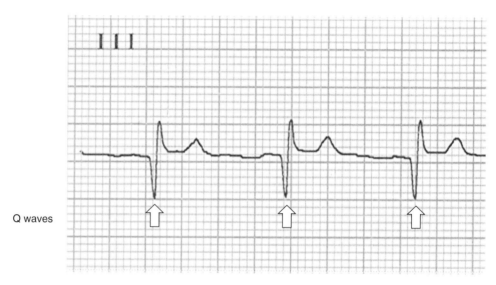

If the *first* wave of the complex is a downward deflection, as in the example, the complex is considered to have a Q wave.

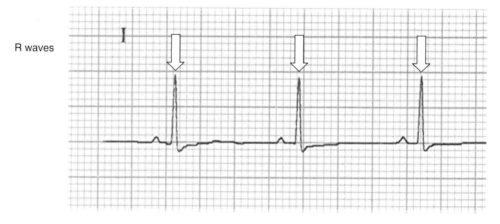

However, if the first wave or deflection is in an upward direction, it is called an R wave. This example does not have a Q wave.

In this example, the first deflection is downward, producing a **Q wave**. The next wave is upward and is called an **R wave**. The QRS complex has both a Q wave and an R wave.

R waves

Q waves

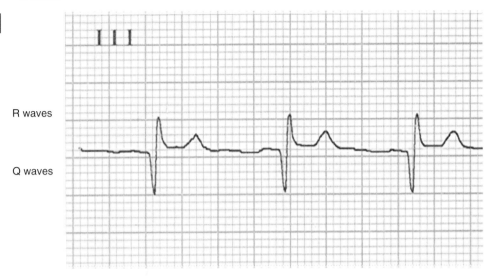

In this example, the first deflection is upward, making it an R wave. The next deflection is downward. This is called an **s wave**. Because the S wave is small, it is given a lowercase s.

R waves

S waves

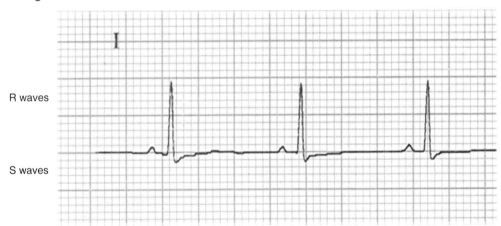

As noted, not all complexes contain all three deflections. In this example, the first deflection is downward. This is a Q wave. The rest of the QRS is also in a downward direction. The complex is referred to as a **QS wave**. This complex has no R wave.

The QRS complex may contain only a single upright wave (an R wave).

Likewise, it may only contain a single downward wave (a QS wave).

Thus, the QRS is still called the QRS complex, even if it does not have all three waves.

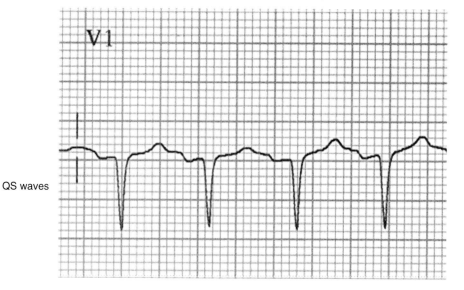

QS waves

This complex contains all three waves.

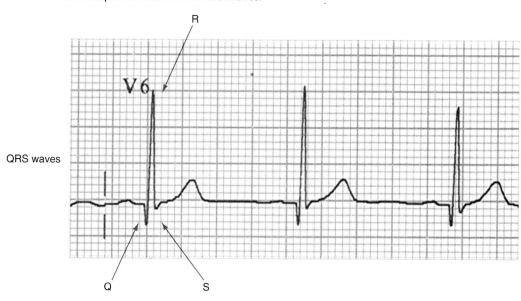

QRS waves

Examples of Naming the Parts of the QRS Complex

The following represent examples of the various combinations of waves that a QRS complex may have. It is interesting to note that although all of the following are QRS complexes, they look different and contain different waves. In some instances, the wave after the R wave may also be in an upward direction. This is known as an R prime or R′ wave.

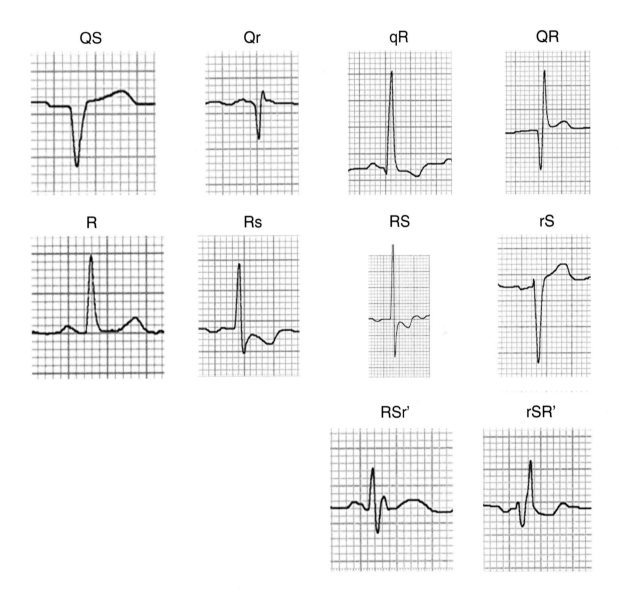

Prominent R waves are usually written with an uppercase R. These examples contain no Q or S waves.

R

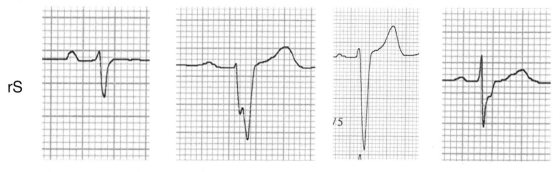

The R waves in these examples are not prominent, so they are written with a lowercase r. The S waves are more prominent and therefore written with an uppercase S.

rS

Prominent R wave, small S wave.

Rs

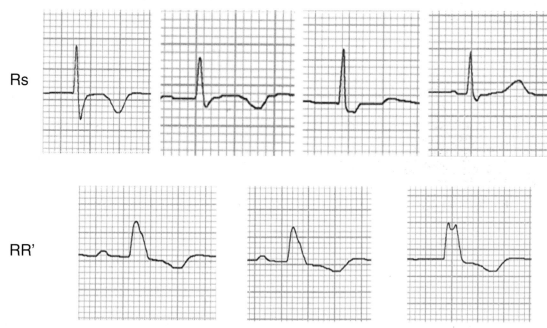

RR'

Ventricular Repolarization (T Wave)

The third deflection on the EKG is the T wave. The T wave represents ventricular repolarization. The ventricles must repolarize or recharge themselves before the next cardiac cycle can begin.

T waves

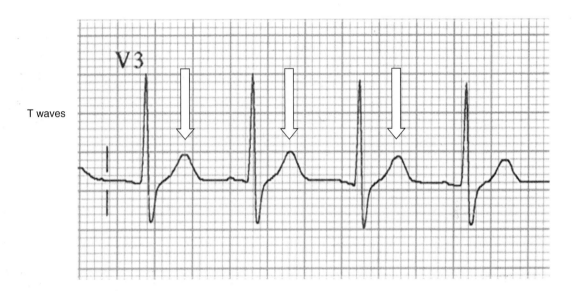

Heart Rate

The EKG provides a skilled reader with a wealth of information about the heart. One of the most basic yet important pieces of information the EKG provides is the heart rate. **The heart rate is defined as the number of beats per minute.** Calculating the heart rate is easy because the EKG is always recorded on graph paper that measures time.

The heart rate is the number of times the heart contracts per minute. The normal range is 60 to 100 beats per minute.

Heart rate is a vital sign. It is almost always clinically relevant.

Sinus rhythm: The normal range is 60 to 100 beats per minute.

Sinus tachycardia: a sinus rate greater than 100 beats per minute. The typical maximum is limited by the patient's age (220 − patient's age).

Sinus bradycardia: a sinus rate less than 60 beats per minute.

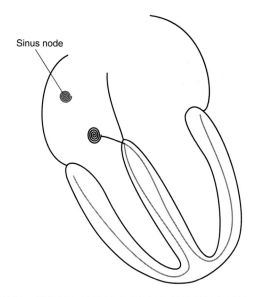

Sinus node

The vertical lines on the EKG are time lines. The lighter vertical lines are 0.04 seconds (or one little box) apart. The darker vertical lines are 0.2 seconds (or one big box) apart.

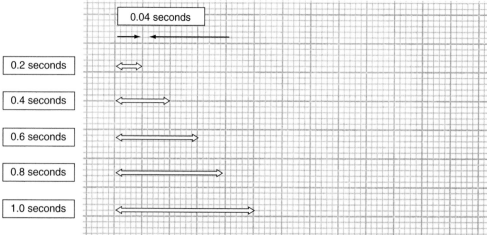

0.04 seconds

0.2 seconds

0.4 seconds

0.6 seconds

0.8 seconds

1.0 seconds

Measurement of the Heart Rate

The most accurate way to measure a heart rate is by measuring the R-R interval. The R-R interval is the distance from one R wave to the next R wave. When measuring the R-R interval, take the beginning of one QRS complex, and measure the number of little boxes up to the beginning of the next QRS complex. Divide this number into 1500. This method of calculating the heart rate is valid if the heart rate is regular.

1500/26 = 58
Heart rate = 58 beats per minute

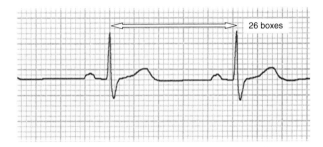

1500/23 = 65
Heart rate = 65 beats per minute

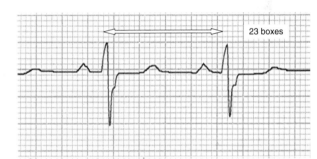

1500/15 = 100
Heart rate = 100 beats per minute

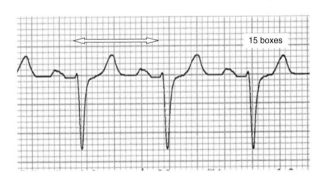

1500/12 = 125
Heart rate = 125 beats per minute

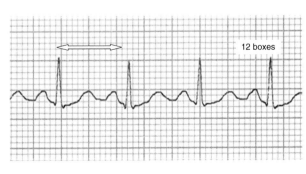

The Heart Rate in Atrial Fibrillation

When the R-R intervals are irregular, the best way to estimate the heart rate is by counting the number of QRS complexes in a 6-second block of time and multiplying that number by 10. The result is the heart rate in beats per minute. The black vertical time lines (seen as the leads change) mark exactly 3 seconds. In the first example below, there are six QRS complexes in the 6-second block. Multiplying six complexes (in 6 seconds) by 10 yields a (heart) ventricular rate of 60 (for 60 seconds).

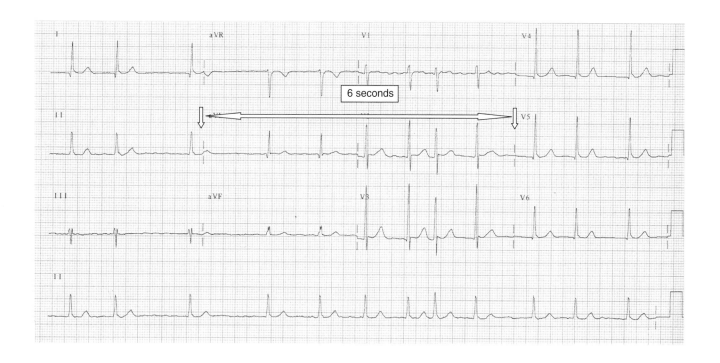

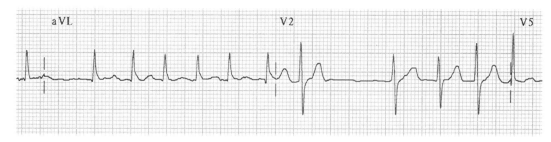

The heart rate is 11 × 10 or 110 beats per minute.

Table of Heart Rates

The table of heart rates shown below is an easy, convenient method for obtaining the heart rate without doing the calculations.

KEY CONCEPT

The heart rate should never be a rough approximation.

Use a chart and calculate the correct heart rate.

Number of Little Boxes	Heart Rate
5	300
6	250
7	214
8	188
9	167
10	150
11	136
12	125
13	115
14	107
15	100
16	94
17	88
18	83
19	79
20	75
21	71
22	68
23	65
24	63
25	60
26	58
27	56
28	54
29	52
30	50
31	48
32	47
33	45
34	44
35	43

Heart Rate

It is important to calculate the heart rate accurately. A heart rate of 136 beats per minute (11 little boxes) differs from a heart rate of 150 beats per minute (10 little boxes). EKG readers have developed several methods to get a quick heart rate, and many commonly use the 300, 150, 100 method. This method is quick but can be inaccurate.

Another important point to remember when calculating the heart rate is to look at all the leads.

1500/14 = 107
Heart rate = 107 beats per minute

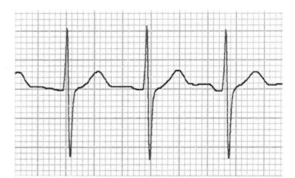

1500/16 = 94
Heart rate = 94 beats per minute

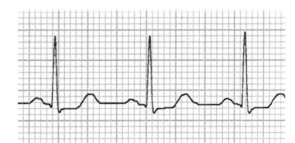

1500/15 = 100
Heart rate = 100 beats per minute

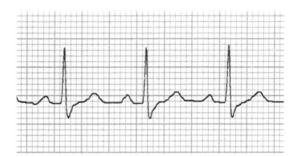

1500/17 = 88
Heart rate = 88 beats per minute

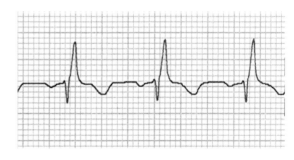

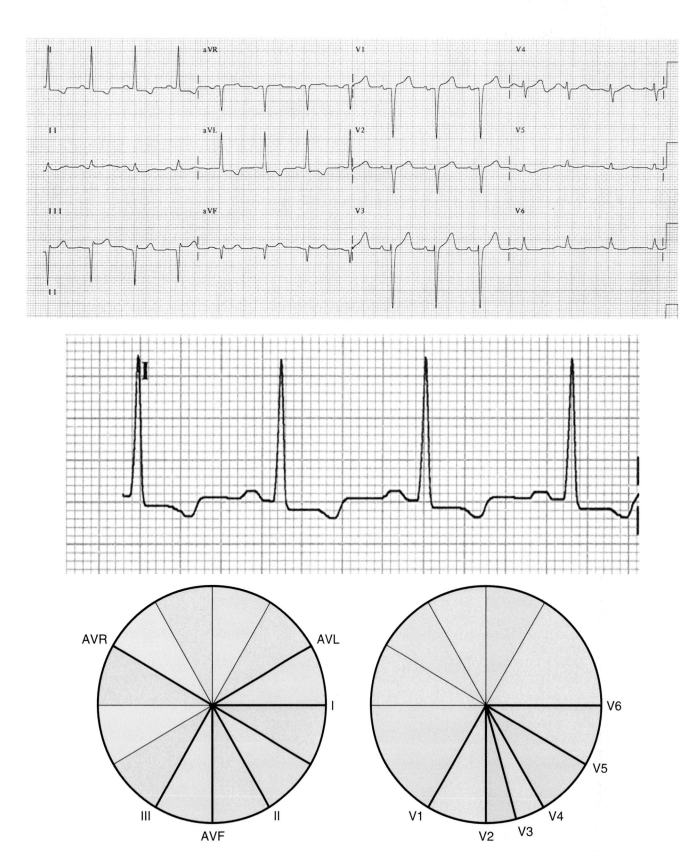

Heart Rate:

Rhythm:

Intervals (measured in the limb leads)

PR: short (< .12)
       normal (.12 to .20)
       long (>0.20 seconds); this is 1st degree AV
       block

QRS: normal (≤0.09 seconds)
       prolonged (.10 or .11); this is intraventricular
       conduction delay (IVCD)
       Bundle Branch Block (.12 seconds or greater)

QT:

P axis: normal
             rightward
             arm-lead reversal or dextrocardia
             junctional rhythm

QRS axis: normal
             left anterior hemiblock
             left posterior hemiblock
             indeterminate

T wave inversion (ischemia or infarction):

II,III,AVF	inferior
I, AVL	lateral
V1, without V2	nonspecific septal
V1 and V2	septal
V3 and V4	anterior
V5 and V6	lateral
V6, without V5	nonspecific lateral

ST Elevation (acute infarction):

II,III,AVF	inferior
I, AVL	lateral
V1, without V2	nonspecific septal
V1 and V2	septal
V3 and V4	anterior
V5 and V6	lateral
V6, without V5.	nonspecific lateral

ST Depression (ischemia or infarction):

I,II,III,AVL,AVF	diffuse subendocardial ischemia or infarction
V2,V3,V4,V5	diffuse subendocardial ischemia or infarction

Q waves (infarction):

II,III,AVF	inferior
I, AVL	lateral
V1, without V2	nonspecific septal
V1 and V2	septal
V3 and V4	anterior
V5 and V6	lateral
V6, without V5	nonspecific lateral

Hypertrophy:

Right atrial: Tall P wave 2.5 mm in II, III, or AVF

Left atrial: Deep negative part of P wave in V1

LVH: R wave in 1 + S wave in III ≥ 25mV
      S wave in V1 + R wave in V5 ≥ 35mV

RVH: Mean QRS either anterior, or rightward

Don't approximate the heart rate. The 300–150–100 method puts the rate at 60 to 75. That's not close enough. The actual rate is 1500/18 or 83 beats per minute. The rhythm is sinus.

Parts of the answer sheets are "grayed out" because these sections have not yet been covered. Answer only the parts that are not highlighted.

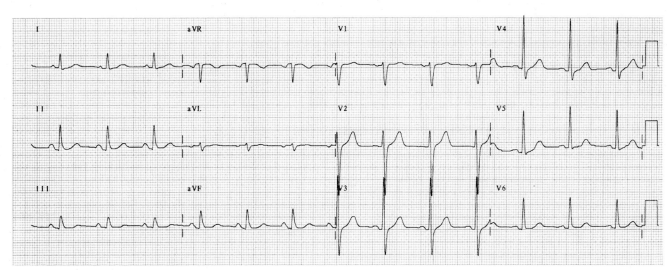

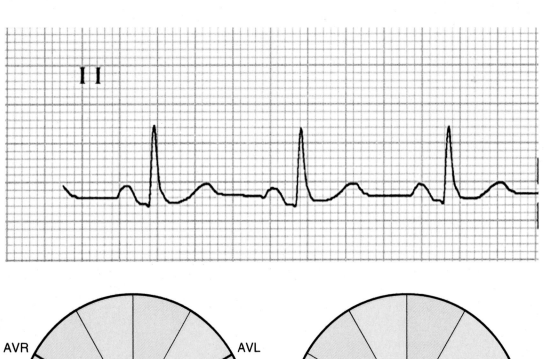

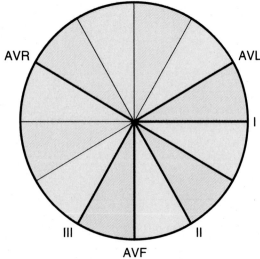

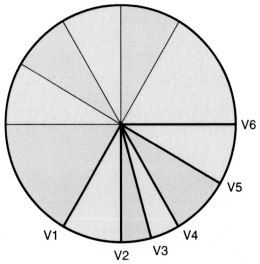

Heart Rate:

Rhythm:

Intervals (measured in the limb leads)

PR: short (< .12)
      normal (.12 to .20)
      long (>0.20 seconds); this is 1st degree AV
      block

QRS: normal (≤0.09 seconds)
       prolonged (.10 or .11); this is intraventricular
       conduction delay (IVCD)
       Bundle Branch Block (.12 seconds or greater)

QT:

ST Elevation (acute infarction):

II,III,AVF	inferior
I, AVL	lateral
V1, without V2	nonspecific septal
V1 and V2	septal
V3 and V4	anterior
V5 and V6	lateral
V6, without V5.	nonspecific lateral

ST Depression (ischemia or infarction):

I,II,III,AVL,AVF	diffuse subendocardial ischemia or infarction
V2,V3,V4,V5	diffuse subendocardial ischemia or infarction

P axis: normal
             rightward
             arm-lead reversal or dextrocardia
             junctional rhythm

QRS axis: normal
               left anterior hemiblock
               left posterior hemiblock
               indeterminate

Q waves (infarction):

II,III,AVF	inferior
I, AVL	lateral
V1, without V2	nonspecific septal
V1 and V2	septal
V3 and V4	anterior
V5 and V6	lateral
V6, without V5	nonspecific lateral

T wave inversion (ischemia or infarction):

II,III,AVF	inferior
I, AVL	lateral
V1, without V2	nonspecific septal
V1 and V2	septal
V3 and V4	anterior
V5 and V6	lateral
V6, without V5	nonspecific lateral

Hypertrophy:

Right atrial: Tall P wave 2.5 mm in II, III, or AVF

Left atrial: Deep negative part of P wave in V1

LVH: R wave in 1 + S wave in III ≥ 25mV
       S wave in V1 + R wave in V5 ≥ 35mV

RVH: Mean QRS either anterior, or rightward

This heart rate is 1500/19, or 79 beats per minute. This is sinus rhythm. It is normal for a "normal" patient. It would not be normal for a patient who was bleeding or in congestive failure, pulmonary edema, or shock. Always correlate EKG findings with the patient. Sometimes a normal finding (sinus rhythm) may be an important clinical clue.

Parts of the answer sheets are "grayed out" because these sections have not yet been covered. Answer only the parts that are not highlighted.

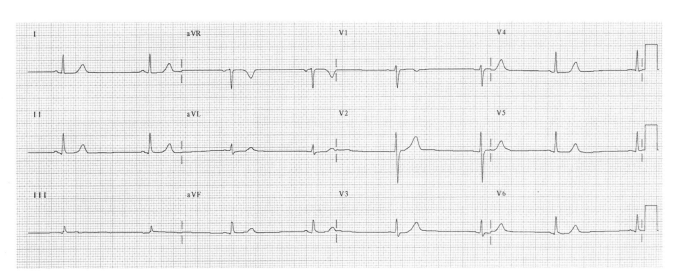

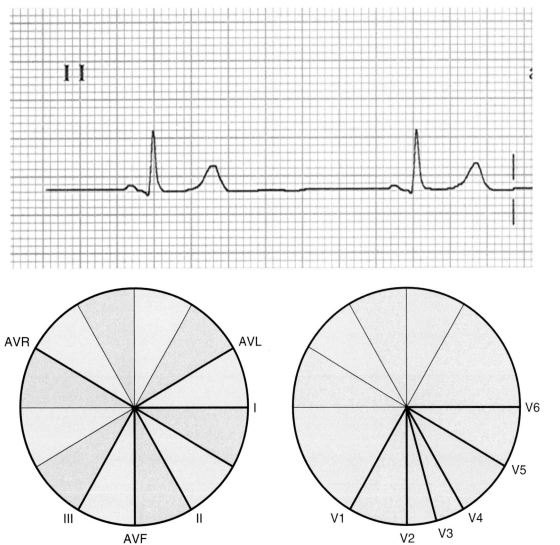

Heart Rate:

Rhythm:

Intervals (measured in the limb leads)

PR: short (< .12)
      normal (.12 to .20)
      long (>0.20 seconds); this is 1st degree AV
      block

QRS: normal (≤0.09 seconds)
       prolonged (.10 or .11); this is intraventricular
       conduction delay (IVCD)
       Bundle Branch Block (.12 seconds or greater)

QT:

P axis: normal
            rightward
            arm-lead reversal or dextrocardia
            junctional rhythm

QRS axis: normal
            left anterior hemiblock
            left posterior hemiblock
            indeterminate

T wave inversion (ischemia or infarction):

II,III,AVF	inferior
I, AVL	lateral
V1, without V2	nonspecific septal
V1 and V2	septal
V3 and V4	anterior
V5 and V6	lateral
V6, without V5	nonspecific lateral

ST Elevation (acute infarction):

II,III,AVF	inferior
I, AVL	lateral
V1, without V2	nonspecific septal
V1 and V2	septal
V3 and V4	anterior
V5 and V6	lateral
V6, without V5.	nonspecific lateral

ST Depression (ischemia or infarction):

I,II,III,AVL,AVF	diffuse subendocardial ischemia or infarction
V2,V3,V4,V5	diffuse subendocardial ischemia or infarction

Q waves (infarction):

II,III,AVF	inferior
I, AVL	lateral
V1, without V2	nonspecific septal
V1 and V2	septal
V3 and V4	anterior
V5 and V6	lateral
V6, without V5	nonspecific lateral

Hypertrophy:

Right atrial: Tall P wave 2.5 mm in II, III, or AVF

Left atrial: Deep negative part of P wave in V1

LVH: R wave in 1 + S wave in III ≥ 25mV
      S wave in V1 + R wave in V5 ≥ 35mV

RVH: Mean QRS either anterior, or rightward

The heart rate is 1500/35 or 43 beats per minute. This is sinus bradycardia. One of the more common causes of sinus bradycardia is the use of a class of drugs called beta blockers. Other causes include sleep, athleticism, and hypothyroidism.

Parts of the answer sheets are "grayed out" because these sections have not yet been covered. Answer only the parts that are not highlighted.

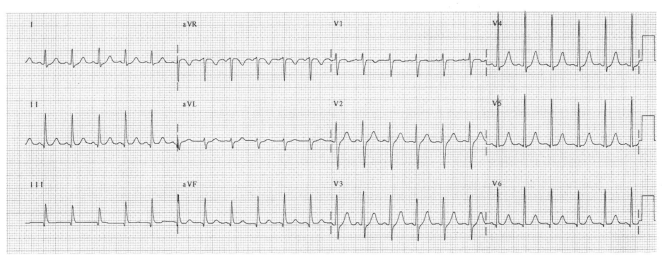

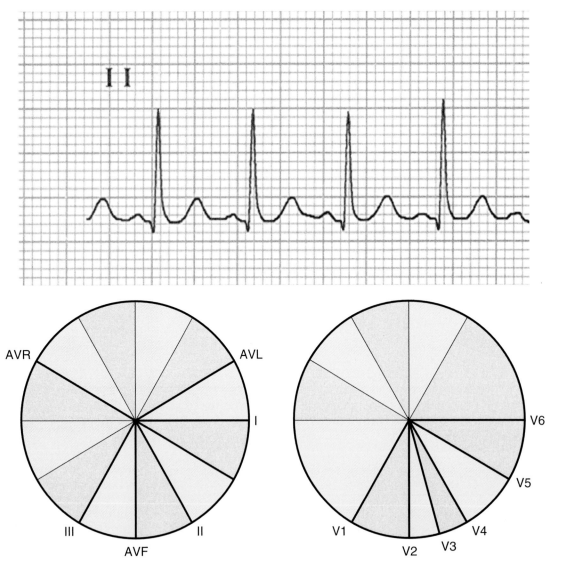

Heart Rate:

Rhythm:

Intervals (measured in the limb leads)

PR: short (< .12)

normal (.12 to .20)

long (>0.20 seconds); this is 1st degree AV block

QRS: normal (≤0.09 seconds)

prolonged (.10 or .11); this is intraventricular conduction delay (IVCD)

Bundle Branch Block (.12 seconds or greater)

QT:

P axis: normal

rightward

arm-lead reversal or dextrocardia

junctional rhythm

QRS axis: normal

left anterior hemiblock

left posterior hemiblock

indeterminate

T wave inversion (ischemia or infarction):

II,III,AVF	inferior
I, AVL	lateral
V1, without V2	nonspecific septal
V1 and V2	septal
V3 and V4	anterior
V5 and V6	lateral
V6, without V5	nonspecific lateral

ST Elevation (acute infarction):

II,III,AVF	inferior
I, AVL	lateral
V1, without V2	nonspecific septal
V1 and V2	septal
V3 and V4	anterior
V5 and V6	lateral
V6, without V5.	nonspecific lateral

ST Depression (ischemia or infarction):

I,II,III,AVL,AVF	diffuse subendocardial ischemia or infarction
V2,V3,V4,V5	diffuse subendocardial ischemia or infarction

Q waves (infarction):

II,III,AVF	inferior
I, AVL	lateral
V1, without V2	nonspecific septal
V1 and V2	septal
V3 and V4	anterior
V5 and V6	lateral
V6, without V5	nonspecific lateral

Hypertrophy:

Right atrial: Tall P wave 2.5 mm in II, III, or AVF

Left atrial: Deep negative part of P wave in V1

LVH: R wave in 1 + S wave in III ≥ 25mV

S wave in V1 + R wave in V5 ≥ 35mV

RVH: Mean QRS either anterior, or rightward

The heart rate is 1500/11 or 136 beats per minute. This is sinus tachycardia. Clinically, the cause of sinus tachycardia should always be identified. This can be one of the most valuable clinical clues on an EKG and should not be overlooked.

Parts of the answer sheets are "grayed out" because these sections have not yet been covered. Answer only the parts that are not highlighted.

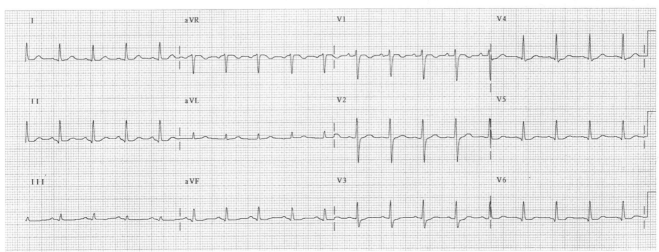

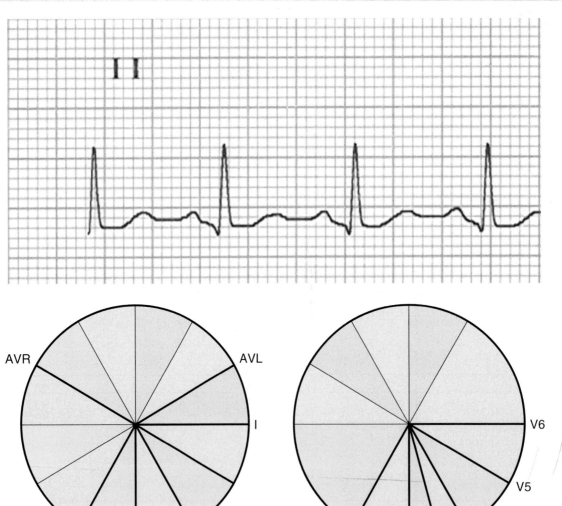

Heart Rate:

Rhythm:

Intervals (measured in the limb leads)

PR: short (< .12)
normal (.12 to .20)
long (>0.20 seconds); this is 1st degree AV block

QRS: normal (≤0.09 seconds)
prolonged (.10 or .11); this is intraventricular conduction delay (IVCD)
Bundle Branch Block (.12 seconds or greater)

QT:

P axis: normal
rightward
arm-lead reversal or dextrocardia
junctional rhythm

QRS axis: normal
left anterior hemiblock
left posterior hemiblock
indeterminate

T wave inversion (ischemia or infarction):

II,III,AVF	inferior
I, AVL	lateral
V1, without V2	nonspecific septal
V1 and V2	septal
V3 and V4	anterior
V5 and V6	lateral
V6, without V5	nonspecific lateral

ST Elevation (acute infarction):

II,III,AVF	inferior
I, AVL	lateral
V1, without V2	nonspecific septal
V1 and V2	septal
V3 and V4	anterior
V5 and V6	lateral
V6, without V5.	nonspecific lateral

ST Depression (ischemia or infarction):

I,II,III,AVL,AVF	diffuse subendocardial ischemia or infarction
V2,V3,V4,V5	diffuse subendocardial ischemia or infarction

Q waves (infarction):

II,III,AVF	inferior
I, AVL	lateral
V1, without V2	nonspecific septal
V1 and V2	septal
V3 and V4	anterior
V5 and V6	lateral
V6, without V5	nonspecific lateral

Hypertrophy:

Right atrial: Tall P wave 2.5 mm in II, III, or AVF

Left atrial: Deep negative part of P wave in V1

LVH: R wave in 1 + S wave in III ≥ 25mV
S wave in V1 + R wave in V5 ≥ 35mV

RVH: Mean QRS either anterior, or rightward

The heart rate is 1500/13 or 115 beats per minute. The rhythm is sinus tachycardia.

Parts of the answer sheets are "grayed out" because these sections have not yet been covered. Answer only the parts that are not highlighted.

Intervals

Now that the heart rate is calculated, the next measurements to be taken and evaluated are the **PR, QRS, and QT intervals.** These intervals are **measured only in the limb leads** (the frontal plane leads: I, II, III, AVR, AVL, and AVF); they are never measured in the precordial leads (the horizontal plane leads: V1, V2, V3, V4, V5, and V6). These intervals are routinely measured on all EKGs.

Like the heart rate, the PR, QRS, and QT intervals are measured (left to right) in **units of time** (seconds) with each little box representing 0.04 seconds.

**Limb leads (I, II, III, AVR, AVL, AVF)
Frontal plane**

**Precordial leads (V1, V2, V3, V4, V5, V6)
Horizontal plane**

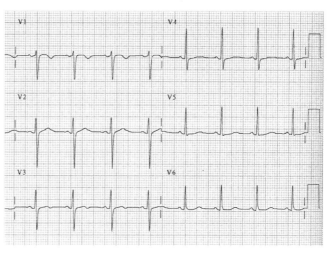

Measure the intervals in the frontal plane above.

Don't measure the intervals in the horizontal plane above.

The PR Interval

The PR interval measures the distance between the beginning of the P wave to the beginning of ventricular depolarization, the QRS complex. The PR interval represents the amount of time it takes for the electrical impulse to travel from the sinus node through the atria into and through the AV node and ends at the beginning of ventricular depolarization. The normal duration of the PR interval is 0.12 seconds to 0.20 seconds.

1. The sinus node fires.
2. The impulse passes through and depolarizes the atrium. As the atrial cells depolarize, they cause the P wave to appear on the EKG.
3. The impulse slowly passes through the AV node, then goes through the bundle of His and the right and left bundles. Finally, it depolarizes the ventricles, which causes the QRS to appear on the EKG.

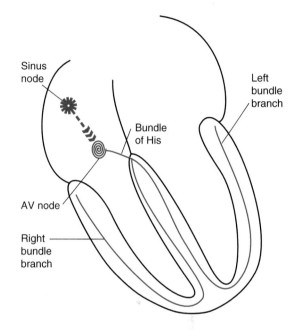

Sinus node

Left bundle branch

Bundle of His

AV node

Right bundle branch

Examples of the PR Interval

The PR interval is measured in the limb leads only and never in the horizontal leads.

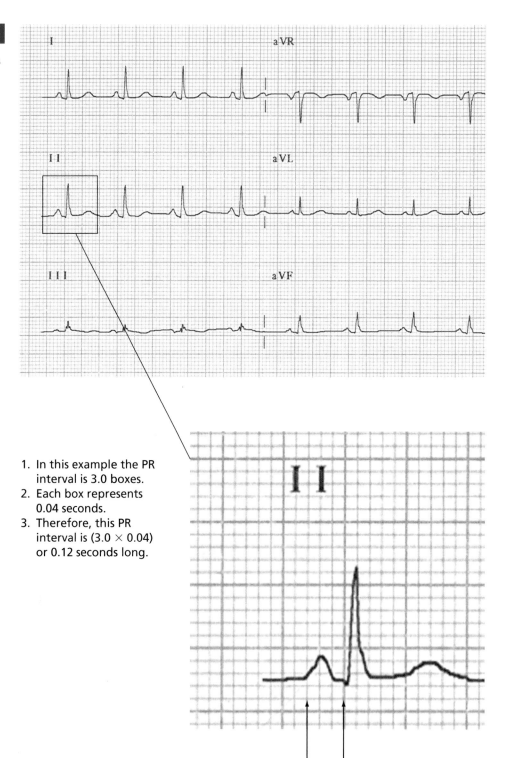

1. In this example the PR interval is 3.0 boxes.
2. Each box represents 0.04 seconds.
3. Therefore, this PR interval is (3.0 × 0.04) or 0.12 seconds long.

The PR interval is measured from the beginning of the P wave to the beginning of the QRS complex.

The PR is measured to the beginning of the QRS, regardless of which wave (q, r, qs) is first.

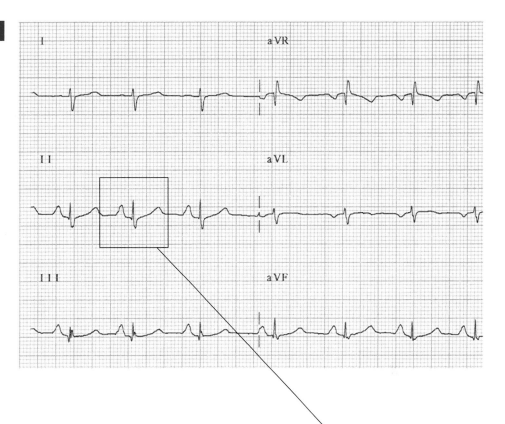

1. In this example the PR interval is 4.0 boxes.
2. Each box represents 0.04 seconds.
3. Therefore, this PR interval is (4.0 × 0.04) or 0.16 seconds long.

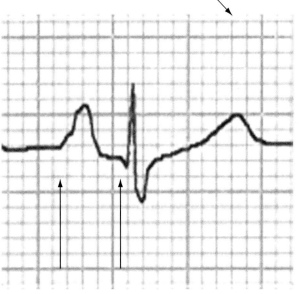

The normal PR interval is 0.12 to 0.20 seconds.

A PR interval longer than 0.20 seconds indicates 1° AV block.

A PR interval shorter than 0.12 seconds indicates accelerated AV conduction and implies the presence of a bypass tract (WPW).

The PR interval is 5 little boxes, or 0.20 seconds.

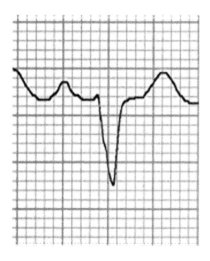

The PR interval is 4 little boxes, or 0.16 seconds.

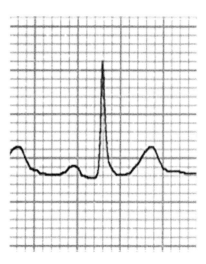

The PR interval is 5.5 little boxes, or 0.22 seconds.

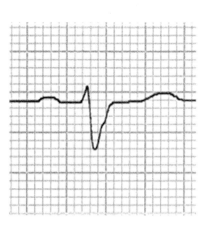

Long PR Intervals: 1° Atrioventricular Block

Disease of the AV node slows conduction through the AV node. Slow conduction through the AV node prolongs the PR interval to **greater than 0.20 seconds.** This is called 1° AV block. Common causes of 1° AV blocks include ischemia, drug toxicity, and degenerative diseases.

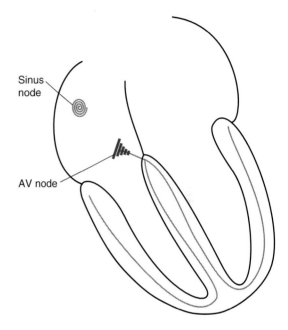

Sinus node

AV node

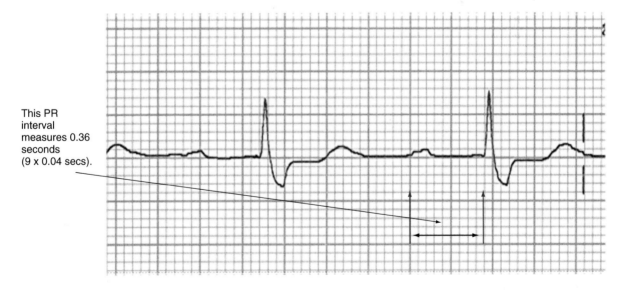

This PR interval measures 0.36 seconds (9 x 0.04 secs).

Short PR Intervals: WPW Syndrome

A PR interval shorter than 0.12 seconds indicates the presence of a shortcut that allows the electrical impulse to bypass the normal AV conduction system. This is called an AV bypass tract, or WPW syndrome (named after Drs. *W*olff, *P*arkinson, and *W*hite). The normal degree of AV block (0.12 to 0.20 seconds) allows a brief period of time for the atrium to fill the ventricle before the ventricle contracts. This short circuit can lead to fatally fast heart rates, as shown below.

Short PR interval here

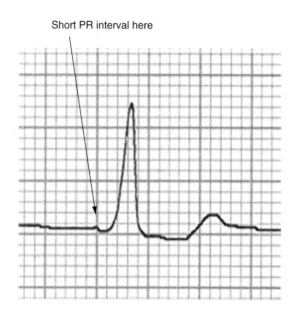

because of shortcut (bypass tract) to the ventricle

AV node

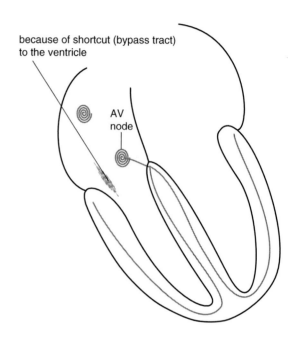

Careful inspection of this arrhythmia shows that the R-R intervals can be 4 little boxes apart. 1500/4 = 375 beats per minute.

The normal AV node cannot conduct at this rate. There must be a faster way that bypasses the normal conduction system (WPW).

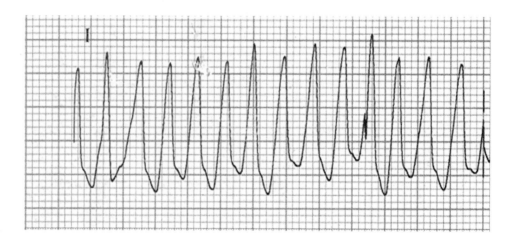

The QRS Interval

The next interval measured is the QRS interval. **The QRS interval measures the distance from the beginning of the QRS complex to the end of the QRS complex.** The QRS interval represents the amount of time it takes for the electrical impulse to depolarize the ventricles. The normal QRS interval is 0.09 seconds or less.

1. The sinus node has fired.
2. The impulse passed through and depolarized the atrium. As the atrial cells depolarized, they caused the P wave to appear on the EKG.
3. The impulse slowly passes through the AV node then goes through the bundle of His and the right and left bundles. Finally, it depolarizes the ventricles.

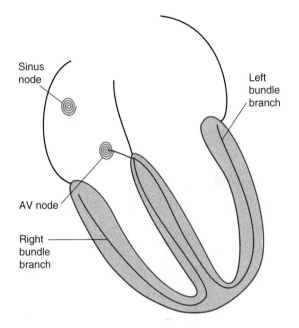

Examples of the QRS Interval

The QRS interval measures the distance from the beginning of the QRS complex to the end of the QRS complex.

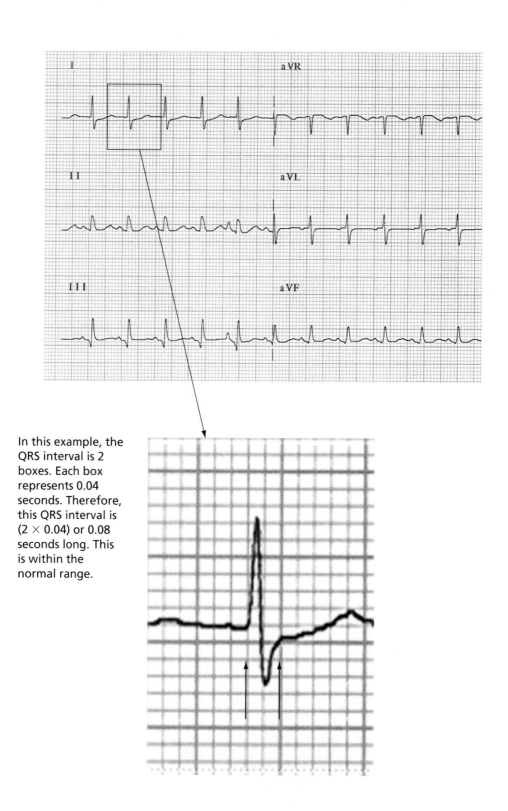

In this example, the QRS interval is 2 boxes. Each box represents 0.04 seconds. Therefore, this QRS interval is (2 × 0.04) or 0.08 seconds long. This is within the normal range.

The QRS interval is measured from the beginning to the end of the complex.

The QRS interval is 3.5 little boxes, or 0.14 seconds.

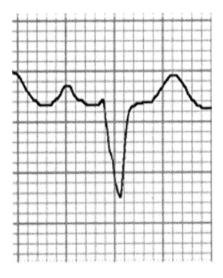

The QRS interval is 2.5 little boxes, or 0.10 seconds.

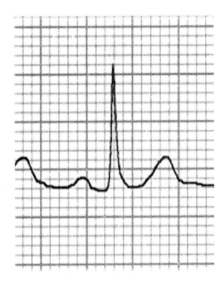

The QRS interval is 3.5 little boxes, or 0.14 seconds.

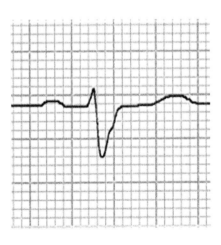

Long QRS Intervals

The normal right and left bundle branches are able to depolarize the normal right and left ventricles in 0.08 to 0.09 seconds, on average. A QRS interval of 0.09 or 0.10 seconds indicates a delay in conduction. This delay is given the awful name of **intraventricular conduction delay (IVCD)**. If the QRS interval reaches 0.12 seconds or longer, then bundle branch block is present. This is discussed more fully in Chapters 9 and 10.

Disease of the bundle branches delays depolarization of the right and left ventricles.

A QRS of 0.08 to 0.09 is normal.

A QRS of 0.10 to 0.11 indicates IVCD.

A QRS of 0.12 or longer indicates bundle branch block.

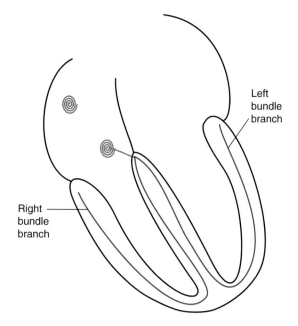

Left bundle branch

Right bundle branch

The QRS interval is 4 little boxes, or 0.16 seconds. This indicates bundle branch block.

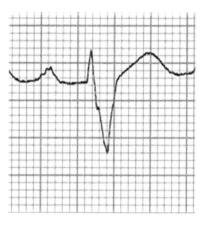

The QT Interval

The last interval to be measured is the QT interval. The QT interval measures the distance from the beginning of the QRS complex to the end of the T wave. The QT represents the time it takes the ventricles to depolarize and then reset or repolarize for the next cycle.

The ventricles depolarize and form the QRS on the EKG.

As soon as the cells depolarize, they begin to reset for the next depolarization.

Depolarization and repolarization require a normal environment of oxygen, potassium, calcium, and autonomic function. This process is also sensitive to drug effects from diuretics, antiarrhythmics, or digitalis.

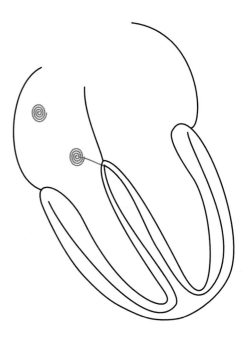

Examples of the QT Interval

The QT interval measures the distance from the beginning of the QRS complex to the end of the T wave.

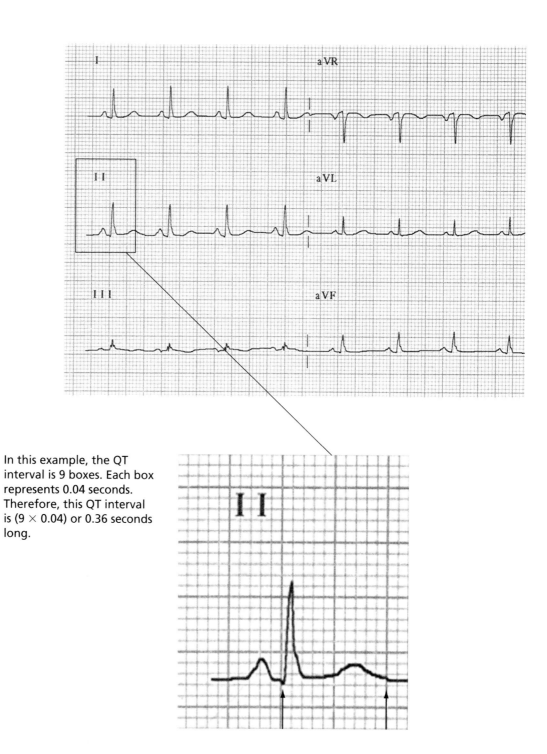

In this example, the QT interval is 9 boxes. Each box represents 0.04 seconds. Therefore, this QT interval is (9 × 0.04) or 0.36 seconds long.

The normal QT interval depends on the heart rate.

A long or short QT interval indicates pathology, typically due to drug effects, toxicity, or electrolyte imbalances.

The QT interval is 10.5 little boxes, or 0.42 seconds.

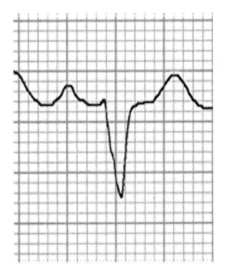

The QT interval is 8 little boxes, or 0.32 seconds.

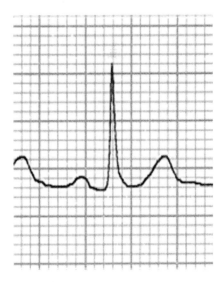

The QT interval is 12 little boxes, or 0.48 seconds.

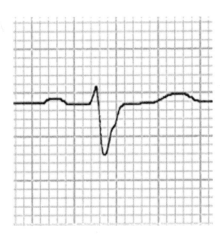

The Corrected QT Interval

The QT interval varies normally according to the heart rate. The faster the heart rate, the shorter the QT interval. The slower the heart rate, the longer the QT interval. Formulas are available to calculate the correct or appropriate QT interval for the patient's heart rate. In practice, it's much simpler to use a table of QT intervals corrected for heart rate.

The normal range of QT intervals depends on the heart rate.

A QT interval in the normal range gives a QTc (corrected QT) in the expected range.

A QT at or above the **long QT** range is definitely abnormal and should be explained.

A QT in the dangerous range should be immediately evaluated, and medications and electrolytes (calcium, potassium, magnesium) should be evaluated.

Heart Rate	Normal Range of the QT		Long QT	Dangerous
	low (QTC 365)	high (QTC 419)	(QTC 440)	(QTC 500)
50	0.40	0.46	0.48	0.55
55	0.38	0.44	0.46	0.52
60	0.37	0.42	0.44	0.50
65	0.35	0.40	0.42	0.48
70	0.34	0.39	0.41	0.46
75	0.33	0.37	0.39	0.45
80	0.32	0.36	0.38	0.43
85	0.31	0.35	0.38	0.42
90	0.30	0.34	0.37	0.41
95	0.29	0.33	0.36	0.40
100	0.28	0.32	0.35	0.39
105	0.28	0.32	0.34	0.38
110	0.27	0.31	0.33	0.37
115	0.26	0.30	0.32	0.36
120	0.26	0.30	0.31	0.35
125	0.25	0.29	0.30	0.35
130	0.25	0.28	0.30	0.34
135	0.24	0.28	0.29	0.33
140	0.24	0.27	0.29	0.33
145	0.23	0.27	0.28	0.32
150	0.23	0.26	0.28	0.32
155	0.23	0.26	0.27	0.31
160	0.22	0.26	0.27	0.31

Indeterminate QT Intervals

Sometimes, it's hard to clearly identify the T wave in the limb leads, making it difficult to measure confidently the QT interval. This difficulty may be due to hypokalemia. When it becomes difficult to see the end of the QT interval, call the QT interval "indeterminate." Always be careful to check the electrolytes. This will be further discussed in Chapter 19.

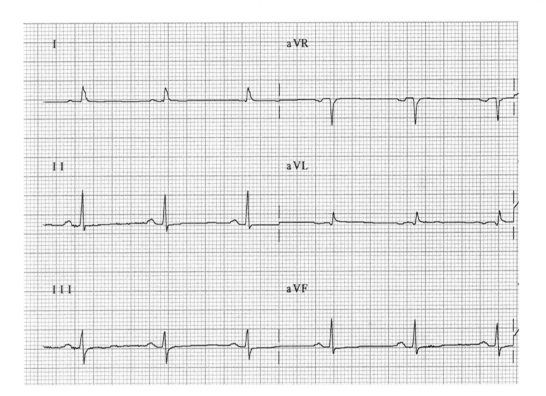

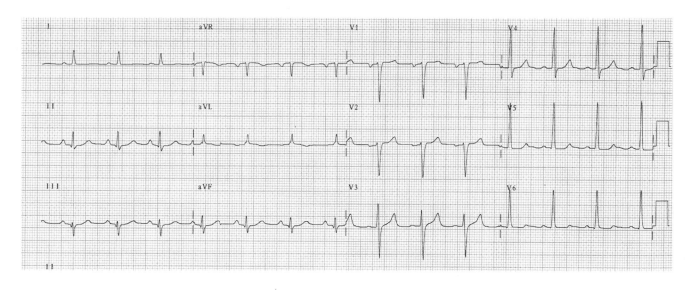

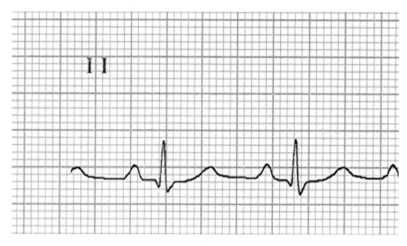

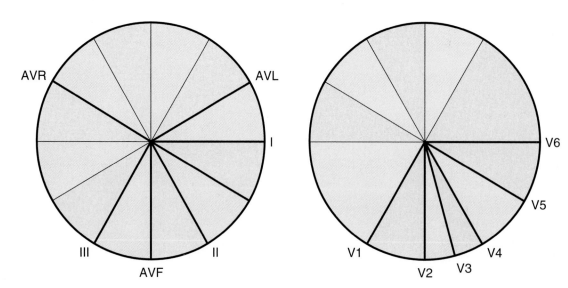

Heart Rate:

Rhythm:

Intervals (measured in the limb leads)

PR: short (< .12)
     normal (.12 to .20)
     long (>0.20 seconds); this is 1st degree AV block

QRS: normal (≤0.09 seconds)
      prolonged (.10 or .11); this is intraventricular conduction delay (IVCD)
      Bundle Branch Block (.12 seconds or greater)

QT:

P axis: normal
           rightward
           arm-lead reversal or dextrocardia
           junctional rhythm

QRS axis: normal
           left anterior hemiblock
           left posterior hemiblock
           indeterminate

T wave inversion (ischemia or infarction):

II,III,AVF	inferior
I, AVL	lateral
V1, without V2	nonspecific septal
V1 and V2	septal
V3 and V4	anterior
V5 and V6	lateral
V6, without V5	nonspecific lateral

ST Elevation (acute infarction):

II,III,AVF	inferior
I, AVL	lateral
V1, without V2	nonspecific septal
V1 and V2	septal
V3 and V4	anterior
V5 and V6	lateral
V6, without V5.	nonspecific lateral

ST Depression (ischemia or infarction):

I,II,III,AVL,AVF	diffuse subendocardial ischemia or infarction
V2,V3,V4,V5	diffuse subendocardial ischemia or infarction

Q waves (infarction):

II,III,AVF	inferior
I, AVL	lateral
V1, without V2	nonspecific septal
V1 and V2	septal
V3 and V4	anterior
V5 and V6	lateral
V6, without V5	nonspecific lateral

Hypertrophy:

Right atrial: Tall P wave 2.5 mm in II, III, or AVF

Left atrial: Deep negative part of P wave in V1

LVH: R wave in 1 + S wave in III ≥ 25mV
      S wave in V1 + R wave in V5 ≥ 35mV

RVH: Mean QRS either anterior, or rightward

The heart rate is 1500/18 or 83 beats per minute. The PR interval measures 4.5 little boxes (4.5 × 0.04), which is 0.18 seconds. This is normal. The QRS interval measures between 2 and 2.5 boxes (2.25 × 0.04), which is 0.09 seconds. (If you measured the QRS as 0.10 seconds, then intraventricular conduction delay (IVCD) is present.) The QT interval measures 8.5 little boxes (8.5 × 0.04) which is 0.34 seconds. From the table in Chapter 5, this QT interval is in the expected range for this heart rate.

Parts of the answer sheets are "grayed out" because these sections have not yet been covered. Answer only the parts that are not highlighted.

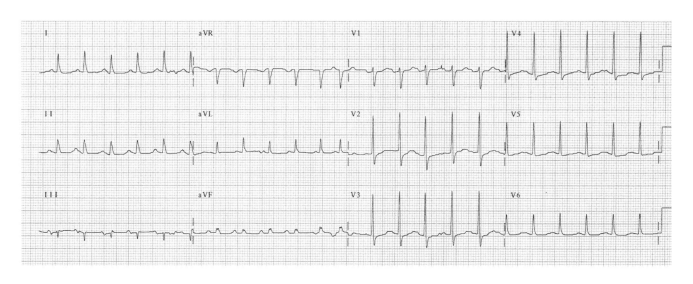

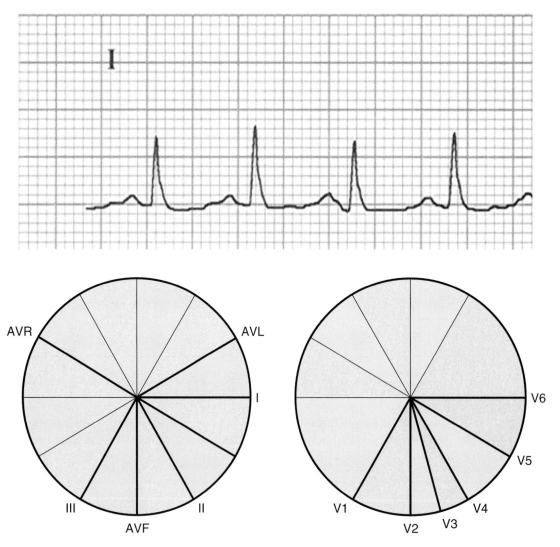

Heart Rate:

Rhythm:

Intervals (measured in the limb leads)

PR: short (< .12)
normal (.12 to .20)
long (>0.20 seconds); this is 1st degree AV
block

QRS: normal (≤0.09 seconds)
prolonged (.10 or .11); this is intraventricular
conduction delay (IVCD)
Bundle Branch Block (.12 seconds or greater)

QT:

P axis: normal
rightward
arm-lead reversal or dextrocardia
junctional rhythm

QRS axis: normal
left anterior hemiblock
left posterior hemiblock
indeterminate

T wave inversion (ischemia or infarction):

II,III,AVF	inferior
I, AVL	lateral
V1, without V2	nonspecific septal
V1 and V2	septal
V3 and V4	anterior
V5 and V6	lateral
V6, without V5	nonspecific lateral

ST Elevation (acute infarction):

II,III,AVF	inferior
I, AVL	lateral
V1, without V2	nonspecific septal
V1 and V2	septal
V3 and V4	anterior
V5 and V6	lateral
V6, without V5.	nonspecific lateral

ST Depression (ischemia or infarction):

I,II,III,AVL,AVF	diffuse subendocardial ischemia or infarction
V2,V3,V4,V5	diffuse subendocardial ischemia or infarction

Q waves (infarction):

II,III,AVF	inferior
I, AVL	lateral
V1, without V2	nonspecific septal
V1 and V2	septal
V3 and V4	anterior
V5 and V6	lateral
V6, without V5	nonspecific lateral

Hypertrophy:

Right atrial: Tall P wave 2.5 mm in II, III, or AVF

Left atrial: Deep negative part of P wave in V1

LVH: R wave in 1 + S wave in III ≥ 25mV
S wave in V1 + R wave in V5 ≥ 35mV

RVH: Mean QRS either anterior, or rightward

The heart rate is 1500/11 or 136 beats per minute. This is sinus tachycardia. It is abnormal, and importantly so. The clinical correlation of the EKG begins with the heart rate. "Begin at the beginning," as Dylan Thomas said. Common causes of sinus tachycardia include shock, hypovolemia (from bleeding, overdiuresis, gastrointestinal loss), asthma medications (sympathomimetics), pain, anxiety, pulmonary embolus, fever, sepsis, anemia, hyperthyroidism. Nothing on the list is insignificant, nothing on the list can be ignored. The PR interval measures 0.16 seconds and is normal. The QT interval cannot be easily measured or even found for that matter. Call this "indeterminate QT interval." *It suggests that the T wave is of low amplitude.* (This is discussed in Chapter 19.) The causes of low-amplitude T waves include hypokalemia. Possibly this patient was on a diuretic and became hypovolemic and hypokalemic as a result. This patient's potassium was 3.1 mEq/L (low).

Parts of the answer sheets are "grayed out" because these sections have not yet been covered. Answer only the parts that are not highlighted.

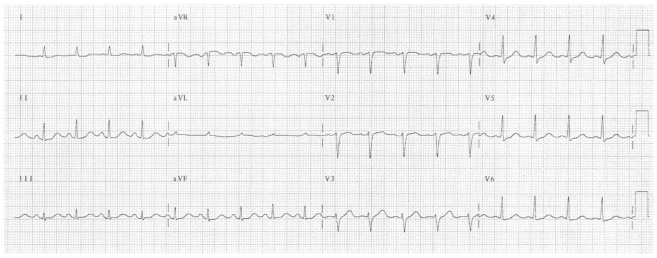

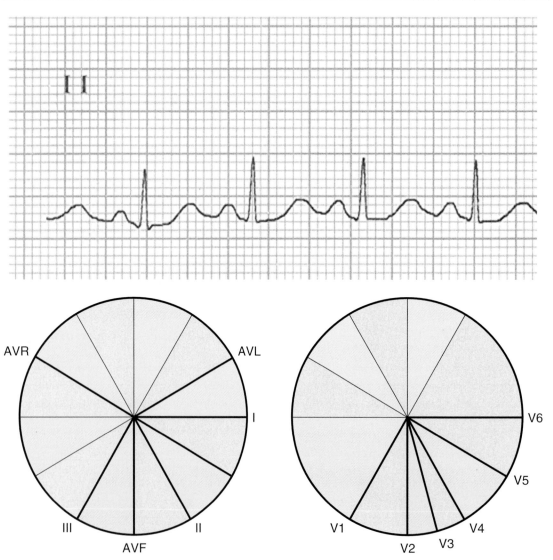

Heart Rate:

Rhythm:

Intervals (measured in the limb leads)

PR: short (< .12)
normal (.12 to .20)
long (>0.20 seconds); this is 1st degree AV block

QRS: normal (≤0.09 seconds)
prolonged (.10 or .11); this is intraventricular conduction delay (IVCD)
Bundle Branch Block (.12 seconds or greater)

QT:

P axis: normal
rightward
arm-lead reversal or dextrocardia
junctional rhythm

QRS axis: normal
left anterior hemiblock
left posterior hemiblock
indeterminate

T wave inversion (ischemia or infarction):

II,III,AVF	inferior
I, AVL	lateral
V1, without V2	nonspecific septal
V1 and V2	septal
V3 and V4	anterior
V5 and V6	lateral
V6, without V5	nonspecific lateral

ST Elevation (acute infarction):

II,III,AVF	inferior
I, AVL	lateral
V1, without V2	nonspecific septal
V1 and V2	septal
V3 and V4	anterior
V5 and V6	lateral
V6, without V5.	nonspecific lateral

ST Depression (ischemia or infarction):

I,II,III,AVL,AVF	diffuse subendocardial ischemia or infarction
V2,V3,V4,V5	diffuse subendocardial ischemia or infarction

Q waves (infarction):

II,III,AVF	inferior
I, AVL	lateral
V1, without V2	nonspecific septal
V1 and V2	septal
V3 and V4	anterior
V5 and V6	lateral
V6, without V5	nonspecific lateral

Hypertrophy:

Right atrial: Tall P wave 2.5 mm in II, III, or AVF

Left atrial: Deep negative part of P wave in V1

LVH: R wave in 1 + S wave in III ≥ 25mV
S wave in V1 + R wave in V5 ≥ 35mV

RVH: Mean QRS either anterior, or rightward

The heart rate is 115 beats per minute. This is sinus tachycardia. Again, the clinical cause of sinus tachycardia is typically important. The PR interval measures 0.14 seconds and is normal. The QRS interval measures 0.08 seconds and is normal. The end of the T wave in lead II crosses the midpoint between the R-R intervals. This is a useful clinical shortcut that indicates the QT interval is probably long for the given heart rate. The QT interval measures 0.32 seconds. From the table in Chapter 5, this QT would correct to a QTc of 0.44 seconds (440 msec) at this heart rate. This is long, and should be evaluated. This is discussed further in Chapter 19. Drugs and electrolyte effects are typically responsible.

Parts of the answer sheets are "grayed out" because these sections have not yet been covered. Answer only the parts that are not highlighted.

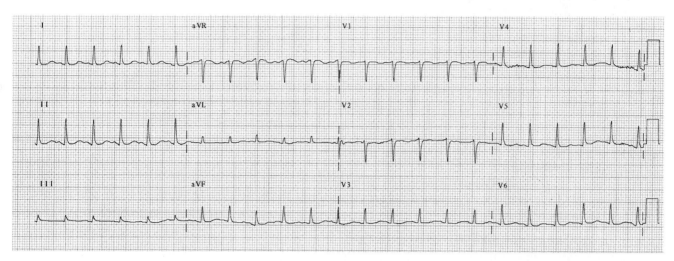

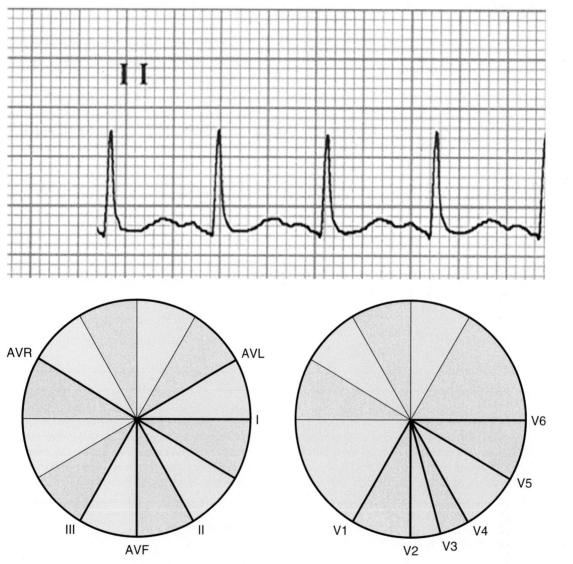

Heart Rate:

Rhythm:

Intervals (measured in the limb leads)

PR: short (< .12)
        normal (.12 to .20)
        long (>0.20 seconds); this is 1st degree AV
        block

QRS: normal (≤0.09 seconds)
        prolonged (.10 or .11); this is intraventricular
        conduction delay (IVCD)
        Bundle Branch Block (.12 seconds or greater)

QT:

P axis: normal
            rightward
            arm-lead reversal or dextrocardia
            junctional rhythm

QRS axis: normal
            left anterior hemiblock
            left posterior hemiblock
            indeterminate

T wave inversion (ischemia or infarction):

II,III,AVF	inferior
I, AVL	lateral
V1, without V2	nonspecific septal
V1 and V2	septal
V3 and V4	anterior
V5 and V6	lateral
V6, without V5	nonspecific lateral

ST Elevation (acute infarction):

II,III,AVF	inferior
I, AVL	lateral
V1, without V2	nonspecific septal
V1 and V2	septal
V3 and V4	anterior
V5 and V6	lateral
V6, without V5.	nonspecific lateral

ST Depression (ischemia or infarction):

I,II,III,AVL,AVF	diffuse subendocardial ischemia or infarction
V2,V3,V4,V5	diffuse subendocardial ischemia or infarction

Q waves (infarction):

II,III,AVF	inferior
I, AVL	lateral
V1, without V2	nonspecific septal
V1 and V2	septal
V3 and V4	anterior
V5 and V6	lateral
V6, without V5	nonspecific lateral

Hypertrophy:

Right atrial: Tall P wave 2.5 mm in II, III, or AVF

Left atrial: Deep negative part of P wave in V1

LVH: R wave in 1 + S wave in III ≥ 25mV
      S wave in V1 + R wave in V5 ≥ 35mV

RVH: Mean QRS either anterior, or rightward

The heart rate is 1500/11 or 136 beats per minute. This is sinus tachycardia. Again, the cause of sinus tachycardia should always be identified. This can be one of the most valuable clinical clues on an EKG and should not be overlooked. The PR interval is 0.12 seconds. The QRS interval measures 0.08 seconds and is normal. The QT interval is 0.32 seconds, which is long for this heart rate. From the table in Chapter 5, this combination of heart rate and QT interval corrects to a QTc of nearly 0.50 seconds (500 msec). Long QT interval can be a manifestation of drug toxicity or electrolyte imbalance. Hypokalemia and hypocalcemia are common causes of long QT interval. Antiarrhythmic drugs, psychotropic drugs, are common drug causes of this. This is discussed further in Chapter 19.

Parts of the answer sheets are "grayed out" because these sections have not yet been covered. Answer only the parts that are not highlighted.

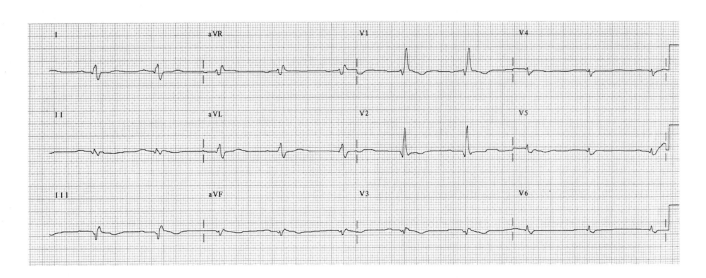

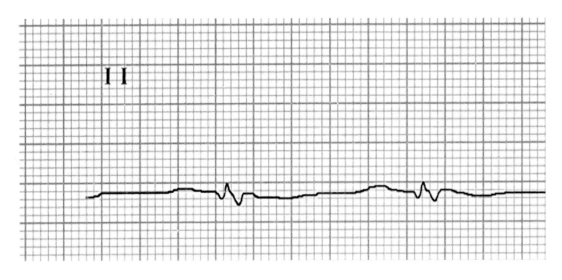

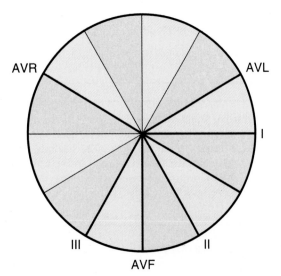

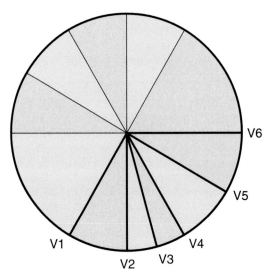

Heart Rate:

Rhythm:

Intervals (measured in the limb leads)

PR: short (< .12)
         normal (.12 to .20)
         long (>0.20 seconds); this is 1st degree AV
         block

QRS: normal (≤0.09 seconds)
         prolonged (.10 or .11); this is intraventricular
         conduction delay (IVCD)
         Bundle Branch Block (.12 seconds or greater)

QT:

P axis: normal
              rightward
              arm-lead reversal or dextrocardia
              junctional rhythm

QRS axis: normal
              left anterior hemiblock
              left posterior hemiblock
              indeterminate

T wave inversion (ischemia or infarction):

II,III,AVF	inferior
I, AVL	lateral
V1, without V2	nonspecific septal
V1 and V2	septal
V3 and V4	anterior
V5 and V6	lateral
V6, without V5	nonspecific lateral

ST Elevation (acute infarction):

II,III,AVF	inferior
I, AVL	lateral
V1, without V2	nonspecific septal
V1 and V2	septal
V3 and V4	anterior
V5 and V6	lateral
V6, without V5.	nonspecific lateral

ST Depression (ischemia or infarction):

I,II,III,AVL,AVF	diffuse subendocardial ischemia or infarction
V2,V3,V4,V5	diffuse subendocardial ischemia or infarction

Q waves (infarction):

II,III,AVF	inferior
I, AVL	lateral
V1, without V2	nonspecific septal
V1 and V2	septal
V3 and V4	anterior
V5 and V6	lateral
V6, without V5	nonspecific lateral

Hypertrophy:

Right atrial: Tall P wave 2.5 mm in II, III, or AVF

Left atrial: Deep negative part of P wave in V1

LVH: R wave in 1 + S wave in III ≥ 25mV
       S wave in V1 + R wave in V5 ≥ 35mV

RVH: Mean QRS either anterior, or rightward

The heart rate is 1500/26 = 58 beats per minute. The PR interval measures 0.24 seconds, which is long and indicates 1° AV block. The causes of 1° AV block include digitalis, primary conduction disease, ischemic heart disease, and other medications. The QRS interval measures 0.14 seconds. This is long and indicates bundle branch block. The further characterization of bundle branch block is discussed in Chapters 9 and 10. The QT interval measures 0.44 seconds but is difficult to measure with confidence. The combination of a heart rate of 58 beats per minute and a QT of 0.44 seconds corresponds to a corrected QT (QTc) of 440 msec. This is again in the long range.

Parts of the answer sheets are "grayed out" because these sections have not yet been covered. Answer only the parts that are not highlighted.

How to Measure Axis

Most books teach EKG interpretation the way third-grade teachers teach multiplication, by memorization. Pattern memorization is a quick and easy way of abandoning any hope of ever understanding what an EKG actually tells us. By memorizing patterns, the student never fully understands the principles behind the 12-lead EKG. This chapter describes axis, which is one scientific method for looking at and interpreting the EKG.

The 12-lead EKG displays the electrical forces of the heart on grid paper. Each electrical force comes from and provides information about a different part of the heart. For 8 to 10 different parts of the heart, there is a corresponding force that produces a wave or complex on the EKG.

Electrical forces, including those represented on the EKG, have two distinct properties: magnitude and direction.

Magnitude describes the size of the force. For example, an electrical force can be huge like a bolt of lightning or minute like a touch of static electricity.

Direction describes where the force is headed. For example, is the lightning bolt coming toward me or going away from me?

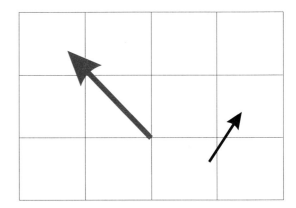

The QRS Axis

Each electrical force, representative of a certain area of the heart, has a normal direction and magnitude.

When a force is abnormal in size or direction, it may indicate that the specific part of the heart producing the force is abnormal. Therefore, learning the heart's normal electrical axis or direction of forces provides a scientific way of understanding and interpreting an EKG.

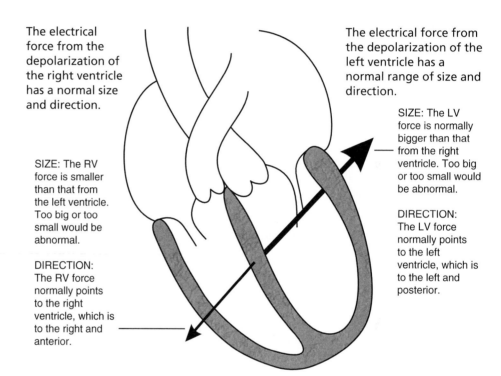

The electrical force from the depolarization of the right ventricle has a normal size and direction.

SIZE: The RV force is smaller than that from the left ventricle. Too big or too small would be abnormal.

DIRECTION: The RV force normally points to the right ventricle, which is to the right and anterior.

The electrical force from the depolarization of the left ventricle has a normal range of size and direction.

SIZE: The LV force is normally bigger than that from the right ventricle. Too big or too small would be abnormal.

DIRECTION: The LV force normally points to the left ventricle, which is to the left and posterior.

The QRS Axis (continued)

The right and left ventricles depolarize at the same time, producing two electrical forces that move in opposite directions. However, because the left ventricle normally produces a larger force, the combined axis points leftward and posterior. Any other direction or magnitude would be considered abnormal.

Only by combining the partial information in each lead with the other leads on the EKG does a complete three-dimensional picture of the electrical forces emerge. The electrical axis is measured for the P wave, the QRS complex, and the T wave, as well as for other forces throughout the book. The remainder of this chapter teaches a method for determining the direction of the electrical force for any of the waves or complexes on the EKG. By mapping out the electrical forces, the student will be able to better understand the information that the EKG provides.

The force that results from the combination of right and left ventricular forces points leftward toward the left ventricle because the left ventricle is much larger than the right ventricle.

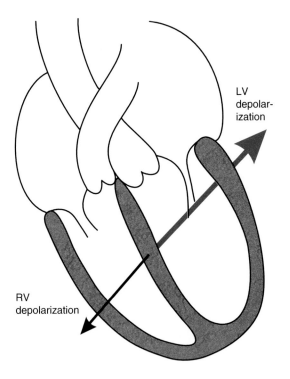

LV depolarization

RV depolarization

The Frontal Plane Axis Diagram

When measuring the axis or direction of any force in the frontal plane, begin by drawing the leads as shown, which represents a frontal view of the heart.

Label the leads as shown.

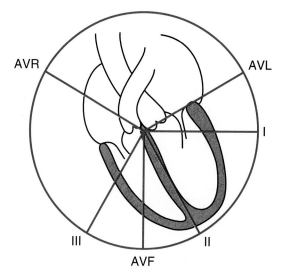

Continue the line segments to the other side of the circle. This results in this diagram.

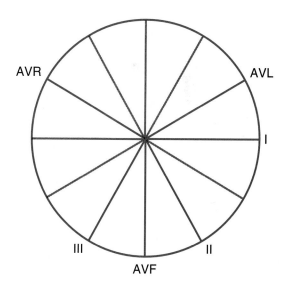

To provide an easy and understandable way to describe direction, label each lead in degrees. Lead I is the starting point at 0°, continuing counterclockwise is considered negative, and continuing clockwise from zero is considered positive. By combining the information from each of these leads (I, II, III, AVR, AVL, and AVF) the direction of any force can be determined. To clarify what the diagram represents, imagine the heart superimposed on top of it. This helps to visualize the direction of the force moving through the heart.

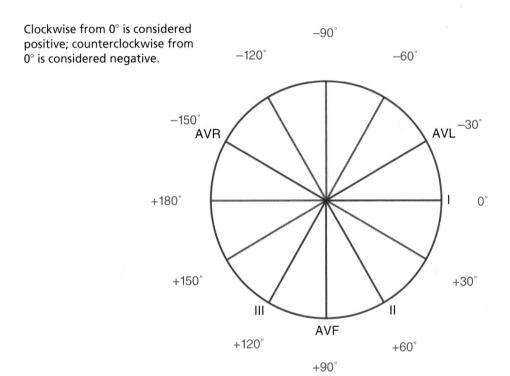

Clockwise from 0° is considered positive; counterclockwise from 0° is considered negative.

The Frontal Plane Leads as Observers

Imagine that at each lead an observer stands looking at the same electrical heart event. Because the observers are standing or looking at the event from different places, they can only describe it from their perspectives. By using each observer's information, we are able to reconstruct an average event to determine the direction of the electrical force.

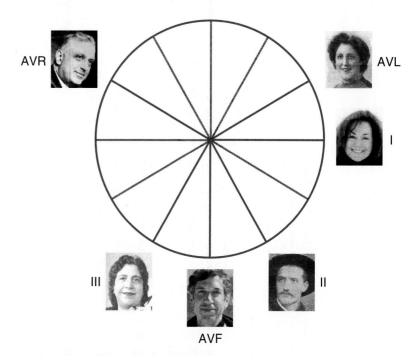

When calculating the axis or direction of any wave or complex, always look at lead I first.

Lead I

The observer is standing at lead I and has the perspective of someone viewing the cardiac events from this location. **A critical point to remember is that the observer standing at lead I evaluates lead I on the EKG but documents her observation on the lead line perpendicular to lead I, which is line AVF, as shown below.** For example, the lead I observer evaluates lead I on the EKG. If the complex in question is upright or positive, the observer sees the force as coming toward her and documents her finding on lead line AVF.

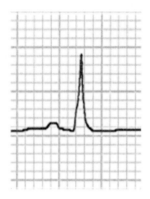

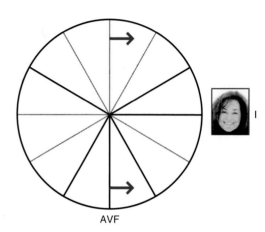

AVF

    If the complex in lead I is negative or downward, the observer sees the force as moving away from her and documents the finding on lead line AVF, as shown in the example below. If lead I observer sees the force as mostly negative, then the force is pointing rightward. Rightward means toward the patient's right. This concept of positive = toward and negative = away is fundamental to understanding the concept of axis.

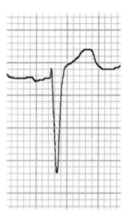

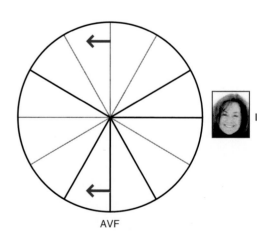

AVF

Examples of Lead I

As stated, the **positive = toward, negative = away** concept is used in the calculation of the P, QRS, ST, and T axes.

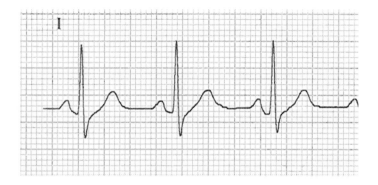

The P wave in lead I is upright or **positive.** Positive = toward, so the P wave must be pointing leftward, because the lead I observer sees the P wave as coming **toward** her.

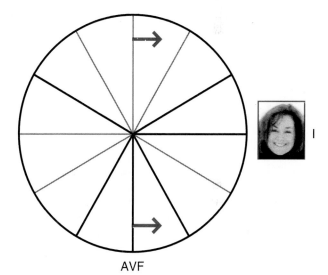

AVF

The ST segment in lead I is pointing downward or **negative.** Negative = away, so the ST segment must be pointing rightward, because the lead I observer sees the ST segment as **going away** from her.

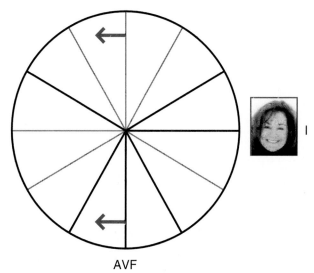

AVF

Lead I: Isoelectric

There are occasions when the complex is neither negative nor positive. This is known as an isoelectric complex (just as positive as it is negative).

In this case, the axis would be perpendicular to the observer, which means the force is neither moving toward nor moving away from the observer.

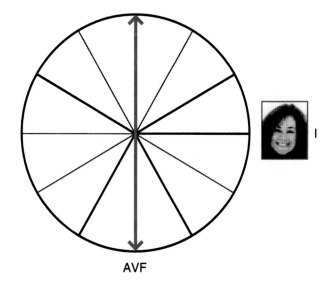

AVF

This QRS is an example of an isoelectric complex. The QRS has as much space under the R wave part of the QRS as does the S wave.

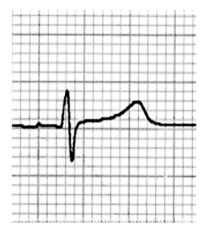

Lead AVF: Positive or Negative

After the axis for lead I is calculated, move on to lead AVF. Again, remember that the AVF observer is evaluating lead AVF but documenting his observations on the line perpendicular to lead AVF, which is line I. Therefore, the AVF observer can provide information about line I and whether the direction of the force is moving toward or away from him.

Look at AVF on an EKG. If the complex is positive, then the force is moving toward the AVF observer, which is illustrated by the arrows.

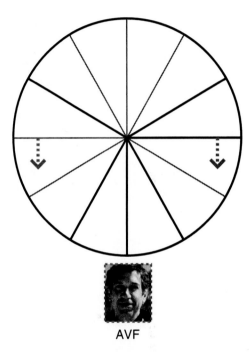

AVF

If the complex is negative in lead I, the force is moving away from the AVF observer, which is illustrated in the diagram by the arrows.

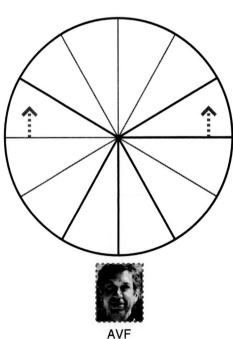

AVF

Lead AVF: Short Examples

The following is an example of using lead AVF to calculate a T-wave axis. The AVF observer is evaluating the T wave in lead AVF. The T wave in this lead is upright or positive, *indicating that the AVF observer sees the force as coming toward him.*

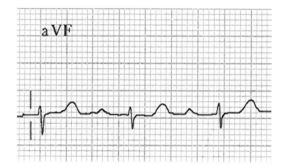

The *T wave* in lead AVF is mostly **positive**. The T wave must be pointing in a downward direction, because the lead AVF observer sees the T wave as coming **toward** him.

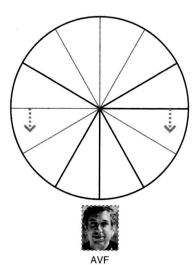

AVF

The *QRS complex* in lead AVF is mostly **negative**. The QRS complex must be pointing in an upward direction, because the lead AVF observer sees the QRS complex as going **away** from him.

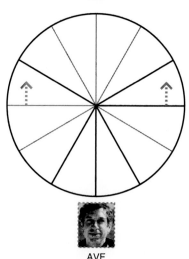

AVF

Lead AVF: Isoelectric

If the P, QRS, or T wave in lead AVF is isoelectric, the axis must be perpendicular to AVF.

The observer sees the force as coming neither toward nor away from him. Rather, the observer sees the force as moving perpendicular to his location.

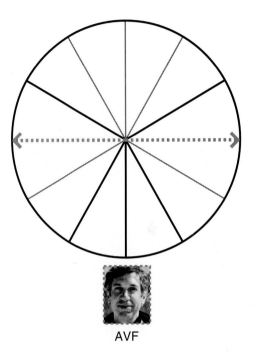

AVF

Calculation of Axis: Example 1

EXAMPLE 1: Find the QRS axis in the frontal plane for this EKG.

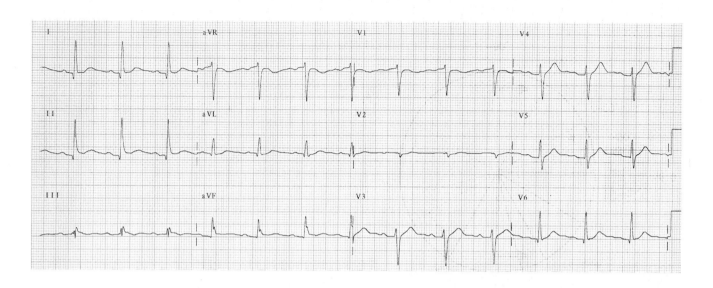

The QRS in lead I is positive.

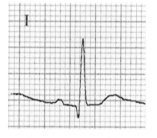

I am the observer at lead I. I see the QRS as mostly upright (positive). I see the QRS as coming **toward** me.

The lead I observer evaluates lead I, but documents her observation on the line perpendicular to lead I, which is line AVF.

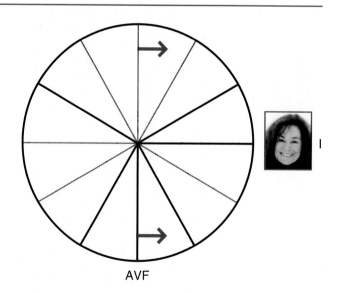

AVF

Example 1 Continued: Lead AVF

EXAMPLE 1 CONTINUED: Find the QRS axis in the frontal plane for this EKG.

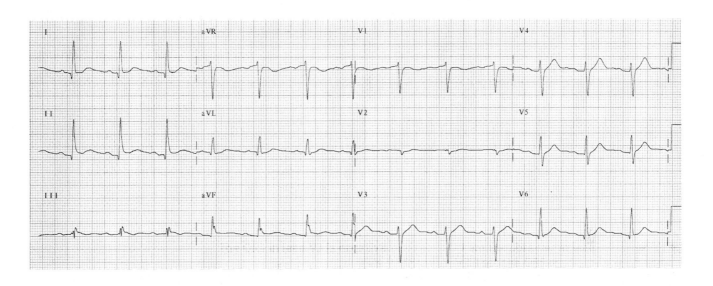

The QRS in lead AVF is positive.

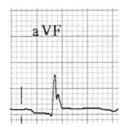

I am the observer at lead AVF. I see the QRS as upright or positive. I see the QRS as coming **toward** me.

The lead AVF observer evaluates lead AVF but documents his observation on the line perpendicular to lead AVF, which is line I.

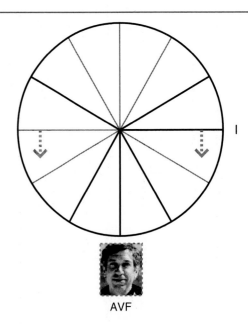

AVF

Example 1 Continued: Combination of Leads

Although the information from leads SI and AVF was drawn on separate diagrams for purposes of illustration, they must be drawn on one diagram to calculate the axis.

The result is that the QRS axis lies below line I and to the left of line AVF, or in the lower left quadrant.

Mathematically, the axis is greater than 0° and less than positive 90°.

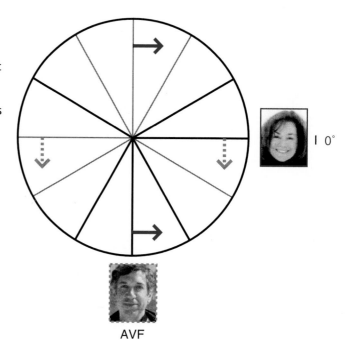

I 0°

AVF

For greater accuracy, the axis can be narrowed further to multiples of 15°, as shown.

To calculate the axis to multiples of 15°, we need to analyze leads II, III, AVR, and AVL.

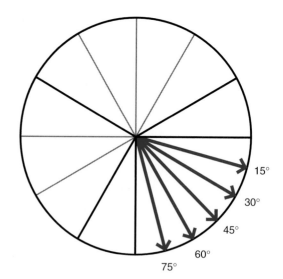

15°

30°

45°

60°

75°

Lead III

To further delineate the axis, we must answer the following question: which way does the axis lie with respect to line AVR? The answer to this question can be found by examining the observer lead perpendicular to lead AVR, which is lead III.

If the complex in lead III is **negative**, the axis lies **away** from lead III.

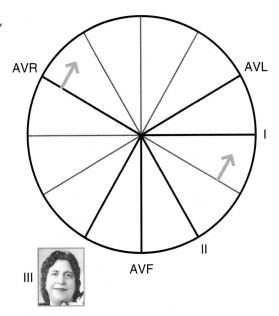

If lead III is **positive**, the axis lies **toward** lead III.

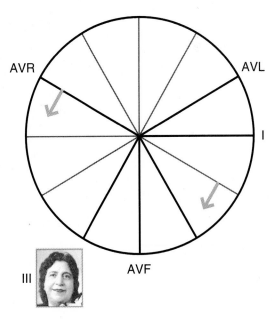

Example 1 Continued: Lead III

Now, continue with Example 1:

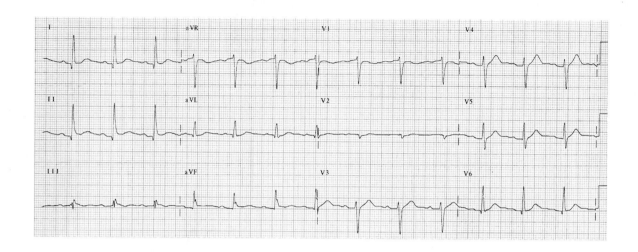

The QRS in lead III is positive.

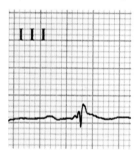

I am the observer at lead III. I see the QRS as upright or positive. I see the QRS as coming toward me.

III

The observer at lead III evaluates lead III on the EKG but documents her observation on the line perpendicular to lead III, which is line AVR.

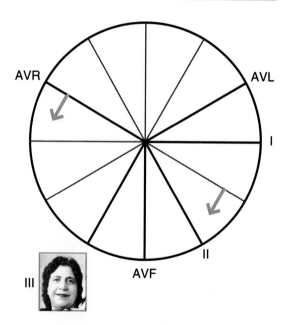

EXAMPLE 1 CONTINUED: SUMMARY

Combine the information from the three leads or observers into one
diagram.

a) Lead I is positive.
b) Lead AVF is positive.
c) Lead III is positive.

Using a, b, and c, from
above, the axis is greater
than +30° and less than
+90°. Because we are
using multiples of 15°,
the axis must be 45°, 60°,
or 75°.

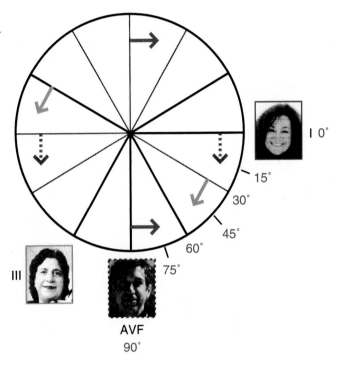

Lead AVL

The last piece of information required to narrow down the axis further in this example is **finding the axis in relation to the line II.**

The answer to this question can be found by examining the observer lead perpendicular to the line lead II, which is lead AVL.

If lead AVL is positive, the axis is toward AVL.

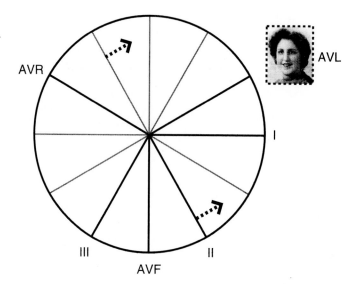

If lead AVL is negative, the axis is away from AVL.

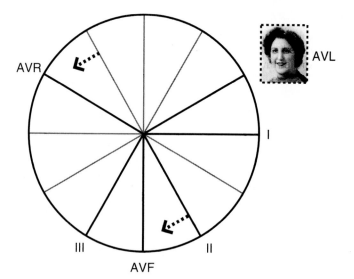

Lead AVL

If lead AVL is isoelectric, the axis is perpendicular to AVL.

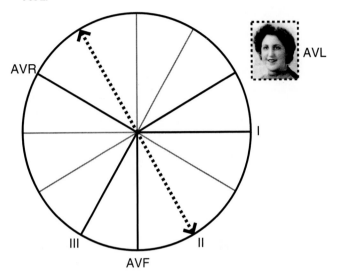

Example 1 Continued: Lead AVL

Now, continue with **Example 1:**

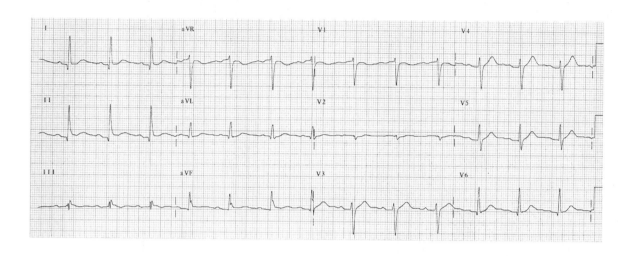

The QRS in lead AVL is positive.

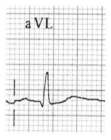

I am the observer at lead AVL. I see the QRS as upright or **positive.** I see the QRS as coming **toward** me.

The observer at lead AVL evaluates lead AVL on the EKG but documents her observation on the line perpendicular to lead AVL, which is line II.

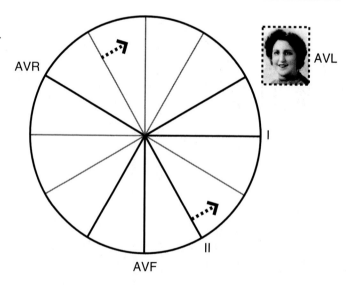

Example I: Conclusion

Combining the information from the four observers or leads into one diagram.

    a) Lead I is positive.
    b) Lead AVF is positive.
    c) Lead III is positive.
    d) Lead AVL is positive.

The axis (the direction of the QRS depolarization in this example) lies at positive 45°.

This one number or description summarizes the observations of the four leads into a single useful concept for direction.

Summary: The electrical force of ventricular depolarization points downward and to the patient's left.

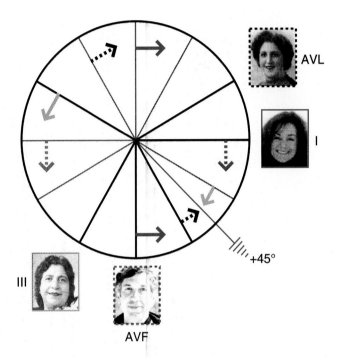

Calculation of Axis: Example 2

EXAMPLE 2: Find the QRS axis in the frontal plane for this EKG.

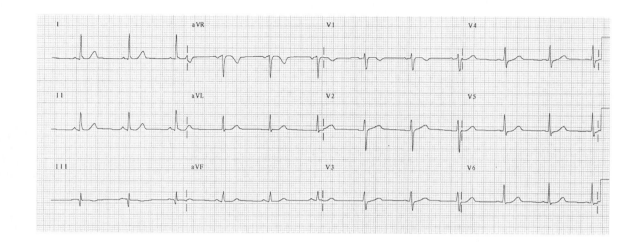

The QRS in lead I is positive.

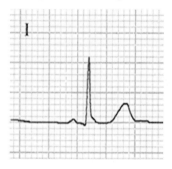

I am the observer at lead I.
I see the QRS as **positive**.
I see the QRS as coming
toward me.

I documented my
observation on the line
perpendicular to lead I,
which is line AVF.

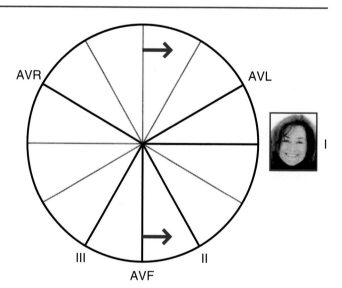

Example 2 Continued: Lead AVF

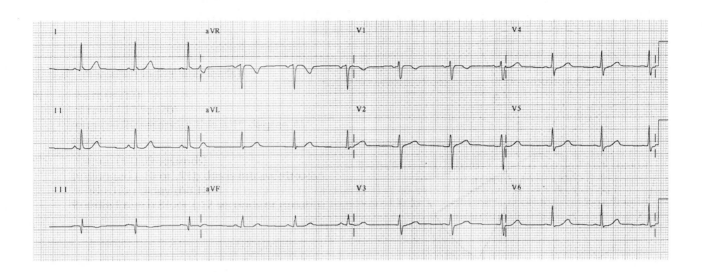

The QRS in lead AVF is positive.

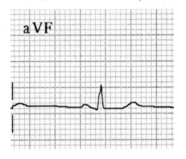

I am the observer at lead AVF. I see the QRS as upright or positive. I see the QRS as coming toward me.

I documented my observation on the line perpendicular to lead AVF, which is line I.

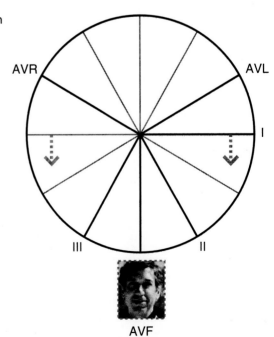

Example 2 Continued: Leads I and AVF

EXAMPLE 2: Combine the information from the first two observers or leads.

Although the information from leads I and AVF was drawn on separate diagrams for purposes of illustration, **the arrows should be drawn on one diagram to calculate the axis.**

The result is that the axis lies below line I and to the left of AVF, or in the lower left quadrant, which is to the patient's left. Mathematically, the axis is greater than 0° and less than +90°.

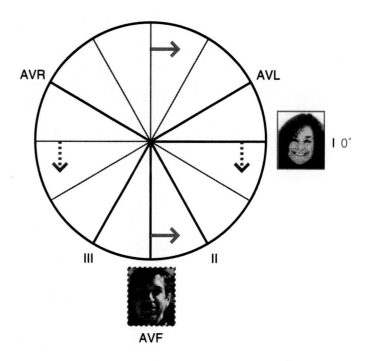

Example 2 Continued: Lead III

EXAMPLE 2: Now, continue with examination of more leads.

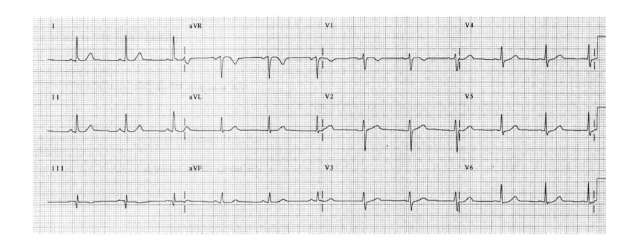

The QRS in lead III is isoelectric.

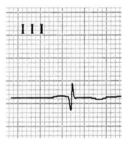

I am the observer at lead III. I see the QRS as neither positive nor negative. I see the QRS as isoelectric. I see the QRS as perpendicular to me.

I documented my observation on the line perpendicular to lead III, which is line AVR.

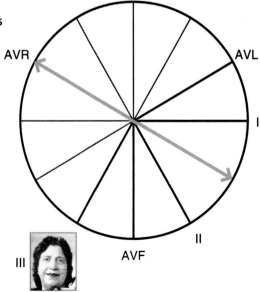

Example 2 Continued: Summary

EXAMPLE 2: Combine the information from the three leads or observers. The axis is positive 30°.

   a) Lead I is positive.
   b) Lead AVF is positive.
   c) Lead III is isoelectric.

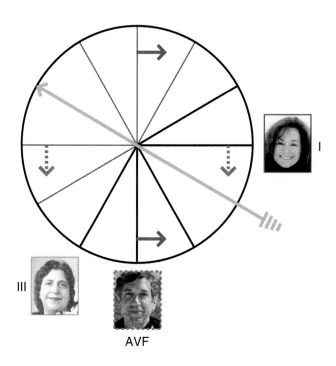

Calculation of Axis: Example 3

EXAMPLE 3: Find the QRS axis in the frontal plane for this EKG.

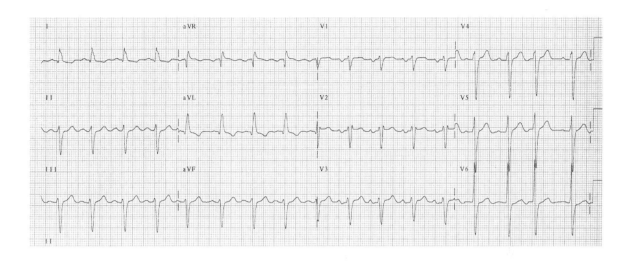

The QRS in lead I is positive.

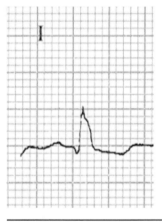

I am the observer at lead I.
I see the QRS as positive.
I see the QRS as coming
toward me.

I documented my
observation on the line
perpendicular to lead I,
which is lead line AVF.

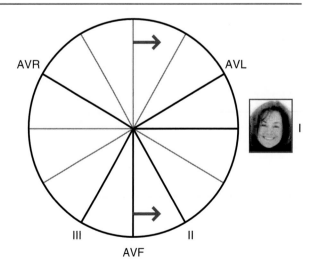

Example 3 Continued: Lead AVF

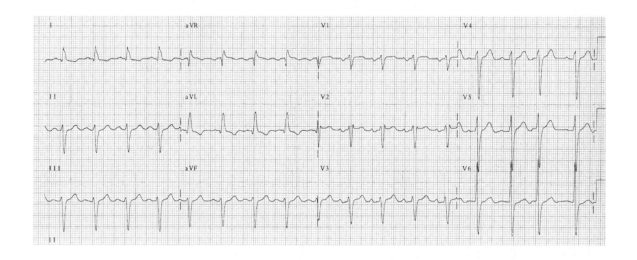

The QRS in lead AVF is negative.

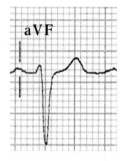

I am the observer at lead AVF. I see the QRS as negative or downward. I see the QRS as going away from me.

I documented my observation on the line perpendicular to lead AVF, which is lead line I.

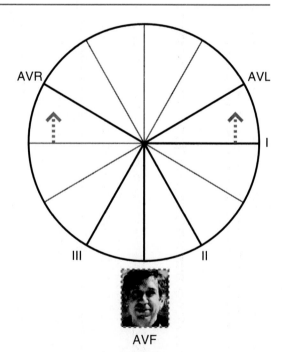

Example 3 Continued: Lead II

EXAMPLE 3: Combine the information from the first two leads.

The axis is less than 0°, but more positive than −90°.

To further delineate the axis, we need to answer the following question: which way does the axis lie with respect to line AVL?

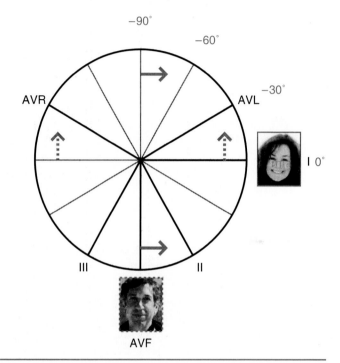

The answer to this question can be found by examining the observer lead perpendicular to lead AVL, which is lead and observer II.

The observer at lead II looks at line AVL. The lead II observer can tell which way the force moves about line AVL.

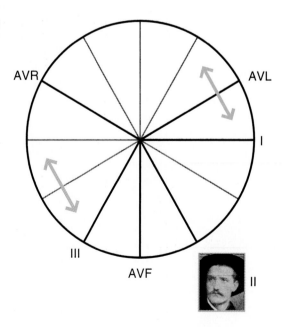

Example 3 Continued: Lead II

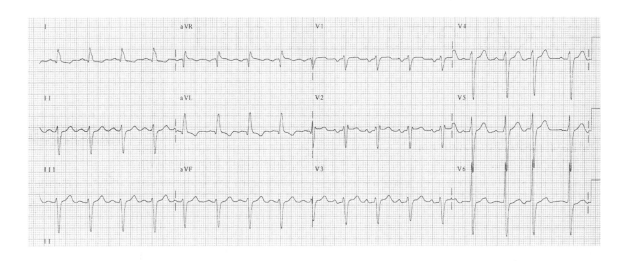

The QRS in lead II is positive.

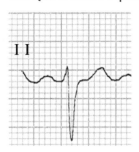

I am the observer at lead II. I see the QRS as negative. I see the QRS as going away from me.

I documented my observation on the line perpendicular to lead II, which is line AVL.

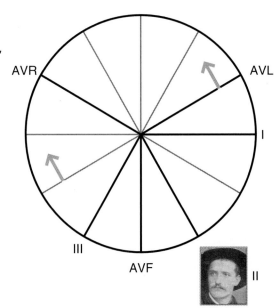

Example 3 Continued: Summary

Combining the information from the three leads narrows the QRS axis to lying at less than −30°, but more positive than −90°.

    a) **Lead I is positive.**
    b) **Lead AVF is negative.**
    c) **Lead II is negative.**

Using a, b, and c from above, the axis is more negative than −30° and less negative than −90°. Because we are using multiples of 15°, the axis must be −45°, −60°, or −75°.

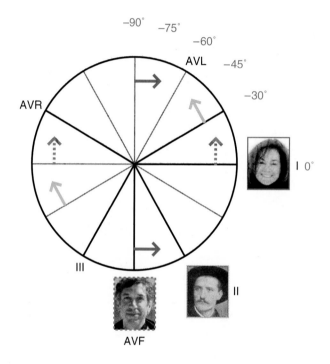

To further delineate the axis, we need to answer the following question: Which way does the axis lie with respect to line III?

The observer at lead AVR looks at line III. The lead AVR observer can tell which way the force moves about line III.

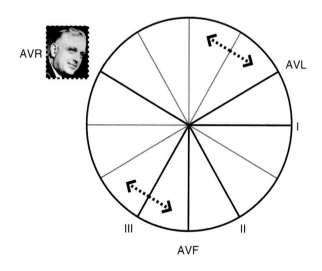

Example 3 Continued: Lead AVR

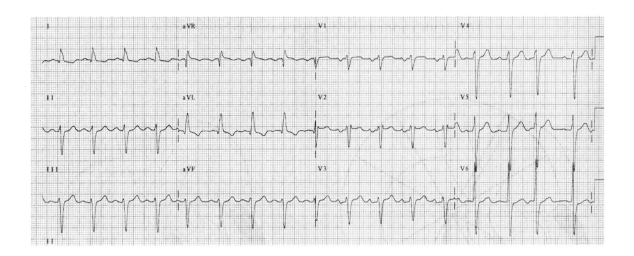

Lead AVR is positive.

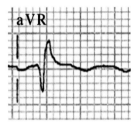

I am the observer at lead AVR. I see the QRS as positive. (Even though the Q and R waves have the same height, the R wave is wider.) I see the QRS as coming toward me.

I documented my observation on the line perpendicular to lead AVR, which is line III.

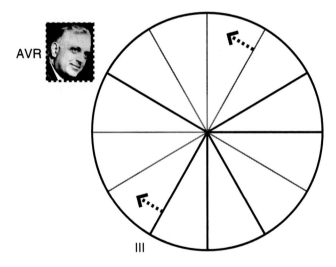

Example 3: Conclusion

Combining the information from the four leads narrows the QRS axis to −75°.

    a) Lead I is positive.
    b) Lead AVF is negative.
    c) Lead II is negative.
    d) Lead AVR is positive.

Using a, b, c, and d from above, the axis is more negative than −60° and more positive than −90°. Because we are using multiples of 15°, the axis must be −75°.

In summary, the QRS depolarization is leftward and superior.

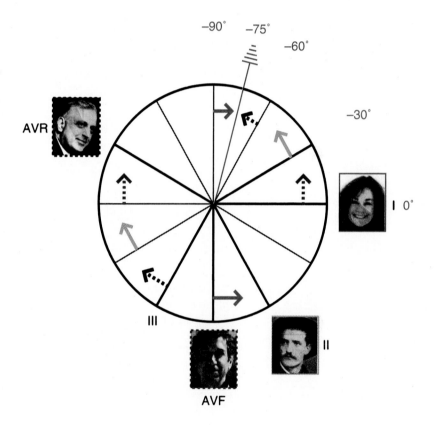

The Horizontal Leads (Precordial or V Leads)

Axes can also be calculated in the horizontal plane. The frontal plane tells us if a force is upward, downward, leftward, or rightward. However, the frontal plane tells us nothing about whether an electrical force is moving frontward (anterior) or backward (posterior). The horizontal leads, which are also called "V" leads or precordial leads, allow calculation with the added dimension of anterior and posterior.

The leads in the horizontal plane are arranged differently from the frontal plane leads.

They are labeled V1 through V6.

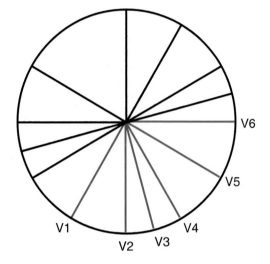

The leads in the horizontal plane are arranged beginning at 3 o'clock, which is 0°. Counterclockwise direction is considered negative. Clockwise direction is considered positive.

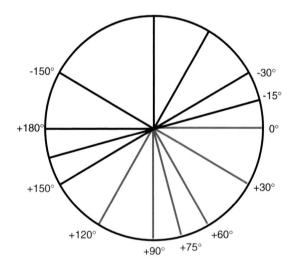

The Horizontal Plane Leads as Observers

Again, as with the frontal plane, imagine that at each V lead there is an observer looking at the same electrical heart event. Because the observers are standing or looking at the event from different places, they can only describe it from their perspectives. Using each observer's information, we are able to reconstruct an average event to determine the direction of the electrical force. Using each observer's information, we are able to construct an average description to determine if the force is moving frontward or backward, rightward or leftward.

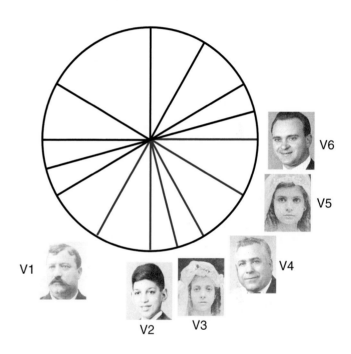

Lead V6

When calculating the horizontal plane, look at lead V6 first. The observer standing at lead V6 evaluates lead V6 on the EKG but documents his observation on the line perpendicular to lead V6, which is lead line V2. Lead V6 tells us whether the average force or axis is coming toward V6 or away from V6, that is, rightward or leftward.

If the force in V6 is **positive**, then the axis or direction of the force must be pointing **toward** V6.

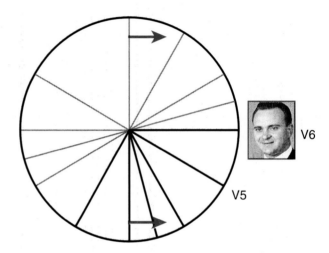

If the force in V6 is **negative**, then the axis or direction of the force must be pointing **away** from V6.

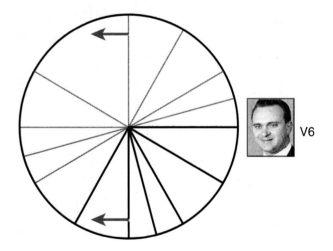

Lead V6: Isoelectric

If the complex in lead V6 is isoelectric, the axis would be perpendicular to lead V6.

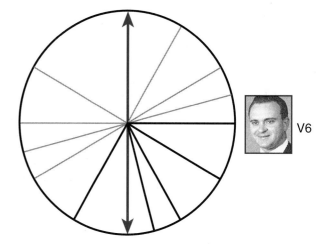

V6

Lead V2

The second lead evaluated in the horizontal plane is V2. The observer standing at lead V2 evaluates V2 but documents his findings on the lead line perpendicular to lead V2, which is lead line V6.

If the complex in lead V2 is **positive** or upright, the axis must be moving **toward** the V2 observer.

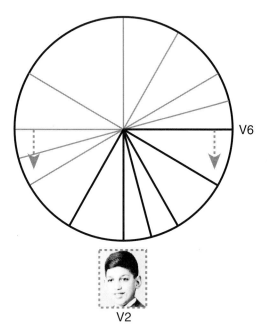

If the complex in lead V2 is **negative** or downward, the axis must be moving **away** from the V2 observer.

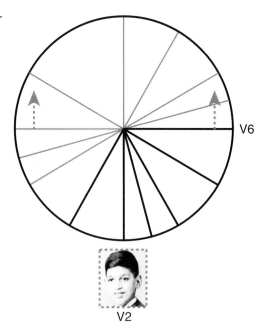

Lead V2: Isoelectric

If V2 is isoelectric, the axis is neither moving toward nor moving away from the V2 observer. Instead, it is directed perpendicular to the observer.

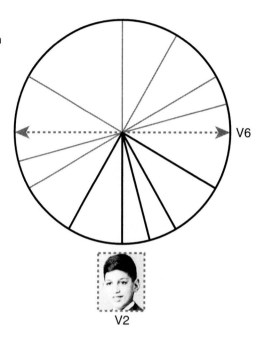

V6

V2

EXAMPLE 4: Find the QRS axis in the horizontal plane for this EKG.

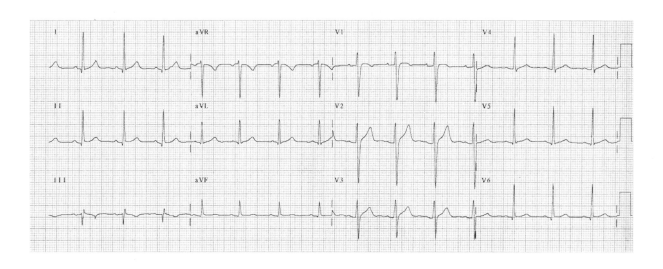

The QRS in lead V6 is positive.

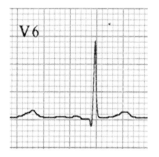

I am the observer at lead V6. I see the QRS as positive. I see the QRS as coming toward me.

The V6 observer evaluates lead V6 on the EKG but documents his observation on the line perpendicular to lead V6, which is lead line V2.

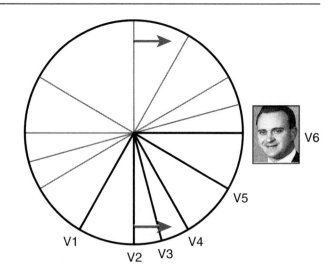

Example 4 Continued: Lead V2

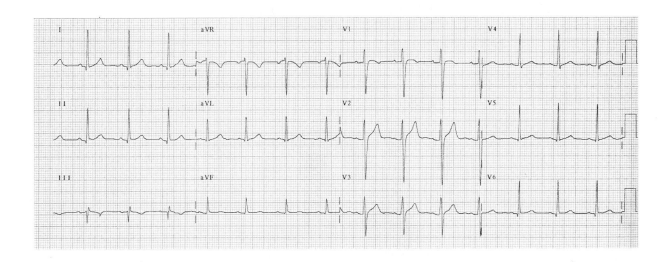

The QRS in lead V2 is negative.

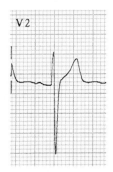

I am the observer at lead V2. I see the QRS as negative. I see the QRS as going away from me.

The V2 observer evaluates lead V2 but documents his observation on the line perpendicular to lead V2, which is line V6.

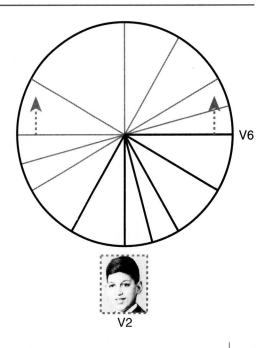

V6

V2

Example 4 Continued: Summary

Although the information from leads V2 and V6 was drawn on separate diagrams for purposes of illustration, they must be drawn on one diagram to calculate the axis.

The result is that the axis lies above V6 and to the right of V2. Mathematically, the axis is greater than −90° and less than 0°, that is, posterior and leftward (toward the patient's left).

The axis lies at less than 0° and more positive than −90°.

To narrow the axis further, we need to calculate where the axis lies with respect to the line perpendicular to V4.

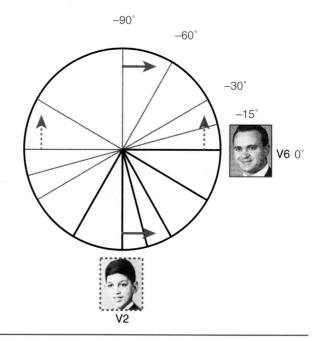

The answer to this question can be found by examining the observer lead at V4.

The observer at lead V4 looks at the force (the QRS in this example) and records the information on the unnamed line (I suggest "grandpa's line") perpendicular to V4.

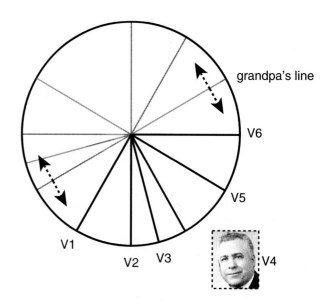

Example 4 Continued: Lead V4

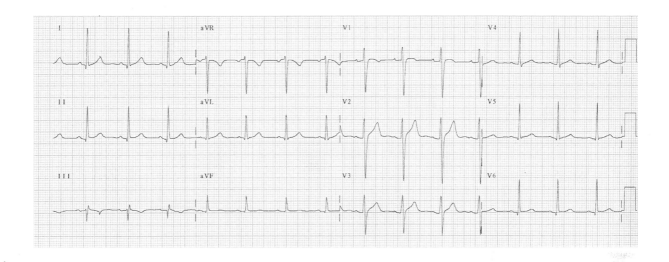

The QRS in lead V4 is positive.

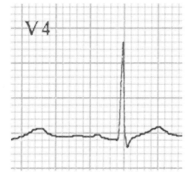

I am the observer at lead V4. I see the QRS as **positive**. I see the QRS as coming **toward** me.

The V4 observer evaluates lead V4 on the EKG but documents his observation on the line perpendicular to lead V4.

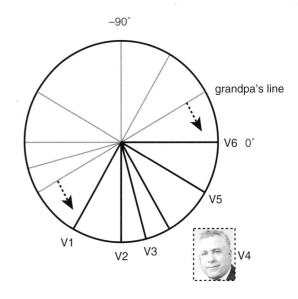

Example 4: Summary

Combining the information and observations from V6, V2, and V4 determines that the axis lies at less than 0° and greater than −15°.

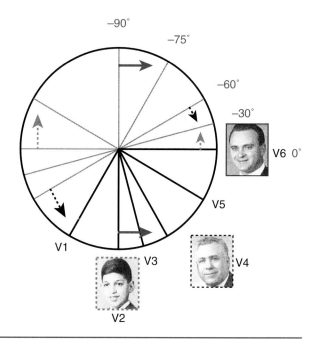

To calculate the axis more closely, we need to find where the axis lies in relation to the line perpendicular to V3. The answer to this question can be found by examining the observer lead at V3.

The observer at lead V3 looks at the force (the QRS in this example) and records the information on the unnamed line perpendicular to V3.

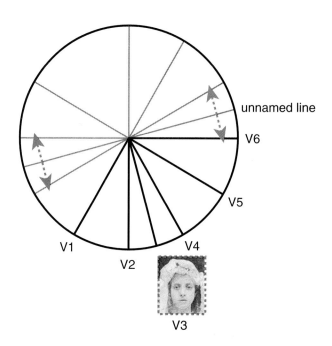

Example 4: Lead V3

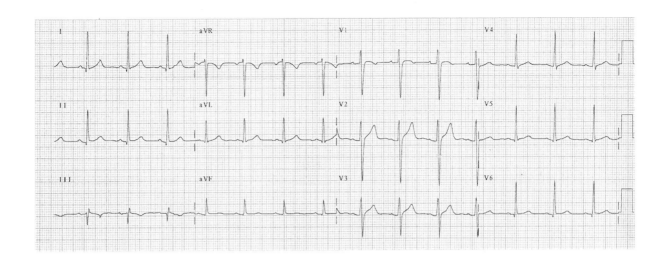

The QRS in lead V3 is negative.

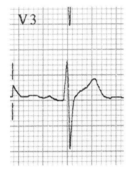

"I am the observer at lead V3. I see the QRS as **negative**. I see the QRS as going **away** from me."

The V3 observer evaluates lead V3 on the EKG but documents his observation on the line perpendicular to V3.

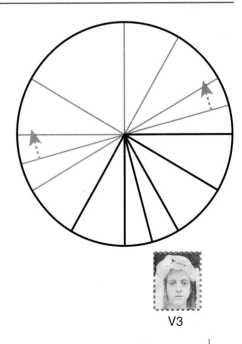

V3

Example 4: Conclusion

Combine all the information and draw it on one diagram.

a) V6 is positive.
b) V2 is negative.
c) V4 is positive.
d) V3 is negative.

The axis in the horizontal plane lies at $-22.5°$.

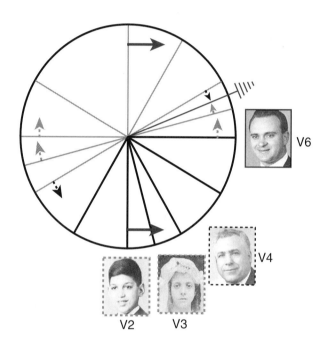

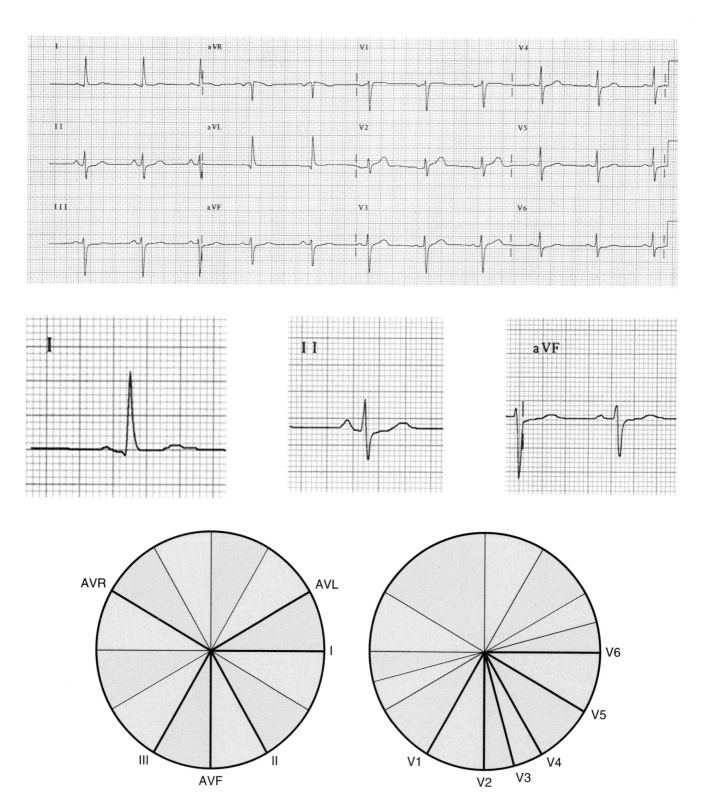

Heart Rate:

Rhythm:

Intervals (measured in the limb leads)

PR: short (< .12)
        normal (.12 to .20)
        long (>0.20 seconds); this is 1st degree AV
        block

QRS: normal (≤0.09 seconds)
        prolonged (.10 or .11); this is intraventricular
        conduction delay (IVCD)
        Bundle Branch Block (.12 seconds or greater)

QT:

P axis: normal
            rightward
            arm-lead reversal or dextrocardia
            junctional rhythm

QRS axis: normal
            left anterior hemiblock
            left posterior hemiblock
            indeterminate

T wave inversion (ischemia or infarction):

II,III,AVF	inferior
I, AVL	lateral
V1, without V2	nonspecific septal
V1 and V2	septal
V3 and V4	anterior
V5 and V6	lateral
V6, without V5	nonspecific lateral

ST Elevation (acute infarction):

II,III,AVF	inferior
I, AVL	lateral
V1, without V2	nonspecific septal
V1 and V2	septal
V3 and V4	anterior
V5 and V6	lateral
V6, without V5.	nonspecific lateral

ST Depression (ischemia or infarction):

I,II,III,AVL,AVF	diffuse subendocardial ischemia or infarction
V2,V3,V4,V5	diffuse subendocardial ischemia or infarction

Q waves (infarction):

II,III,AVF	inferior
I, AVL	lateral
V1, without V2	nonspecific septal
V1 and V2	septal
V3 and V4	anterior
V5 and V6	lateral
V6, without V5	nonspecific lateral

Hypertrophy:

Right atrial: Tall P wave 2.5 mm in II, III, or AVF

Left atrial: Deep negative part of P wave in V1

LVH: R wave in 1 + S wave in III ≥ 25mV
      S wave in V1 + R wave in V5 ≥ 35mV

RVH: Mean QRS either anterior, or rightward

The heart rate is 63 beats per minute. The PR interval measures 0.16 seconds. The QRS interval measures 0.10 seconds. This indicates intraventricular conduction delay (IVCD). This is further discussed in Chapters 9 and 10. The QT interval measures 0.40 seconds, although it is hard to measure with confidence. This is due to the low amplitude of the T waves. Low-amplitude T waves are a very important clue on the EKG to the possible presence of an electrolyte disturbance such as hypokalemia. This is discussed in Chapter 19. When it is difficult to measure the QT interval, look at the amplitude of the T wave, and, if appropriate, check the patient's electrolytes. The P axis in the frontal plane is +60°. In the frontal plane, the mean QRS is positive in leads I and AVL, but negative in leads III, AVR, and AVF. It is isoelectric in lead II. This combination gives an axis of −30°. In the horizontal plane, the mean QRS is negative in lead V1, isoelectric in lead V2, and positive in lead V6. This combination gives a mean QRS axis of 0°. Continuing, the frontal plane T wave is positive in leads I, II, III, and AVF. It is negative in AVR and isoelectric in lead AVL. This combination gives a frontal plane T axis of +60°. In the horizontal plane, the T wave is positive in leads V2 through V6 and probably isoelectric in lead V1. This gives a horizontal plane T axis of +30°. If it take more than 2 seconds to decide if a wave is positive or negative, then it is probably isoelectric.

Parts of the answer sheets are "grayed out" because these sections have not yet been covered. Answer only the parts that are not highlighted.

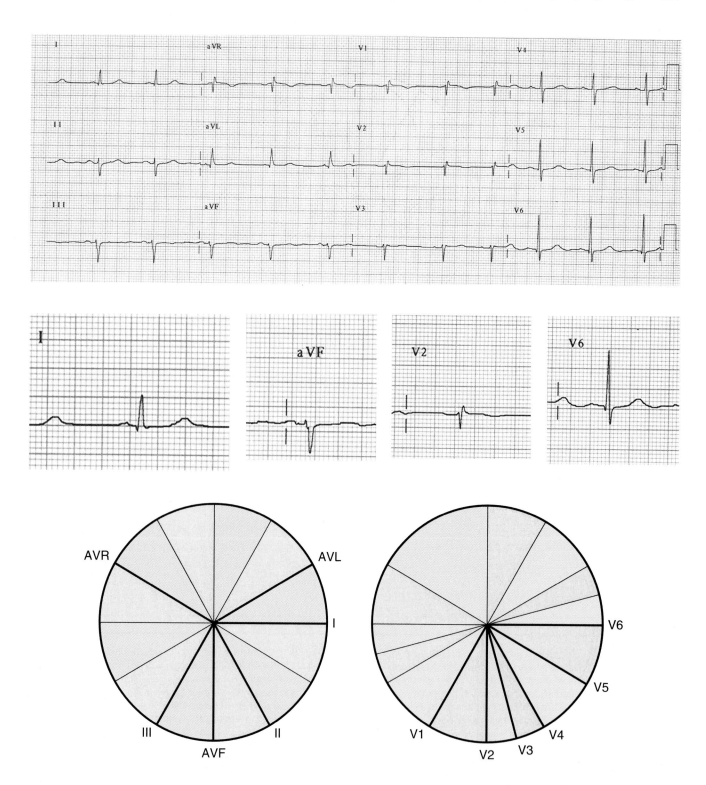

Heart Rate:

Rhythm:

Intervals (measured in the limb leads)

PR: short (< .12)
normal (.12 to .20)
long (>0.20 seconds); this is 1st degree AV block

QRS: normal (≤0.09 seconds)
prolonged (.10 or .11); this is intraventricular conduction delay (IVCD)
Bundle Branch Block (.12 seconds or greater)

QT:

P axis: normal
rightward
arm-lead reversal or dextrocardia
junctional rhythm

QRS axis: normal
left anterior hemiblock
left posterior hemiblock
indeterminate

T wave inversion (ischemia or infarction):

II,III,AVF	inferior
I, AVL	lateral
V1, without V2	nonspecific septal
V1 and V2	septal
V3 and V4	anterior
V5 and V6	lateral
V6, without V5	nonspecific lateral

ST Elevation (acute infarction):

II,III,AVF	inferior
I, AVL	lateral
V1, without V2	nonspecific septal
V1 and V2	septal
V3 and V4	anterior
V5 and V6	lateral
V6, without V5.	nonspecific lateral

ST Depression (ischemia or infarction):

I,II,III,AVL,AVF	diffuse subendocardial ischemia or infarction
V2,V3,V4,V5	diffuse subendocardial ischemia or infarction

Q waves (infarction):

II,III,AVF	inferior
I, AVL	lateral
V1, without V2	nonspecific septal
V1 and V2	septal
V3 and V4	anterior
V5 and V6	lateral
V6, without V5	nonspecific lateral

Hypertrophy:

Right atrial: Tall P wave 2.5 mm in II, III, or AVF

Left atrial: Deep negative part of P wave in V1

LVH: R wave in 1 + S wave in III ≥ 25mV
S wave in V1 + R wave in V5 ≥ 35mV

RVH: Mean QRS either anterior, or rightward

The heart rate is 65 beats per minute. The PR interval measures 0.16 seconds. The QRS interval measures 0.08 seconds. The QT interval measures 0.44 seconds. This is long. The P wave is positive in leads I, II, III, AVL, and AVF. It is negative in AVR. This combination gives a P axis of +45°. *Reasonable people should not disagree by more than 15°. Thus if the P wave in lead L is considered isoelectric, it will make the P axis + 60°.* In the frontal plane, the mean QRS is positive in leads I and AVL. It is negative in leads II, III, and AVF. It is negative in lead AVR. This combination gives a mean QRS axis of −45°. A reader who calls the QRS in lead AVR isoelectric would obtain a mean QRS axis of −60°. *Because the result does not change the interpretation, don't nitpick. Save nitpicking for when it really counts.* In the horizontal plane, the mean QRS axis is negative in leads V1, V2, and V3. It is positive in leads V4, V5, and V6. This combination gives a mean QRS axis of −22.5°. *Don't be frightened by the numbers. The reason for calculating axis in this part of the book is that you need to visualize in exactly what direction things are happening.* The frontal plane T axis is positive in I, II, AVL, and AVF. It is negative in AVR and isoelectric in lead III. This gives a frontal plane T axis of +30°. In the horizontal plane, the T wave is negative in V1, isoelectric in lead V2, and positive in leads V3 through V6. This gives a horizontal T axis of 0°.

Parts of the answer sheets are "grayed out" because these sections have not yet been covered. Answer only the parts that are not highlighted.

Worksheet 6-3

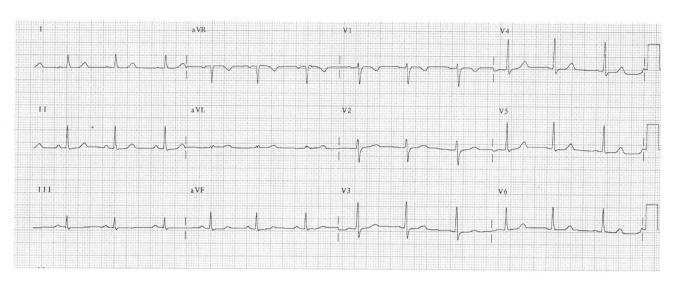

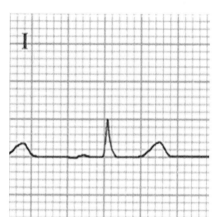

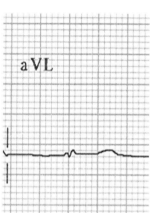

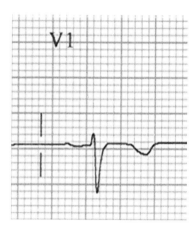

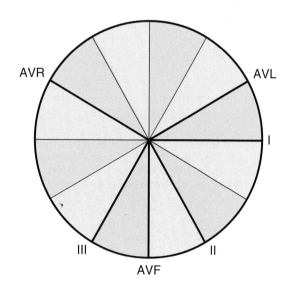

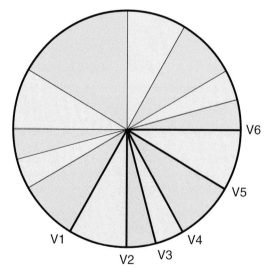

Heart Rate:

Rhythm:

ST Elevation (acute infarction):

II,III,AVF	inferior
I, AVL	lateral
V1, without V2	nonspecific septal
V1 and V2	septal
V3 and V4	anterior
V5 and V6	lateral
V6, without V5.	nonspecific lateral

Intervals (measured in the limb leads)

PR: short (< .12)
    normal (.12 to .20)
    long (>0.20 seconds); this is 1st degree AV
    block

QRS: normal (≤0.09 seconds)
    prolonged (.10 or .11); this is intraventricular
    conduction delay (IVCD)
    Bundle Branch Block (.12 seconds or greater)

QT:

ST Depression (ischemia or infarction):

I,II,III,AVL,AVF	diffuse subendocardial ischemia or infarction
V2,V3,V4,V5	diffuse subendocardial ischemia or infarction

P axis: normal
    rightward
    arm-lead reversal or dextrocardia
    junctional rhythm

QRS axis: normal
    left anterior hemiblock
    left posterior hemiblock
    indeterminate

Q waves (infarction):

II,III,AVF	inferior
I, AVL	lateral
V1, without V2	nonspecific septal
V1 and V2	septal
V3 and V4	anterior
V5 and V6	lateral
V6, without V5	nonspecific lateral

T wave inversion (ischemia or infarction):

II,III,AVF	inferior
I, AVL	lateral
V1, without V2	nonspecific septal
V1 and V2	septal
V3 and V4	anterior
V5 and V6	lateral
V6, without V5	nonspecific lateral

Hypertrophy:

Right atrial: Tall P wave 2.5 mm in II, III, or AVF

Left atrial: Deep negative part of P wave in V1

LVH: R wave in 1 + S wave in III ≥ 25mV
    S wave in V1 + R wave in V5 ≥ 35mV

RVH: Mean QRS either anterior, or rightward

The heart rate is 75 beats per minute. The PR interval measures 0.16 seconds. The QRS interval measures 0.08 seconds. The QT interval measures 0.36 seconds. In the frontal plane, the P wave is positive in leads I, II, III, and AVF. It is negative in lead AVR but isoelectric in lead AVL. This combination gives a P axis of +60°. In the frontal plane, the mean QRS is positive in leads I, II, III, and AVF. It is negative in AVR but isoelectric in AVL. *If you consider AVL positive, you are probably so overly compulsive that you have no friends. . . . loosen up.* This combination gives a mean QRS of +60°. In the horizontal plane, the mean QRS axis is negative in V1 and V2, but positive in leads V3 through V6. This combination gives a mean QRS axis of −7.5°. Continuing, in the frontal plane, the T axis is positive in leads I, II, AVL, and AVF. It is negative in AVR and isoelectric in III. This combination gives a mean T axis of +30° in the frontal plane. In the horizontal plane, the T axis is negative in V1 but positive in V2 through V6. This combination gives a mean horizontal T axis of +15°.

Parts of the answer sheets are "grayed out" because these sections have not yet been covered. Answer only the parts that are not highlighted.

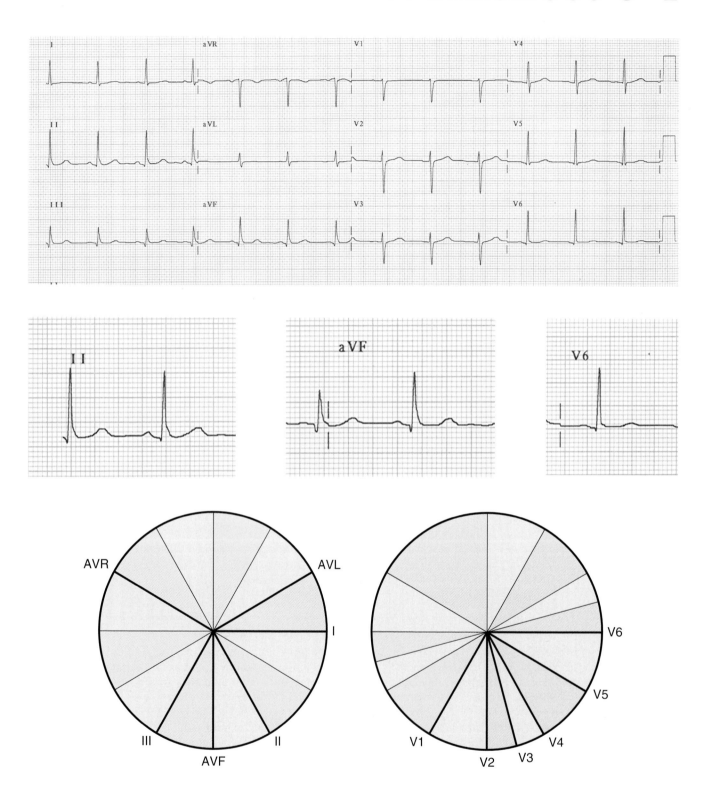

Heart Rate:

Rhythm:

ST Elevation (acute infarction):

II,III,AVF	inferior
I, AVL	lateral
V1, without V2	nonspecific septal
V1 and V2	septal
V3 and V4	anterior
V5 and V6	lateral
V6, without V5.	nonspecific lateral

Intervals (measured in the limb leads)

PR: short (< .12)
       normal (.12 to .20)
       long (>0.20 seconds); this is 1st degree AV block

QRS: normal (≤0.09 seconds)
       prolonged (.10 or .11); this is intraventricular conduction delay (IVCD)
       Bundle Branch Block (.12 seconds or greater)

QT:

ST Depression (ischemia or infarction):

I,II,III,AVL,AVF	diffuse subendocardial ischemia or infarction
V2,V3,V4,V5	diffuse subendocardial ischemia or infarction

P axis: normal
           rightward
           arm-lead reversal or dextrocardia
           junctional rhythm

QRS axis: normal
           left anterior hemiblock
           left posterior hemiblock
           indeterminate

Q waves (infarction):

II,III,AVF	inferior
I, AVL	lateral
V1, without V2	nonspecific septal
V1 and V2	septal
V3 and V4	anterior
V5 and V6	lateral
V6, without V5	nonspecific lateral

T wave inversion (ischemia or infarction):

II,III,AVF	inferior
I, AVL	lateral
V1, without V2	nonspecific septal
V1 and V2	septal
V3 and V4	anterior
V5 and V6	lateral
V6, without V5	nonspecific lateral

Hypertrophy:

Right atrial: Tall P wave 2.5 mm in II, III, or AVF

Left atrial: Deep negative part of P wave in V1

LVH: R wave in 1 + S wave in III ≥ 25mV
      S wave in V1 + R wave in V5 ≥ 35mV

RVH: Mean QRS either anterior, or rightward

The heart rate is 75 beats per minute. The PR interval measures 0.16 seconds. The QRS interval measures 0.09 seconds. The QT interval measures 0.40 seconds. (*Remember: The PR, QRS, and QT interval are measured only in the limb leads, never in the V leads.*) In the frontal plane, the P wave is positive in leads I, II, III, and AVF. It is negative in lead AVR but isoelectric in lead AVL. This combination gives a P axis of +60°. In the frontal plane, the mean QRS axis is positive in leads I, II, III, AVL, and AVF. It is negative in lead AVR. This combination gives a mean QRS axis of +45°. In the horizontal plane, the mean QRS is negative in leads V1, V2, and V3. It is positive in leads V4, V5, and V6. This combination gives a mean QRS axis of −22.5°. Continuing, in the frontal plane, the T axis is positive in leads I, II, III, and AVF. It is negative in lead AVR but isoelectric in AVL. This combination gives a frontal plane T axis of +60°. In the horizontal plane, the T axis is isoelectric in lead V1 but positive in leads V2 through V6. This combination gives a mean T axis of +30°.

Parts of the answer sheets are "grayed out" because these sections have not yet been covered. Answer only the parts that are not highlighted.

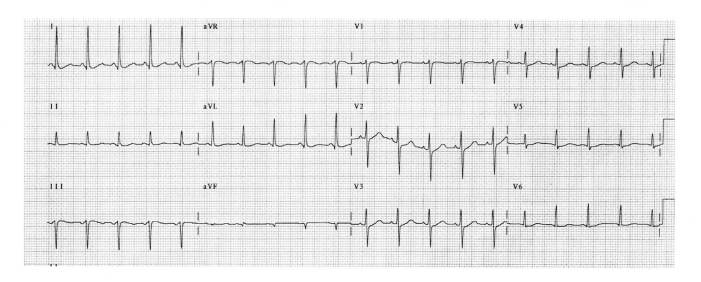

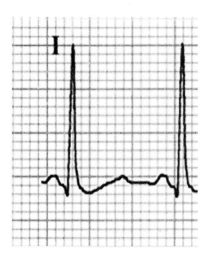

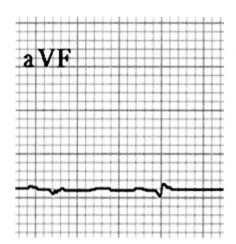

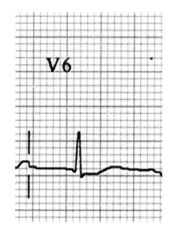

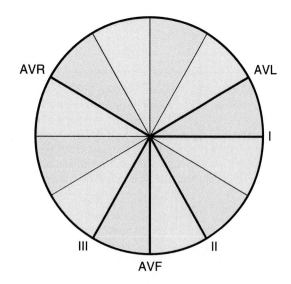

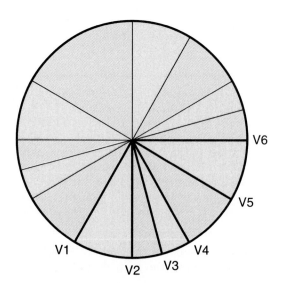

Heart Rate:

Rhythm:

Intervals (measured in the limb leads)

PR: short (< .12)
        normal (.12 to .20)
        long (>0.20 seconds); this is 1st degree AV block

QRS: normal (≤0.09 seconds)
        prolonged (.10 or .11); this is intraventricular conduction delay (IVCD)
        Bundle Branch Block (.12 seconds or greater)

QT:

P axis: normal
            rightward
            arm-lead reversal or dextrocardia
            junctional rhythm

QRS axis: normal
            left anterior hemiblock
            left posterior hemiblock
            indeterminate

T wave inversion (ischemia or infarction):

II,III,AVF	inferior
I, AVL	lateral
V1, without V2	nonspecific septal
V1 and V2	septal
V3 and V4	anterior
V5 and V6	lateral
V6, without V5	nonspecific lateral

ST Elevation (acute infarction):

II,III,AVF	inferior
I, AVL	lateral
V1, without V2	nonspecific septal
V1 and V2	septal
V3 and V4	anterior
V5 and V6	lateral
V6, without V5.	nonspecific lateral

ST Depression (ischemia or infarction):

I,II,III,AVL,AVF	diffuse subendocardial ischemia or infarction
V2,V3,V4,V5	diffuse subendocardial ischemia or infarction

Q waves (infarction):

II,III,AVF	inferior
I, AVL	lateral
V1, without V2	nonspecific septal
V1 and V2	septal
V3 and V4	anterior
V5 and V6	lateral
V6, without V5	nonspecific lateral

Hypertrophy:

Right atrial: Tall P wave 2.5 mm in II, III, or AVF

Left atrial: Deep negative part of P wave in V1

LVH: R wave in 1 + S wave in III ≥ 25mV
      S wave in V1 + R wave in V5 ≥ 35mV

RVH: Mean QRS either anterior, or rightward

The heart rate is 115 beats per minute. This is probably sinus tachycardia. The PR interval measures 0.09 seconds, which is short and indicates accelerated AV conduction, or a nonsinus mechanism. The QRS interval measures 0.09 seconds. The QT interval measures 0.32 seconds. This is long. The QT is difficult to measure with confidence, because the T wave is of such low amplitude. (*Remember that hypokalemia can cause low-amplitude T waves. Could this patient be on diuretics, and be tachycardic due to hypovolemia, and have low-amplitude T waves due to hypokalemia? Always put all the little clues together. Ignore nothing. Check the history, check the patient, check the labs.*) The P axis is positive in leads I, II, and AVL, but negative in III and AVR. It is isoelectric in lead AVF. This gives a P axis of 0°. In the frontal plane, the mean QRS axis is positive in I, II, and AVL. It is negative in leads III, AVR, and probably AVF. (*The QRS changes slightly in lead AVF sometimes with respiration, as it moves the location of the heart.*) This combination gives a frontal plane QRS axis of −15°. In the horizontal plane, the mean QRS axis is negative in leads V1, V2, and V3 but positive in leads V4, V5, and V6. This combination gives a mean QRS axis of −22.5°. Continuing with the T wave, in the frontal plane the T wave is positive in lead I but otherwise cannot be localized with confidence. This T axis is therefore *indeterminate.* In the horizontal plane, the T axis is +30°.

Parts of the answer sheets are "grayed out" because these sections have not yet been covered. Answer only the parts that are not highlighted.

Worksheet 6-6

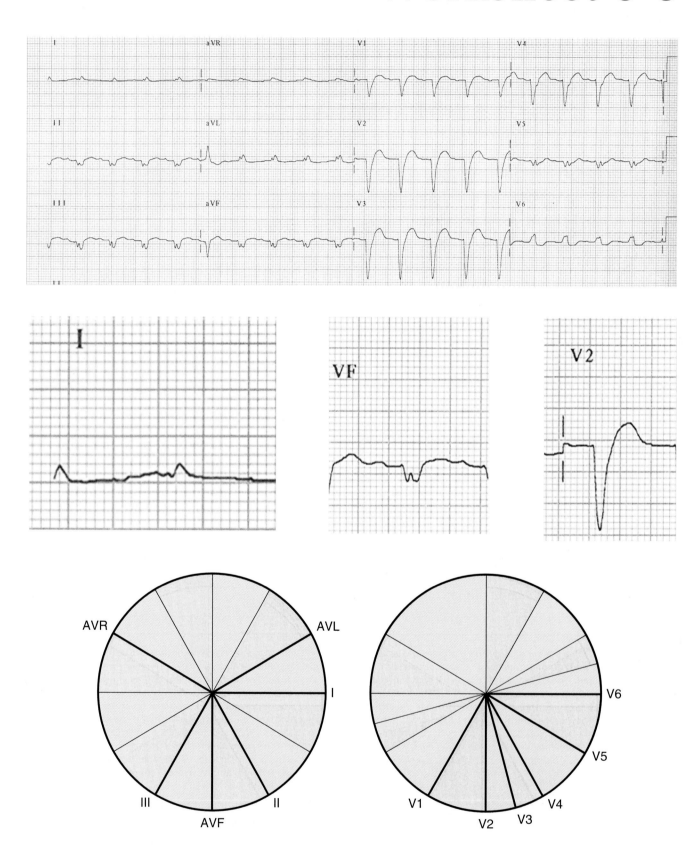

Heart Rate:

Rhythm:

Intervals (measured in the limb leads)

PR: short (< .12)
        normal (.12 to .20)
        long (>0.20 seconds); this is 1st degree AV
        block

QRS: normal (≤0.09 seconds)
        prolonged (.10 or .11); this is intraventricular
        conduction delay (IVCD)
        Bundle Branch Block (.12 seconds or greater)

QT:

P axis: normal
            rightward
            arm-lead reversal or dextrocardia
            junctional rhythm

QRS axis: normal
            left anterior hemiblock
            left posterior hemiblock
            indeterminate

T wave inversion (ischemia or infarction):

II,III,AVF	inferior
I, AVL	lateral
V1, without V2	nonspecific septal
V1 and V2	septal
V3 and V4	anterior
V5 and V6	lateral
V6, without V5	nonspecific lateral

ST Elevation (acute infarction):

II,III,AVF	inferior
I, AVL	lateral
V1, without V2	nonspecific septal
V1 and V2	septal
V3 and V4	anterior
V5 and V6	lateral
V6, without V5.	nonspecific lateral

ST Depression (ischemia or infarction):

| I,II,III,AVL,AVF | diffuse subendocardial ischemia or infarction |
| V2,V3,V4,V5 | diffuse subendocardial ischemia or infarction |

Q waves (infarction):

II,III,AVF	inferior
I, AVL	lateral
V1, without V2	nonspecific septal
V1 and V2	septal
V3 and V4	anterior
V5 and V6	lateral
V6, without V5	nonspecific lateral

Hypertrophy:

Right atrial: Tall P wave 2.5 mm in II, III, or AVF

Left atrial: Deep negative part of P wave in V1

LVH: R wave in 1 + S wave in III ≥ 25mV
      S wave in V1 + R wave in V5 ≥ 35mV

RVH: Mean QRS either anterior, or rightward

The heart rate is 107 and indicates sinus tachycardia. The PR interval measures 0.20 seconds. The QRS interval measures 0.12 seconds. (Bundle branch block is discussed in Chapters 9 and 10.) In the frontal plane, the P axis is +90°. In the frontal plane, the mean QRS axis is isoelectric in lead I and negative in lead AVF. This combination gives a mean QRS axis of −90°. (If the reader called lead I positive, this would give an axis of −75° instead of −90°.) In the horizontal plane, the QRS is negative in V1 through V4. It is isoelectric in lead V5 and positive in lead V6. This combination gives a mean QRS axis of −60°. *In this EKG, the T wave and ST segment merge into one. It is difficult to decide where the ST ends and the T wave begins. In that case, it is useful to treat the combination of the ST and T wave as one force and calculate the axis of the combination force.* Continuing, the ST-T axis in the frontal plane is isoelectric in lead I and positive in lead AVF. This gives a mean ST-T axis of +90°. In the horizontal plane, the ST-T axis is positive in leads V1 through V4. It is isoelectric in lead V5 and negative in lead V6. This combination gives an ST-T axis of +120° in the horizontal plane.

Parts of the answer sheets are "grayed out" because these sections have not yet been covered. Answer only the parts that are not highlighted.

Worksheet 6-7

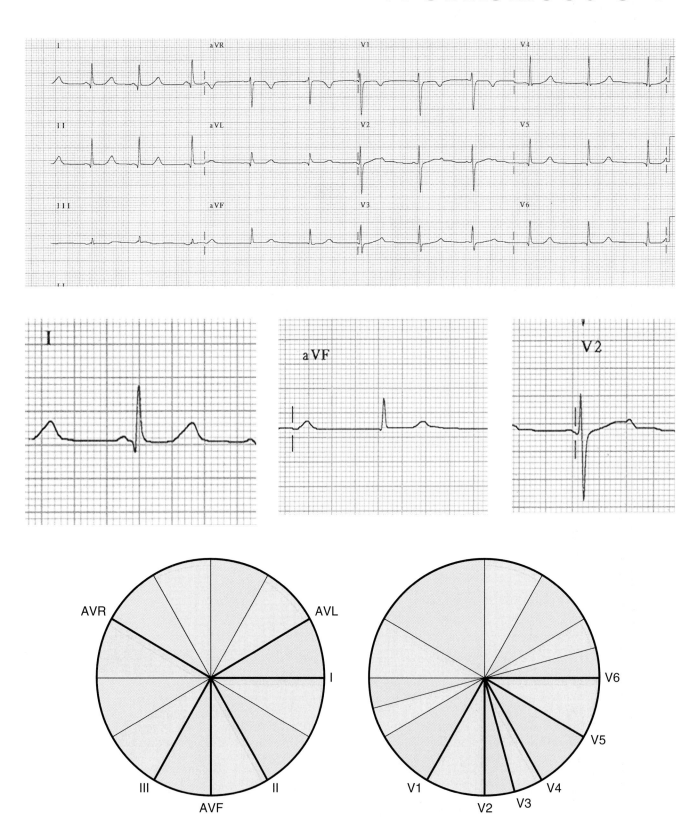

Heart Rate:

Rhythm:

ST Elevation (acute infarction):

II,III,AVF	inferior
I, AVL	lateral
V1, without V2	nonspecific septal
V1 and V2	septal
V3 and V4	anterior
V5 and V6	lateral
V6, without V5.	nonspecific lateral

Intervals (measured in the limb leads)

PR: short (< .12)
     normal (.12 to .20)
     long (>0.20 seconds); this is 1st degree AV
     block

QRS: normal (≤0.09 seconds)
      prolonged (.10 or .11); this is intraventricular
      conduction delay (IVCD)
      Bundle Branch Block (.12 seconds or greater)

QT:

ST Depression (ischemia or infarction):

I,II,III,AVL,AVF	diffuse subendocardial ischemia or infarction
V2,V3,V4,V5	diffuse subendocardial ischemia or infarction

P axis: normal
            rightward
            arm-lead reversal or dextrocardia
            junctional rhythm

QRS axis: normal
            left anterior hemiblock
            left posterior hemiblock
            indeterminate

Q waves (infarction):

II,III,AVF	inferior
I, AVL	lateral
V1, without V2	nonspecific septal
V1 and V2	septal
V3 and V4	anterior
V5 and V6	lateral
V6, without V5	nonspecific lateral

T wave inversion (ischemia or infarction):

II,III,AVF	inferior
I, AVL	lateral
V1, without V2	nonspecific septal
V1 and V2	septal
V3 and V4	anterior
V5 and V6	lateral
V6, without V5	nonspecific lateral

Hypertrophy:

Right atrial: Tall P wave 2.5 mm in II, III, or AVF

Left atrial: Deep negative part of P wave in V1

LVH: R wave in 1 + S wave in III ≥ 25mV
     S wave in V1 + R wave in V5 ≥ 35mV

RVH: Mean QRS either anterior, or rightward

The heart rate is 75 beats per minute. The rhythm is sinus. The PR interval measures 0.10 seconds and is short. The QRS interval measures 0.08 seconds. The QT interval measures 0.44 seconds, which is long. In the frontal plane, the P axis is positive in lead I but is otherwise difficult to see with confidence. Therefore, the P axis is indeterminate. (*A short PR interval and an indeterminate P axis suggest junctional rhythm.*) In the frontal plane, the mean QRS axis is positive in leads I, II, III, AVL, and AVF. It is negative in lead AVR. The combination gives a mean QRS axis of +45°. In the horizontal plane, the QRS is negative in V1 and V2 but positive in leads V3 through V6. This combination gives a mean QRS axis of −7.5°. Continuing with the T axis, in the frontal plane, the T axis is positive in leads I, II, AVL, and AVF. It is negative in lead AVR and isoelectric in lead III. This combination gives a mean T axis of +30° (or −15° if the reader called the T negative in III). In the horizontal plane, the T axis is +15°.

Parts of the answer sheets are "grayed out" because these sections have not yet been covered. Answer only the parts that are not highlighted.

The P Wave Axis

P axis

Right atrial abnormality

Junctional rhythm

Dextrocardia

Depolarization of the right atrium and left atrium causes an electrical force that appears on the EKG as a P wave. **The P wave axis describes the direction and magnitude of this force.** The electrical impulse normally travels through the atria toward the AV node in a direction that is downward and to the left.

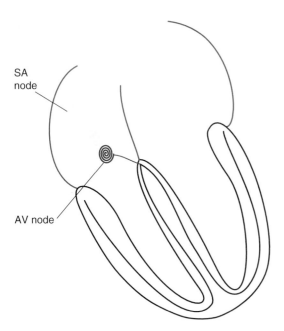

The electrical impulse starts at the SA node, travels across the atrium, and arrives at the AV node.

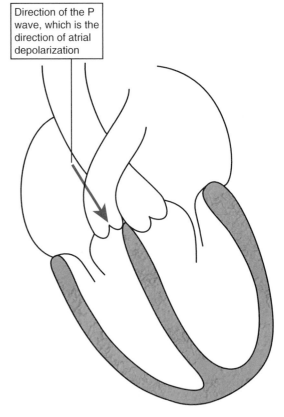

Direction of the P wave, which is the direction of atrial depolarization

The P wave axis should normally point downward and leftward.

The Normal P Axis

A normal range for the P wave axis in the frontal plane is anywhere from −30° to +75°. The normal P axis electrical depolarization should point in this range.

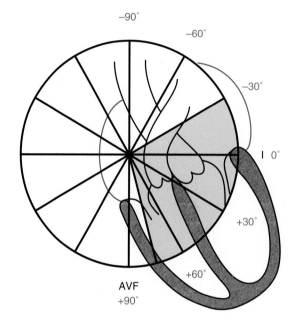

Right Atrial Abnormality

Enlargement or hypertrophy of the right atrium changes the P axis to a rightward direction. A P axis of +90° to +105° suggests right atrial enlargement (bigger chamber) or hypertrophy (thicker walls). A P axis of +90° to +105° indicates right atrial abnormality (RAA).

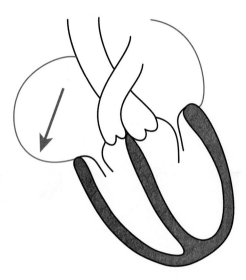

Enlargement of the right atrium produces a bigger electrical force in the right atrium and so moves the P axis to the right.

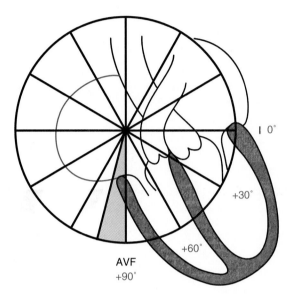

A P axis of +90° to +105° indicates right atrial abnormality.

Junctional Rhythm

Junctional rhythm depolarizes the atria from the AV node upward. This changes the P wave axis from downward to upward. A P wave axis of −45° to −120° suggests junctional rhythm.

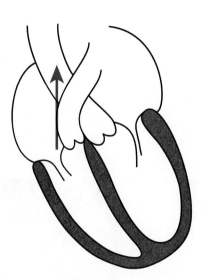

Depolarization of the atria from the AV node junction occurs in an upward direction.

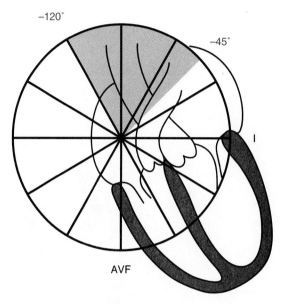

The P axis can point anywhere from −45° to −120° in junctional rhythm.

Dextrocardia

A P axis that points rightward with an axis greater than +105 degrees or less than −120° suggests dextrocardia. Dextrocardia is a congenital condition in which the contents of the thorax and abdomen are reversed in placement in a mirror image from normal. A P axis that points rightward with an axis greater than +105° or less than −120° could also occur when the right and left arm leads are accidentally reversed.

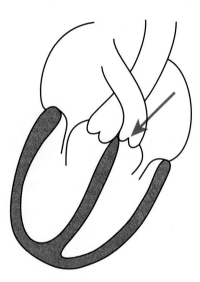

Depolarization of the atria from the left towards the right occurs in dextrocardia, or accidental misplacement of the arm leads on the patient.

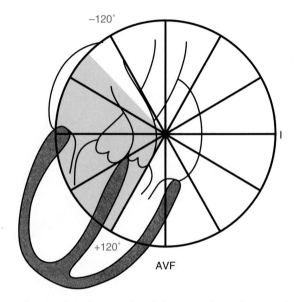

The P axis points to the right, anywhere from less than −120° to greater than +105°.

SUMMARY OF THE P AXIS

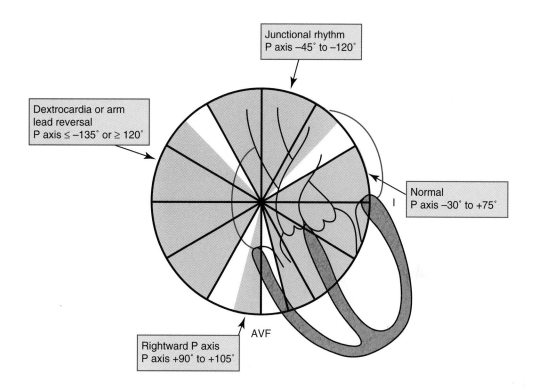

Junctional rhythm
P axis −45˚ to −120˚

Dextrocardia or arm
lead reversal
P axis ≤ −135˚ or ≥ 120˚

Normal
P axis −30˚ to +75˚

I

AVF

Rightward P axis
P axis +90˚ to +105˚

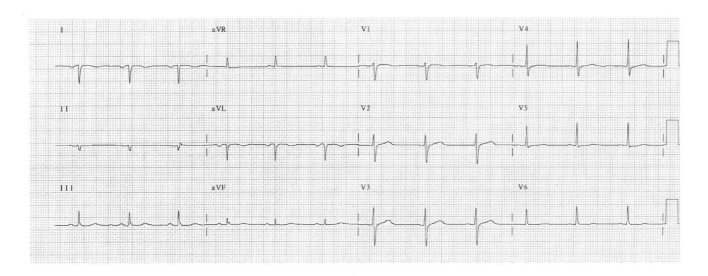

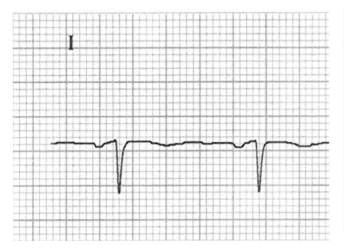

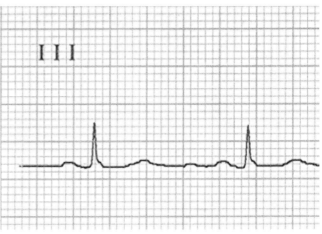

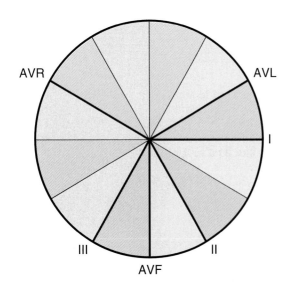

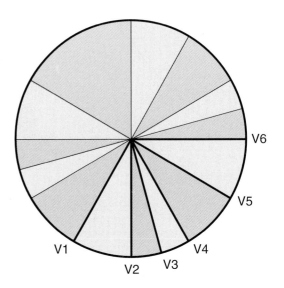

Heart Rate:

Rhythm:

Intervals (measured in the limb leads)

PR: short (< .12)
normal (.12 to .20)
long (>0.20 seconds); this is 1st degree AV block

QRS: normal (≤0.09 seconds)
prolonged (.10 or .11); this is intraventricular conduction delay (IVCD)
Bundle Branch Block (.12 seconds or greater)

QT:

P axis: normal
rightward
arm-lead reversal or dextrocardia
junctional rhythm

QRS axis: normal
left anterior hemiblock
left posterior hemiblock
indeterminate

T wave inversion (ischemia or infarction):

II,III,AVF	inferior
I, AVL	lateral
V1, without V2	nonspecific septal
V1 and V2	septal
V3 and V4	anterior
V5 and V6	lateral
V6, without V5	nonspecific lateral

ST Elevation (acute infarction):

II,III,AVF	inferior
I, AVL	lateral
V1, without V2	nonspecific septal
V1 and V2	septal
V3 and V4	anterior
V5 and V6	lateral
V6, without V5.	nonspecific lateral

ST Depression (ischemia or infarction):

I,II,III,AVL,AVF	diffuse subendocardial ischemia or infarction
V2,V3,V4,V5	diffuse subendocardial ischemia or infarction

Q waves (infarction):

II,III,AVF	inferior
I, AVL	lateral
V1, without V2	nonspecific septal
V1 and V2	septal
V3 and V4	anterior
V5 and V6	lateral
V6, without V5	nonspecific lateral

Hypertrophy:

Right atrial: Tall P wave 2.5 mm in II, III, or AVF

Left atrial: Deep negative part of P wave in V1

LVH: R wave in 1 + S wave in III ≥ 25mV
S wave in V1 + R wave in V5 ≥ 35mV

RVH: Mean QRS either anterior, or rightward

The heart rate is 71 beats per minute. The rhythm is sinus. The PR interval is best seen in lead III and measures 0.16 seconds, which is normal. The QRS interval is 0.08 seconds, which is also normal. The QT interval is best seen in lead III and measures 0.36 seconds, which is normal. The P axis is +150°, because the P wave is negative in I but positive in AVF and isoelectric in lead II. The P axis of +150° is abnormal and suggests dextrocardia or misplacement of the right and left arm leads. In dextrocardia, the QRS complexes would decrease in size from lead V1 to lead V6, because the leads are being placed further and further away from the heart. On this EKG, the QRS complexes are normal from lead V1 to lead V6, so dextrocardia is not present. The person taking this EKG accidentally misplaced the right and left arm leads. This happens. You should be able to recognize this and order another EKG.

Parts of the answer sheets are "grayed out" because these sections have not yet been covered. Answer only the parts that are not highlighted.

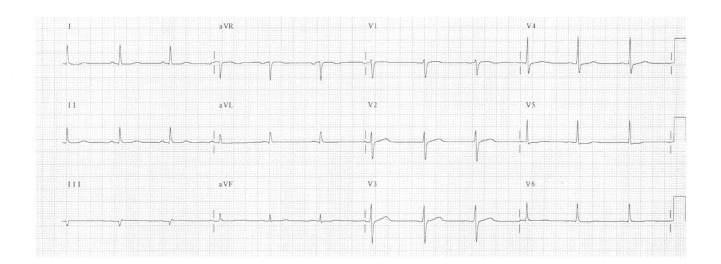

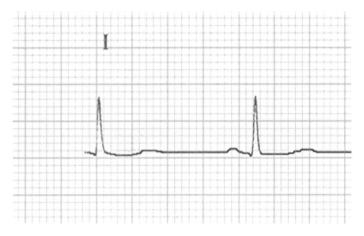

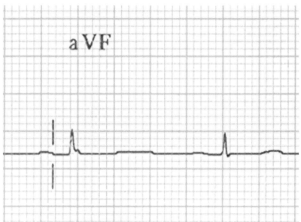

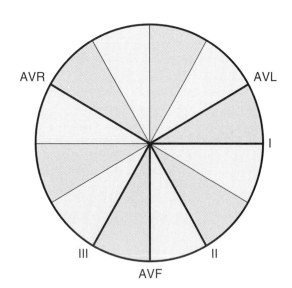

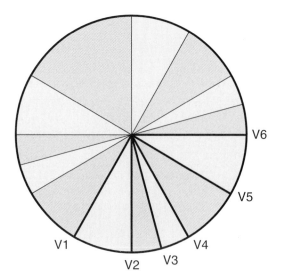

Heart Rate:

Rhythm:

Intervals (measured in the limb leads)

PR: short (< .12)
        normal (.12 to .20)
        long (>0.20 seconds); this is 1st degree AV
        block

QRS: normal (≤0.09 seconds)
        prolonged (.10 or .11); this is intraventricular
        conduction delay (IVCD)
        Bundle Branch Block (.12 seconds or greater)

QT:

ST Elevation (acute infarction):

II, III, AVF	inferior
I, AVL	lateral
V1, without V2	nonspecific septal
V1 and V2	septal
V3 and V4	anterior
V5 and V6	lateral
V6, without V5.	nonspecific lateral

ST Depression (ischemia or infarction):

I, II, III, AVL, AVF	diffuse subendocardial ischemia or infarction
V2, V3, V4, V5	diffuse subendocardial ischemia or infarction

P axis: normal
               rightward
               arm-lead reversal or dextrocardia
               junctional rhythm

QRS axis: normal
               left anterior hemiblock
               left posterior hemiblock
               indeterminate

Q waves (infarction):

II, III, AVF	inferior
I, AVL	lateral
V1, without V2	nonspecific septal
V1 and V2	septal
V3 and V4	anterior
V5 and V6	lateral
V6, without V5	nonspecific lateral

T wave inversion (ischemia or infarction):

II, III, AVF	inferior
I, AVL	lateral
V1, without V2	nonspecific septal
V1 and V2	septal
V3 and V4	anterior
V5 and V6	lateral
V6, without V5	nonspecific lateral

Hypertrophy:

Right atrial: Tall P wave 2.5 mm in II, III, or AVF

Left atrial: Deep negative part of P wave in V1

LVH: R wave in 1 + S wave in III ≥ 25mV
        S wave in V1 + R wave in V5 ≥ 35mV

RVH: Mean QRS either anterior, or rightward

The heart rate is 68 beats per minute. The rhythm is sinus. The PR interval measures 0.16 seconds in lead AVF and is normal. The QRS interval measures 0.08 seconds and is normal. The QT interval measures 0.38 seconds and is normal. The P axis is +60°, because it is positive in leads I and AVF and isoelectric in lead AVL. If you call the P wave in lead AVL positive, then the P-axis would be +45°, which is normal. If you call the P wave negative in lead AVL, then the P axis would be +75°, which is also normal. If it takes more than 5 seconds to decide whether a complex in a lead is positive or negative, it is probably isoelectric. This EKG is taken from the same patient as the EKG on the previous patient, with the right and left arm leads now correctly placed. Notice that leads V1 to V6 are unaffected by misplacement of the arm leads. The mean QRS axis is +15° and the T axis is +75°.

Parts of the answer sheets are "grayed out" because these sections have not yet been covered. Answer only the parts that are not highlighted.

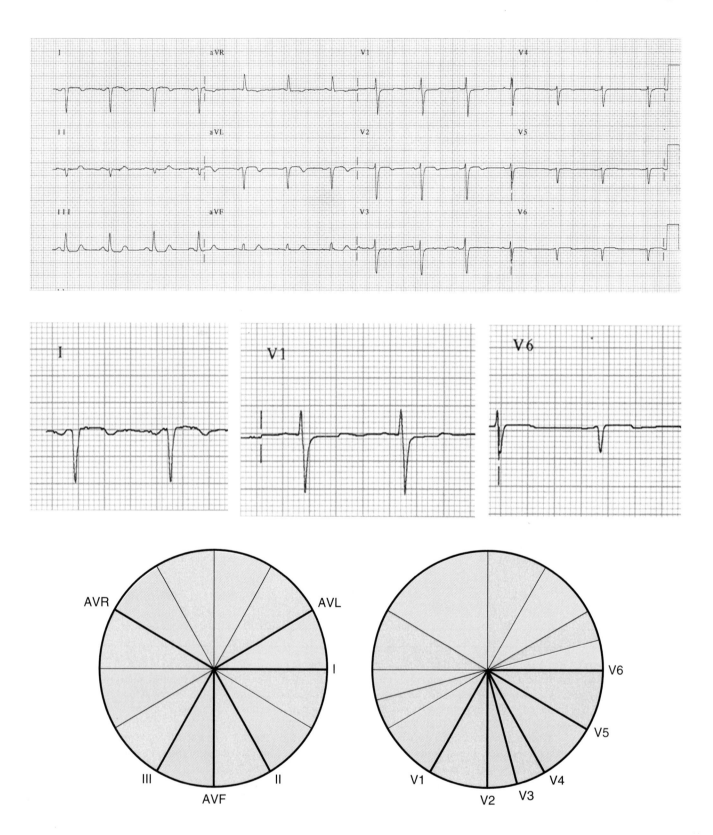

Heart Rate:

Rhythm:

Intervals (measured in the limb leads)

PR: short (< .12)
      normal (.12 to .20)
      long (>0.20 seconds); this is 1st degree AV
      block

QRS: normal (≤0.09 seconds)
      prolonged (.10 or .11); this is intraventricular
      conduction delay (IVCD)
      Bundle Branch Block (.12 seconds or greater)

QT:

P axis: normal
              rightward
              arm-lead reversal or dextrocardia
              junctional rhythm

QRS axis: normal
              left anterior hemiblock
              left posterior hemiblock
              indeterminate

T wave inversion (ischemia or infarction):

II,III,AVF	inferior
I, AVL	lateral
V1, without V2	nonspecific septal
V1 and V2	septal
V3 and V4	anterior
V5 and V6	lateral
V6, without V5	nonspecific lateral

ST Elevation (acute infarction):

II,III,AVF	inferior
I, AVL	lateral
V1, without V2	nonspecific septal
V1 and V2	septal
V3 and V4	anterior
V5 and V6	lateral
V6, without V5.	nonspecific lateral

ST Depression (ischemia or infarction):

I,II,III,AVL,AVF	diffuse subendocardial ischemia or infarction
V2,V3,V4,V5	diffuse subendocardial ischemia or infarction

Q waves (infarction):

II,III,AVF	inferior
I, AVL	lateral
V1, without V2	nonspecific septal
V1 and V2	septal
V3 and V4	anterior
V5 and V6	lateral
V6, without V5	nonspecific lateral

Hypertrophy:

Right atrial: Tall P wave 2.5 mm in II, III, or AVF

Left atrial: Deep negative part of P wave in V1

LVH: R wave in 1 + S wave in III ≥ 25mV
      S wave in V1 + R wave in V5 ≥ 35mV

RVH: Mean QRS either anterior, or rightward

The heart rate is 83 beats per minute. The PR interval is 0.14 seconds. The QRS interval measures 0.08 seconds. The QT interval measures 0.34 seconds. These are all normal. The P axis is +135°, because the P wave is positive in AVF, II, and AVR but negative in lead I. This P axis is consistent with either right and left arm lead reversal or dextrocardia. Looking at the V leads, the QRS complexes diminish in size from V1 to V6, as though the leads are getting further and further away from the heart. This patient has dextrocardia. The mean QRS axis is +165°, and the T axis is +90°.

Parts of the answer sheets are "grayed out" because these sections have not yet been covered. Answer only the parts that are not highlighted.

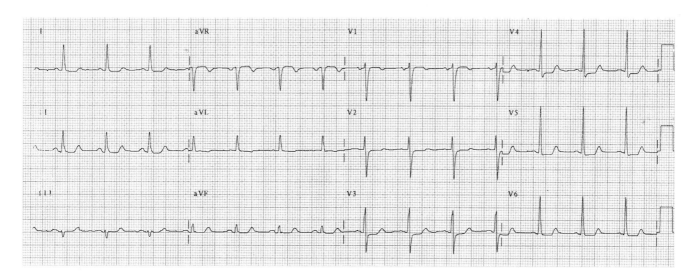

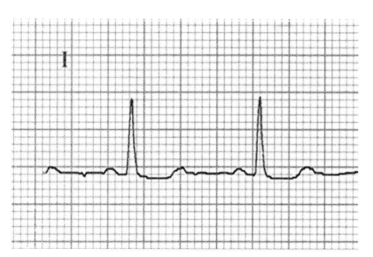

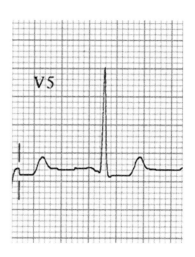

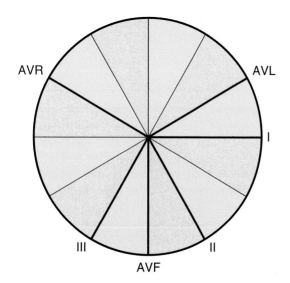

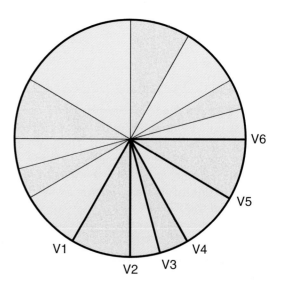

Heart Rate:

Rhythm:

Intervals (measured in the limb leads)

PR: short (< .12)
       normal (.12 to .20)
       long (>0.20 seconds); this is 1st degree AV block

QRS: normal (≤0.09 seconds)
       prolonged (.10 or .11); this is intraventricular conduction delay (IVCD)
       Bundle Branch Block (.12 seconds or greater)

QT:

P axis: normal
               rightward
               arm-lead reversal or dextrocardia
               junctional rhythm

QRS axis: normal
               left anterior hemiblock
               left posterior hemiblock
               indeterminate

T wave inversion (ischemia or infarction):

II,III,AVF	inferior
I, AVL	lateral
V1, without V2	nonspecific septal
V1 and V2	septal
V3 and V4	anterior
V5 and V6	lateral
V6, without V5	nonspecific lateral

ST Elevation (acute infarction):

II,III,AVF	inferior
I, AVL	lateral
V1, without V2	nonspecific septal
V1 and V2	septal
V3 and V4	anterior
V5 and V6	lateral
V6, without V5.	nonspecific lateral

ST Depression (ischemia or infarction):

I,II,III,AVL,AVF	diffuse subendocardial ischemia or infarction
V2,V3,V4,V5	diffuse subendocardial ischemia or infarction

Q waves (infarction):

II,III,AVF	inferior
I, AVL	lateral
V1, without V2	nonspecific septal
V1 and V2	septal
V3 and V4	anterior
V5 and V6	lateral
V6, without V5	nonspecific lateral

Hypertrophy:

Right atrial: Tall P wave 2.5 mm in II, III, or AVF

Left atrial: Deep negative part of P wave in V1

LVH: R wave in 1 + S wave in III ≥ 25mV
      S wave in V1 + R wave in V5 ≥ 35mV

RVH: Mean QRS either anterior, or rightward

The heart rate is 83 beats per minute. The PR interval measures 0.14 seconds, which is normal. The QRS interval measures 0.08 seconds, which is normal. The QT interval measures 0.34 seconds, which is normal. The P axis is +60°, because the P wave is positive in leads I and AVF and isoelectric in lead AVL. Again, don't waste time deciding whether the P wave is positive (making the P axis +45°), negative (making the P axis +75°) or isoelectric in lead AVL. It would change nothing. The P axis is normal. This EKG was taken from the same patient as the previous EKG. This time, the arm leads, the leg leads, and all the V leads were replaced onto the patient in a mirror-image fashion from right to left. This normalizes the P, QRS, and T axes if there is no other underlying pathology. Continuing, the mean QRS axis is +15°, and the T axis is +60°.

Parts of the answer sheets are "grayed out" because these sections have not yet been covered. Answer only the parts that are not highlighted.

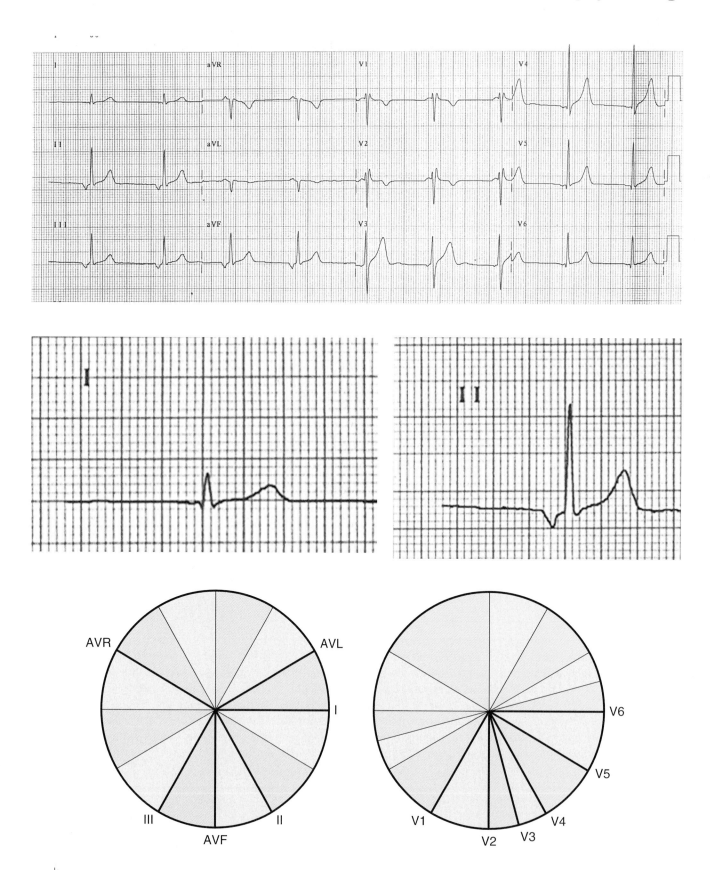

Heart Rate:

Rhythm:

ST Elevation (acute infarction):

II,III,AVF	inferior
I, AVL	lateral
V1, without V2	nonspecific septal
V1 and V2	septal
V3 and V4	anterior
V5 and V6	lateral
V6, without V5.	nonspecific lateral

Intervals (measured in the limb leads)

PR: short (< .12)
        normal (.12 to .20)
        long (>0.20 seconds); this is 1st degree AV block

QRS: normal (≤0.09 seconds)
        prolonged (.10 or .11); this is intraventricular conduction delay (IVCD)
        Bundle Branch Block (.12 seconds or greater)

QT:

ST Depression (ischemia or infarction):

| I,II,III,AVL,AVF | diffuse subendocardial ischemia or infarction |
| V2,V3,V4,V5 | diffuse subendocardial ischemia or infarction |

P axis: normal
            rightward
            arm-lead reversal or dextrocardia
            junctional rhythm

QRS axis: normal
            left anterior hemiblock
            left posterior hemiblock
            indeterminate

Q waves (infarction):

II,III,AVF	inferior
I, AVL	lateral
V1, without V2	nonspecific septal
V1 and V2	septal
V3 and V4	anterior
V5 and V6	lateral
V6, without V5	nonspecific lateral

T wave inversion (ischemia or infarction):

II,III,AVF	inferior
I, AVL	lateral
V1, without V2	nonspecific septal
V1 and V2	septal
V3 and V4	anterior
V5 and V6	lateral
V6, without V5	nonspecific lateral

Hypertrophy:

Right atrial: Tall P wave 2.5 mm in II, III, or AVF

Left atrial: Deep negative part of P wave in V1

LVH: R wave in 1 + S wave in III ≥ 25mV
      S wave in V1 + R wave in V5 ≥ 35mV

RVH: Mean QRS either anterior, or rightward

The heart rate is 50 beats per minute. The PR interval is 0.12 seconds. The QRS interval measures 0.08 seconds. The QT interval measures 0.40 seconds, which is borderline short from the table in Chapter 5. Causes of short QT include hypercalcemia and digitalis toxicity. The P axis is −90°, indicating junctional rhythm. Digitalis toxicity causes junctional rhythm (Chapter 19).

An overly rapid look at this EKG, ignoring the P wave axis and the QT interval, would miss important clues for digitalis toxicity.

Parts of the answer sheets are "grayed out" because these sections have not yet been covered. Answer only the parts that are not highlighted.

Hemiblock

Intraventricular conduction disturbances occur when there is a delay or loss of electrical conduction through the normal conduction pathway. There are several types of intraventricular conduction abnormalities. The most common are left bundle branch block, right bundle branch block, and hemiblock.

Normally, the electrical impulse is generated in the sinus node and proceeds through the atria, initiating atrial depolarization.

The impulse continues to transverse the atrioventricular (AV) node and travels through the bundle of His and down the right and left bundle branches, resulting in ventricular depolarization.

When a bundle branch block is present, the electrical impulse is unable to pass through one or both of the defective bundle branches, interfering with normal ventricular depolarization.

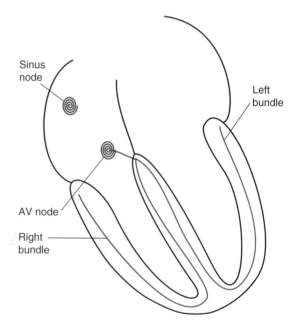

Sinus node

Left bundle

AV node

Right bundle

The Left Bundle Branch

The right and left bundle branches differ anatomically. The right bundle branch consists of one branch and is responsible for depolarization of the right ventricle. **The left bundle branch consists of two branches: the left anterior superior branch and the left inferior posterior branch.** These branches are responsible for depolarization of the left ventricle, including the septum.

Hemiblock occurs when one of these branches is unable to conduct the electrical impulse, interfering with normal left ventricular depolarization.

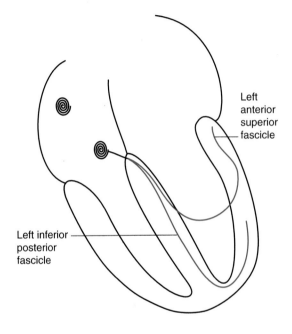

Left anterior superior fascicle

Left inferior posterior fascicle

Left Anterior Hemiblock

Left anterior hemiblock occurs when there is decreased conductivity of the left anterior-superior fascicle of the left bundle branch. **It is diagnosed by evaluating the mean QRS axis in the frontal plane.** *Left anterior hemiblock shifts the mean QRS axis upward and leftward.* This occurs because the electrical impulse from the left inferior-superior fascicle spreads superiorly and to the left to depolarize the entire left ventricle because the left anterior branch is unable to do so.

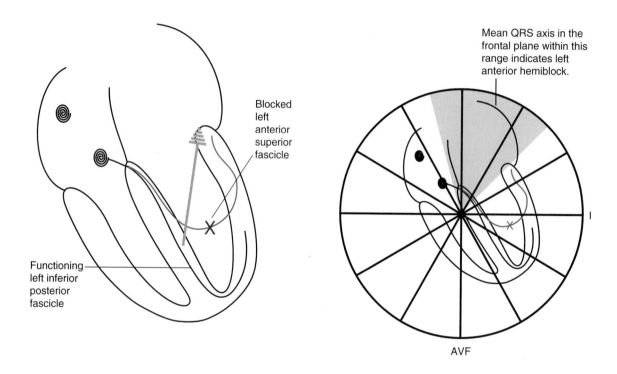

Blocked left anterior superior fascicle

Functioning left inferior posterior fascicle

Mean QRS axis in the frontal plane within this range indicates left anterior hemiblock.

I

AVF

Example of Left Anterior Hemiblock

In this example, the mean plane QRS axis is −60°, indicating the presence of left anterior hemiblock.

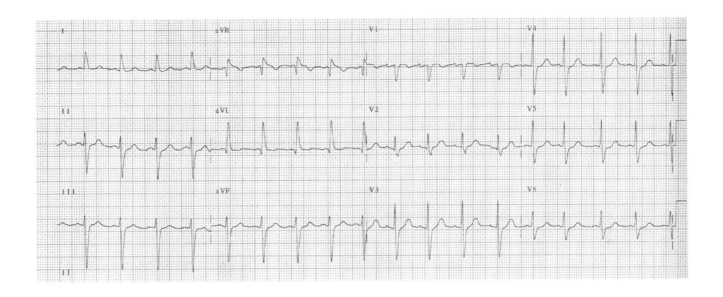

In this example:

1. The mean QRS is positive in leads I and AVL.
2. The mean QRS is negative in leads II, III, and AVF. AVR is isoelectric.
3. Therefore, the mean frontal plane QRS axis is −60°.

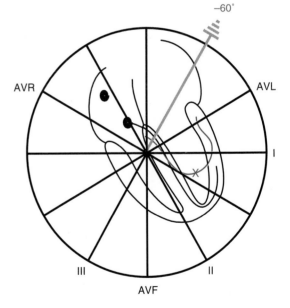

SUMMARY OF LEFT ANTERIOR HEMIBLOCK

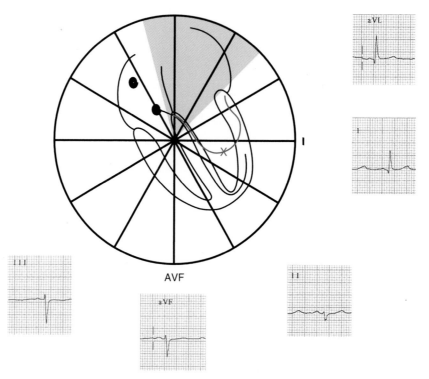

Concept: Left anterior hemiblock moves the QRS axis superiorly and usually leftward.

Axis: The mean QRS axis in the frontal plane is −45° to −105°.

Pattern: Leads II, III, and AVF are typically negative, with a small r wave and a larger S wave. Leads I and AVL are positive, with a small q wave and a larger R wave.

Left Anterior Hemiblock: Lead Pattern

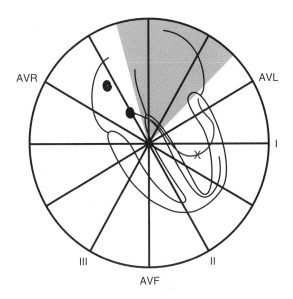

Leads II, III, AVF
(negative)

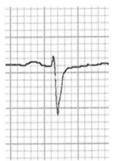

Leads I, AVL
(positive)

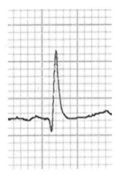

Left Posterior Hemiblock

The second type of hemiblock is called left posterior hemiblock. Left posterior hemiblock occurs when there is delayed or incomplete conduction through the left posterior-inferior division of the left bundle branch. Left posterior hemiblock shifts the mean QRS axis inferiorly and to the right. Left posterior hemiblock is also diagnosed by examining the mean QRS axis in the frontal plane.

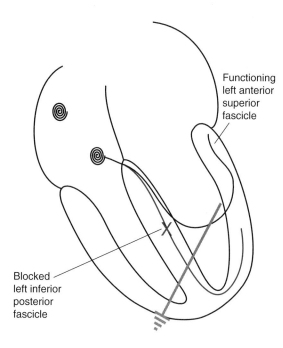

Functioning left anterior superior fascicle

Blocked left inferior posterior fascicle

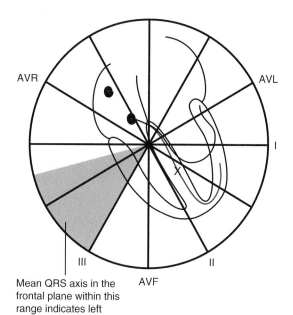

Mean QRS axis in the frontal plane within this range indicates left inferior posterior hemiblock.

Example of Left Posterior Hemiblock

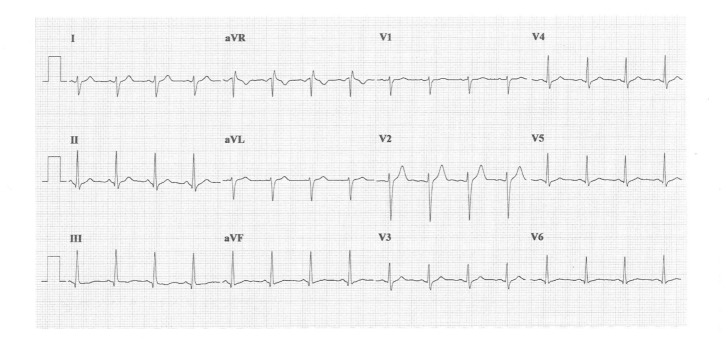

Left posterior hemiblock produces a mean QRS axis of +120° to +165°.

In this example, the mean QRS axis is positive in leads II, III, and AVF but negative in leads I and AVL. AVR is called isoelectric.

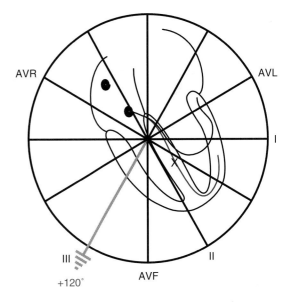

SUMMARY OF LEFT POSTERIOR HEMIBLOCK

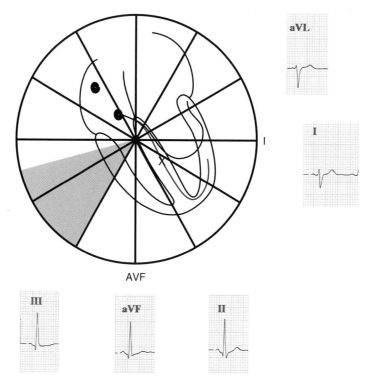

Concept: Left posterior hemiblock moves the QRS axis inferiorly and rightward.

Axis: The mean QRS axis in the frontal plane is +120° to +165°.

Pattern: Leads II, III, and AVF are typically positive, with a small q wave and a larger R wave. Leads I and AVL are negative, with a small r wave and a larger S wave.

Left Posterior Hemiblock: Lead Pattern

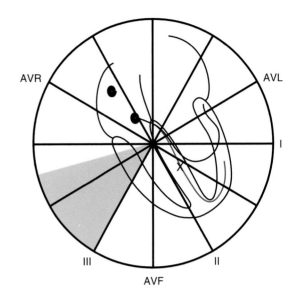

Leads II, III, AVF
(positive)

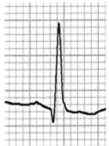

Leads I, AVL
(negative)

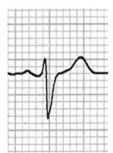

SUMMARY OF HEMIBLOCK

Left anterior hemiblock mean QRS axis: −45° to −105°.

Left posterior hemiblock mean QRS axis: +120° to +165°.

I

AVF

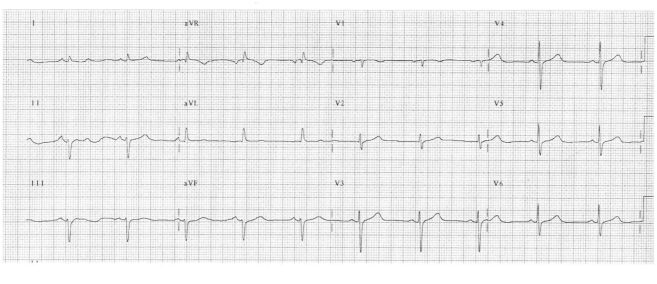

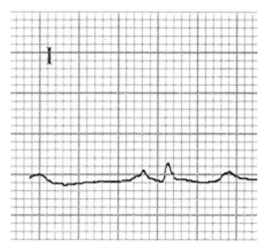

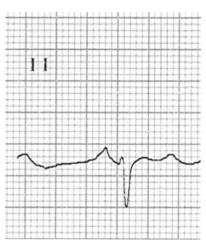

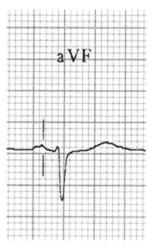

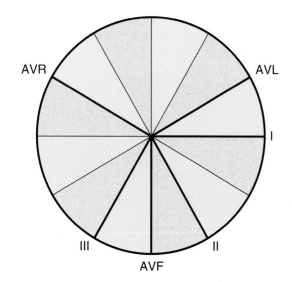

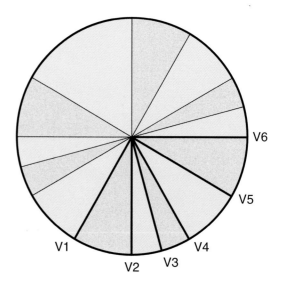

Heart Rate:

Rhythm:

Intervals (measured in the limb leads)

PR: short (< .12)
      normal (.12 to .20)
      long (>0.20 seconds); this is 1st degree AV
      block

QRS: normal (≤0.09 seconds)
      prolonged (.10 or .11); this is intraventricular
      conduction delay (IVCD)
      Bundle Branch Block (.12 seconds or greater)

QT:

P axis:	normal
	rightward
	arm-lead reversal or dextrocardia
	junctional rhythm
QRS axis:	normal
	left anterior hemiblock
	left posterior hemiblock
	indeterminate

T wave inversion (ischemia or infarction):

II,III,AVF	inferior
I, AVL	lateral
V1, without V2	nonspecific septal
V1 and V2	septal
V3 and V4	anterior
V5 and V6	lateral
V6, without V5	nonspecific lateral

ST Elevation (acute infarction):

II,III,AVF	inferior
I, AVL	lateral
V1, without V2	nonspecific septal
V1 and V2	septal
V3 and V4	anterior
V5 and V6	lateral
V6, without V5.	nonspecific lateral

ST Depression (ischemia or infarction):

I,II,III,AVL,AVF	diffuse subendocardial ischemia or infarction
V2,V3,V4,V5	diffuse subendocardial ischemia or infarction

Q waves (infarction):

II,III,AVF	inferior
I, AVL	lateral
V1, without V2	nonspecific septal
V1 and V2	septal
V3 and V4	anterior
V5 and V6	lateral
V6, without V5	nonspecific lateral

Hypertrophy:

Right atrial: Tall P wave 2.5 mm in II, III, or AVF

Left atrial: Deep negative part of P wave in V1

LVH: R wave in 1 + S wave in III ≥ 25mV
      S wave in V1 + R wave in V5 ≥ 35mV

RVH: Mean QRS either anterior, or rightward

The heart rate is 63 beats per minute. The rhythm is sinus. The PR interval measures 0.16 seconds, which is normal. The QRS interval is 0.09 seconds, which is also normal. The QT interval measures 0.40 seconds, which is normal. The P axis is +75° and is normal. **The mean QRS axis is −75°, because the QRS is negative in II but positive in I and AVR. The QRS is abnormal and lies within the diagnostic range of left anterior hemiblock (LAHB).**

Parts of the answer sheets are "grayed out" because these sections have not yet been covered. Answer only the parts that are not highlighted.

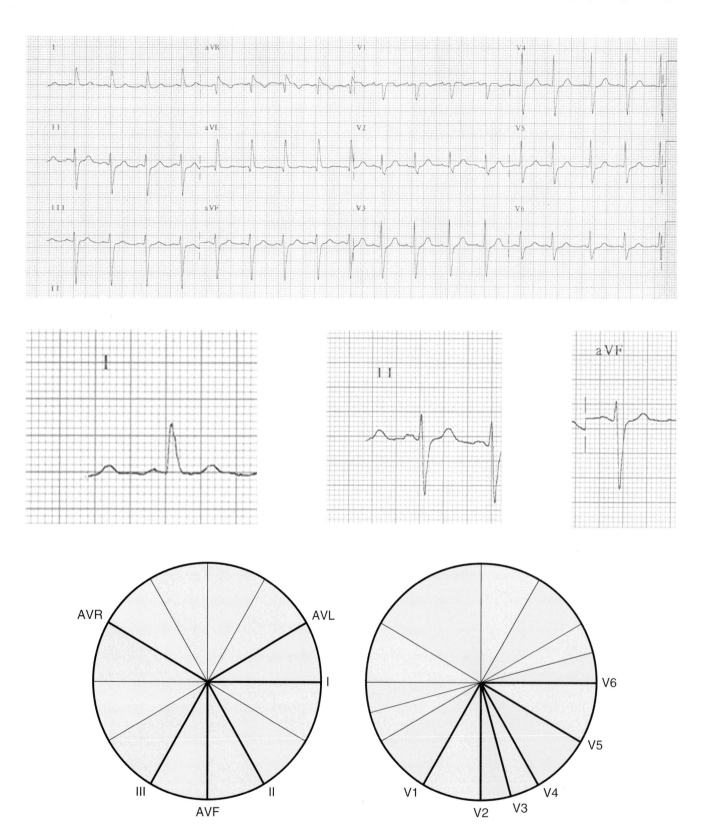

Heart Rate:

Rhythm:

Intervals (measured in the limb leads)

PR: short (< .12)
       normal (.12 to .20)
       long (>0.20 seconds); this is 1st degree AV
       block

QRS: normal (≤0.09 seconds)
       prolonged (.10 or .11); this is intraventricular
       conduction delay (IVCD)
       Bundle Branch Block (.12 seconds or greater)

QT:

P axis: normal
             rightward
             arm-lead reversal or dextrocardia
             junctional rhythm

QRS axis: normal
             left anterior hemiblock
             left posterior hemiblock
             indeterminate

T wave inversion (ischemia or infarction):

II,III,AVF	inferior
I, AVL	lateral
V1, without V2	nonspecific septal
V1 and V2	septal
V3 and V4	anterior
V5 and V6	lateral
V6, without V5	nonspecific lateral

ST Elevation (acute infarction):

II,III,AVF	inferior
I, AVL	lateral
V1, without V2	nonspecific septal
V1 and V2	septal
V3 and V4	anterior
V5 and V6	lateral
V6, without V5.	nonspecific lateral

ST Depression (ischemia or infarction):

I,II,III,AVL,AVF	diffuse subendocardial ischemia or infarction
V2,V3,V4,V5	diffuse subendocardial ischemia or infarction

Q waves (infarction):

II,III,AVF	inferior
I, AVL	lateral
V1, without V2	nonspecific septal
V1 and V2	septal
V3 and V4	anterior
V5 and V6	lateral
V6, without V5	nonspecific lateral

Hypertrophy:

Right atrial: Tall P wave 2.5 mm in II, III, or AVF

Left atrial: Deep negative part of P wave in V1

LVH: R wave in 1 + S wave in III ≥ 25mV
      S wave in V1 + R wave in V5 ≥ 35mV

RVH: Mean QRS either anterior, or rightward

The heart rate is 107 beats per minute. The rhythm is sinus tachycardia. The PR interval measures 0.12 seconds and is normal. The QRS interval measures 0.10 seconds and is abnormal. The QRS interval of 0.10 seconds indicates intraventricular conduction delay (IVCD). The QT interval measures 0.32 seconds and is normal. The P axis is +75° because it is positive in leads I, II, III, and AVF but negative in AVL. **The mean QRS axis is −60°, because it is negative in II, III, and AVF but positive in I and AVL.** (It can be difficult to assess AVR as being positive or isoelectric. If it takes longer than a few seconds to decide, it is probably isoelectric.) This QRS axis is abnormal and falls within the diagnostic range of left anterior hemiblock.

Parts of the answer sheets are "grayed out" because these sections have not yet been covered. Answer only the parts that are not highlighted.

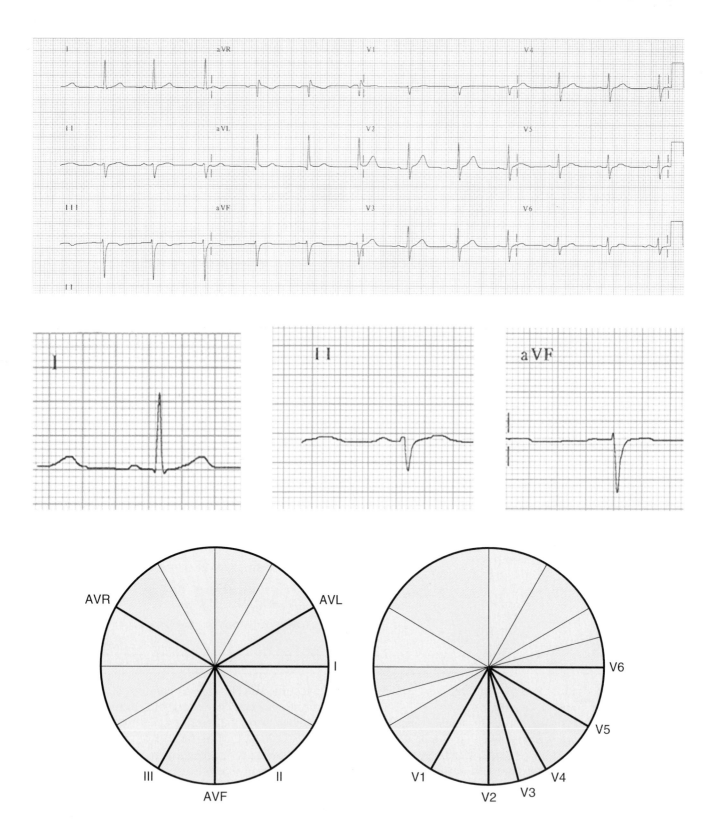

Heart Rate:

Rhythm:

Intervals (measured in the limb leads)

PR: short (< .12)
     normal (.12 to .20)
     long (>0.20 seconds); this is 1st degree AV
     block

QRS: normal (≤0.09 seconds)
     prolonged (.10 or .11); this is intraventricular
     conduction delay (IVCD)
     Bundle Branch Block (.12 seconds or greater)

QT:

P axis: normal
           rightward
           arm-lead reversal or dextrocardia
           junctional rhythm

QRS axis: normal
           left anterior hemiblock
           left posterior hemiblock
           indeterminate

T wave inversion (ischemia or infarction):

II,III,AVF	inferior
I, AVL	lateral
V1, without V2	nonspecific septal
V1 and V2	septal
V3 and V4	anterior
V5 and V6	lateral
V6, without V5	nonspecific lateral

ST Elevation (acute infarction):

II,III,AVF	inferior
I, AVL	lateral
V1, without V2	nonspecific septal
V1 and V2	septal
V3 and V4	anterior
V5 and V6	lateral
V6, without V5.	nonspecific lateral

ST Depression (ischemia or infarction):

| I,II,III,AVL,AVF | diffuse subendocardial ischemia or infarction |
| V2,V3,V4,V5 | diffuse subendocardial ischemia or infarction |

Q waves (infarction):

II,III,AVF	inferior
I, AVL	lateral
V1, without V2	nonspecific septal
V1 and V2	septal
V3 and V4	anterior
V5 and V6	lateral
V6, without V5	nonspecific lateral

Hypertrophy:

Right atrial: Tall P wave 2.5 mm in II, III, or AVF

Left atrial: Deep negative part of P wave in V1

LVH: R wave in 1 + S wave in III ≥ 25mV
      S wave in V1 + R wave in V5 ≥ 35mV

RVH: Mean QRS either anterior, or rightward

The heart rate varies from 71 to 75 beats per minute. This is sinus rhythm. The PR interval measures 0.18 seconds in lead AVF. The QRS interval measures 0.09 seconds. The QT interval measures 0.36 seconds, which is normal. The P axis is +60° in the frontal plane, which is normal. **The mean QRS axis in the frontal plane is −45°. This is abnormal and indicates left anterior hemiblock (LAHB).** The T axis in the frontal plane is +15°.

Parts of the answer sheets are "grayed out" because these sections have not yet been covered. Answer only the parts that are not highlighted.

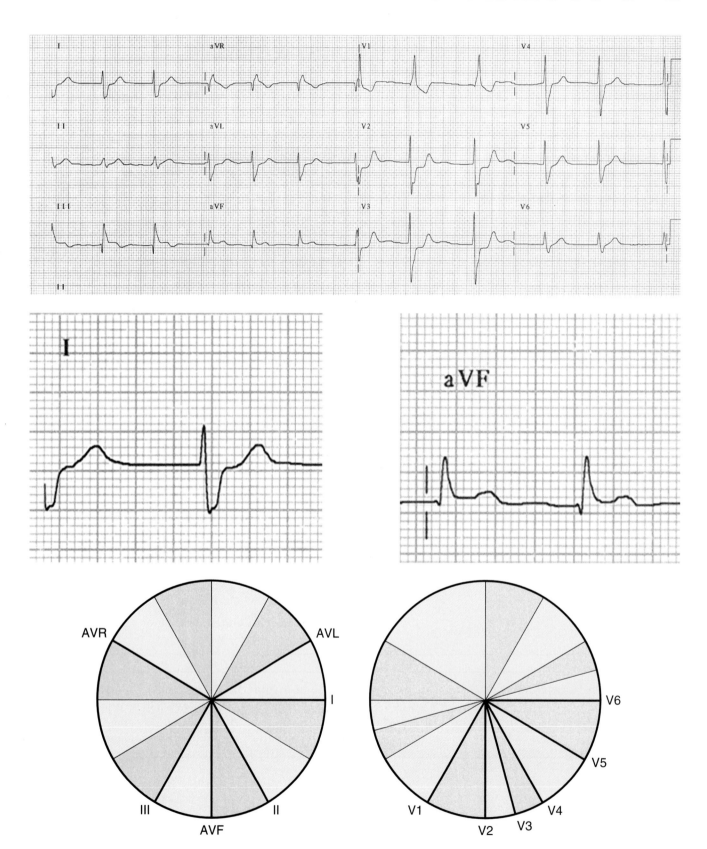

Heart Rate:

Rhythm:

Intervals (measured in the limb leads)

PR: short (< .12)
normal (.12 to .20)
long (>0.20 seconds); this is 1st degree AV block

QRS: normal (≤0.09 seconds)
prolonged (.10 or .11); this is intraventricular conduction delay (IVCD)
Bundle Branch Block (.12 seconds or greater)

QT:

P axis: normal
rightward
arm-lead reversal or dextrocardia
junctional rhythm

QRS axis: normal
left anterior hemiblock
left posterior hemiblock
indeterminate

T wave inversion (ischemia or infarction):

II,III,AVF	inferior
I, AVL	lateral
V1, without V2	nonspecific septal
V1 and V2	septal
V3 and V4	anterior
V5 and V6	lateral
V6, without V5	nonspecific lateral

ST Elevation (acute infarction):

II,III,AVF	inferior
I, AVL	lateral
V1, without V2	nonspecific septal
V1 and V2	septal
V3 and V4	anterior
V5 and V6	lateral
V6, without V5.	nonspecific lateral

ST Depression (ischemia or infarction):

| I,II,III,AVL,AVF | diffuse subendocardial ischemia or infarction |
| V2,V3,V4,V5 | diffuse subendocardial ischemia or infarction |

Q waves (infarction):

II,III,AVF	inferior
I, AVL	lateral
V1, without V2	nonspecific septal
V1 and V2	septal
V3 and V4	anterior
V5 and V6	lateral
V6, without V5	nonspecific lateral

Hypertrophy:

Right atrial: Tall P wave 2.5 mm in II, III, or AVF

Left atrial: Deep negative part of P wave in V1

LVH: R wave in 1 + S wave in III ≥ 25mV
S wave in V1 + R wave in V5 ≥ 35mV

RVH: Mean QRS either anterior, or rightward

The ventricular rate is 60 beats per minute. The rhythm is irregularly irregular, indicating atrial fibrillation. The PR interval is undefined in atrial fibrillation. The QRS interval measures 0.14 seconds. This is abnormal and indicates bundle branch block. (Chapters 9 and 10 discuss bundle branch block.) The QT interval measures 0.40 seconds. The P axis is undefined. **The mean QRS axis is +135°, because the *overall QRS complex* is negative in I and AVl but positive in II, III, AVR, and AVF. This QRS axis is abnormal and lies within the diagnostic range of left posterior hemiblock (LPHB). The T axis is +30°.**

Parts of the answer sheets are "grayed out" because these sections have not yet been covered. Answer only the parts that are not highlighted.

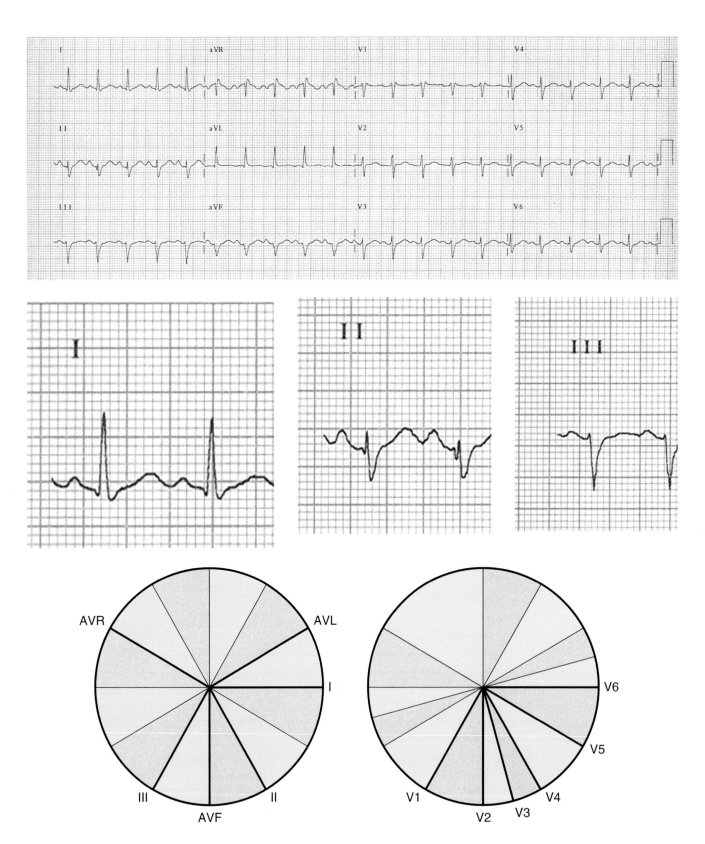

Heart Rate:

Rhythm:

Intervals (measured in the limb leads)

PR: short (< .12)
      normal (.12 to .20)
      long (>0.20 seconds); this is 1st degree AV
      block

QRS: normal (≤0.09 seconds)
      prolonged (.10 or .11); this is intraventricular
      conduction delay (IVCD)
      Bundle Branch Block (.12 seconds or greater)

QT:

P axis: normal
           rightward
           arm-lead reversal or dextrocardia
           junctional rhythm

QRS axis: normal
           left anterior hemiblock
           left posterior hemiblock
           indeterminate

T wave inversion (ischemia or infarction):

II,III,AVF	inferior
I, AVL	lateral
V1, without V2	nonspecific septal
V1 and V2	septal
V3 and V4	anterior
V5 and V6	lateral
V6, without V5	nonspecific lateral

ST Elevation (acute infarction):

II,III,AVF	inferior
I, AVL	lateral
V1, without V2	nonspecific septal
V1 and V2	septal
V3 and V4	anterior
V5 and V6	lateral
V6, without V5.	nonspecific lateral

ST Depression (ischemia or infarction):

I,II,III,AVL,AVF	diffuse subendocardial ischemia or infarction
V2,V3,V4,V5	diffuse subendocardial ischemia or infarction

Q waves (infarction):

II,III,AVF	inferior
I, AVL	lateral
V1, without V2	nonspecific septal
V1 and V2	septal
V3 and V4	anterior
V5 and V6	lateral
V6, without V5	nonspecific lateral

Hypertrophy:

Right atrial: Tall P wave 2.5 mm in II, III, or AVF

Left atrial: Deep negative part of P wave in V1

LVH: R wave in 1 + S wave in III ≥ 25mV
     S wave in V1 + R wave in V5 ≥ 35mV

RVH: Mean QRS either anterior, or rightward

The heart rate is 125 beats per minute. This is sinus tachycardia. The PR interval measures 0.16 seconds, which is normal. The QRS interval measures 0.10 seconds, which is abnormal. This indicates intraventricular conduction delay (IVCD). The QT interval measures 0.34 seconds, which is abnormally long for this heart rate. The corrected QT interval is above 440 ms and is approaching the dangerous range. The P axis is normal at +60°. *As a shortcut, when the P wave is positive in leads I and AVF, classify it as normal, without calculating the axis further.* Continuing, the mean QRS axis is −45°, because the QRS complex is positive in I and AVl and negative in II, III, and AVF. Lead AVR is probably negative. This QRS axis is abnormal and lies within the diagnostic range of left anterior hemiblock. The frontal plane T axis is +45°.

Parts of the answer sheets are "grayed out" because these sections have not yet been covered. Answer only the parts that are not highlighted.

Right Bundle Branch Block

Right bundle branch block **(RBBB)** occurs when there is a dysfunction of the right bundle branch interfering with normal impulse conduction and right ventricular depolarization. Right intraventricular conduction delay (RIVCD) slows the QRS interval of 0.10 to 0.11 seconds. RBBB slows the QRS interval to at least 0.12 seconds. **A QRS interval of 0.12 seconds or longer defines the presence of bundle branch block.**

Normally, the electrical impulse begins in the **sinus node**.

It proceeds through the atria, initiating atrial depolarization.

The impulse continues and transverses the **AV node** and travels into the **bundle of His**.

Finally, it travels quickly down the **right and left bundle branches** and spreads the impulse, causing ventricular depolarization, which we see as the QRS complex.

Any loss of conduction in either of the bundles slows the process of ventricular depolarization and increases the normal QRS interval of 0.08 to 0.09 seconds.

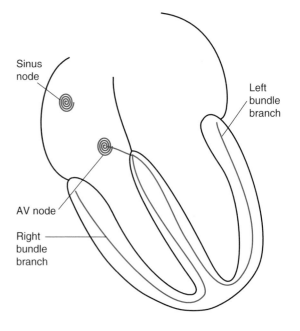

Sinus node

Left bundle branch

AV node

Right bundle branch

The Normal QRS Interval

Determining which bundle branch is blocked requires an analysis of the entire QRS complex. The **normal QRS complex** can be thought of as a combination of two forces known as the **initial force** and the **main force.** The initial force occurs at the beginning of the QRS complex and lasts 0.02 seconds. The main force can be defined as the remainder of the normal QRS complex and lasts 0.06 seconds. The key words are "normal QRS." **A QRS interval of 0.09 seconds or less indicates that conduction through both the right and the left bundles is occurring normally.**

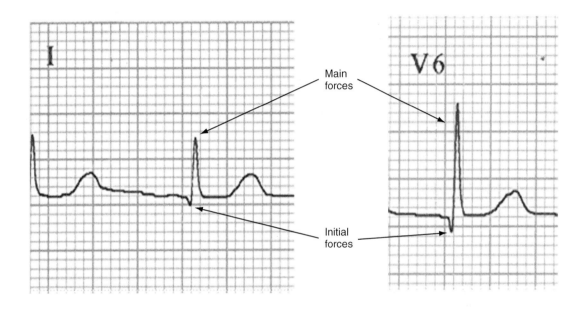

Main forces

Initial forces

The Normal QRS: Initial Forces

Depolarization of the septum causes the initial part of the QRS. **The left bundle branch normally depolarizes the ventricular septum in a left to right direction.** The initial force should normally produce an axis that points toward the ventricular septum, which is rightward.

In the horizontal plane, this produces an initial small q wave in lead I.

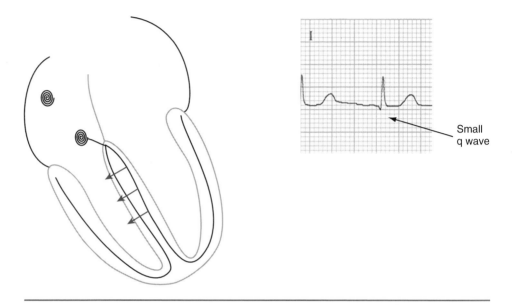

Small q wave

In the horizontal plane, septal depolarization produces initial forces that are anterior and rightward. This is represented on the EKG as an initial r wave in V1 and an initial q wave in V6.

In the horizontal plane, this produces an initial small q wave in lead V6, and an initial small r wave in lead V1.

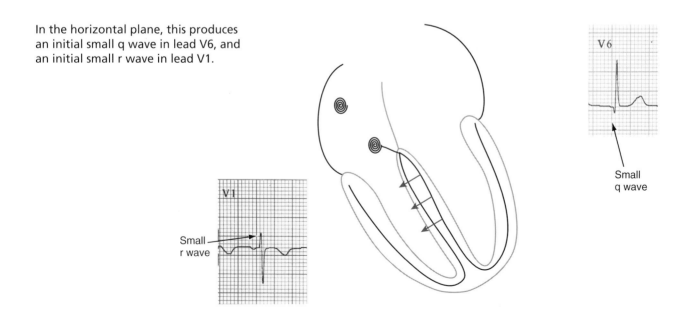

Small q wave

Small r wave

The Normal QRS: Main Forces

The main force of the normal QRS complex represents simultaneous right and left ventricular depolarization by the right and left bundle branches. Because the left ventricle has a much greater mass than the right ventricle, the main force points toward the left ventricle.

In the frontal plane, the main force points leftward and produces a larger R wave in lead I.

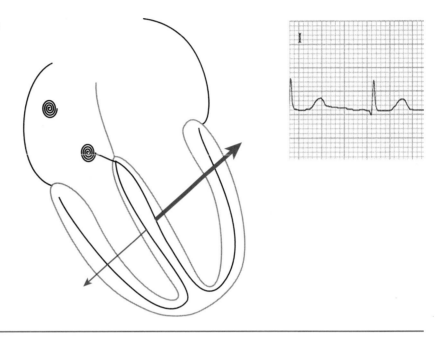

In the horizontal plane, the main force points posterior and leftward. It produces an S wave in lead VI and an R wave in lead V6.

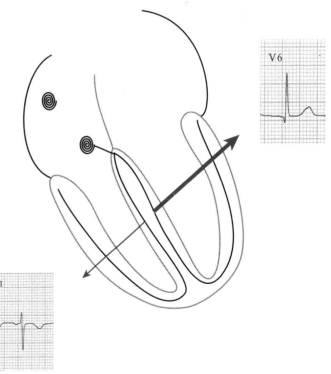

Right Bundle Branch Block: Late or Terminal Forces

In RBBB the right bundle branch is broken. The normal left bundle branch quickly depolarizes the septum and left ventricle (in 0.08 or 0.09 seconds). After 0.08 seconds, the left bundle takes on the additional burden of depolarizing the right ventricle. The left bundle has no direct access to the right ventricle, so it takes longer for the impulse to find and depolarize the right ventricle. This lengthens the QRS interval in RBBB to 0.12 seconds.

As a result, the QRS interval is widened to 0.12 seconds.

The last part of the QRS represents electrical activity in the right ventricle.

In the frontal plane, the late (or terminal) force points rightward toward the right ventricle.

This produces an S wave at the end of the QRS in lead I.

In the horizontal plane the late (or terminal) force points anterior and rightward toward the right ventricle.

This produces an S wave at the end of V6 and an R or R' at the end of V1 or V2.

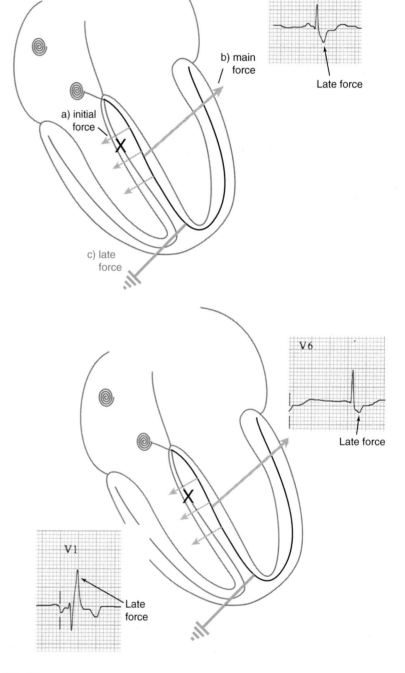

a) initial force

b) main force

c) late force

I
Late force

V6
Late force

V1
Late force

SUMMARY OF RIGHT BUNDLE BRANCH BLOCK: FRONTAL PLANE CONCEPT

It takes longer to depolarize the ventricles when the right bundle branch doesn't work, which lengthens the QRS to 0.12 seconds or longer. The last part of the QRS points rightward to the tardy right ventricle.

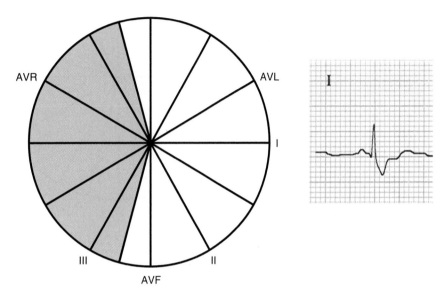

Concept: RBBB causes a wide 0.12 second QRS. The last part of the QRS points rightward toward the right ventricle.

Axis: The late or terminal QRS axis in the frontal plane is < −90°, or > +90°.

Pattern: The QRS is 0.12 sec and
The last part of the QRS in lead I is an S wave.

SUMMARY OF RIGHT BUNDLE BRANCH BLOCK: HORIZONTAL PLANE CONCEPT

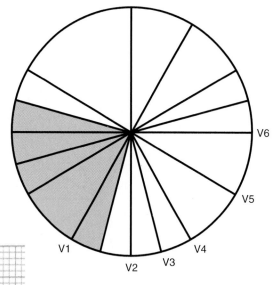

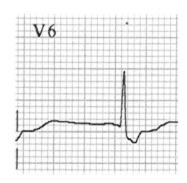

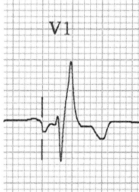

Concept: RBBB causes a QRS complex to measure 0.12 seconds or greater. The last part of the QRS points to the right ventricle, which is anterior and rightward.

Axis: The late or terminal QRS axis in the frontal plane is < −150°, or > +90°.

Pattern: The QRS is 0.12 sec, and
The QRS complex in lead V1 ends in an R wave and an S wave in V6.

SUMMARY OF RIGHT BUNDLE BRANCH BLOCK: LAST PART OF THE QRS PATTERN

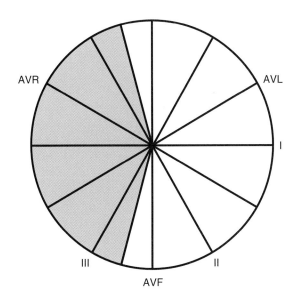
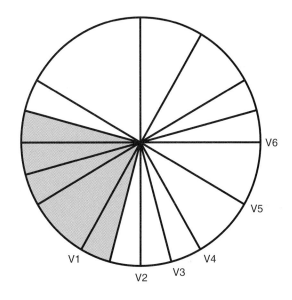

Leads I, V6

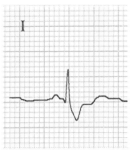

Lead VI

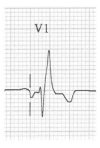

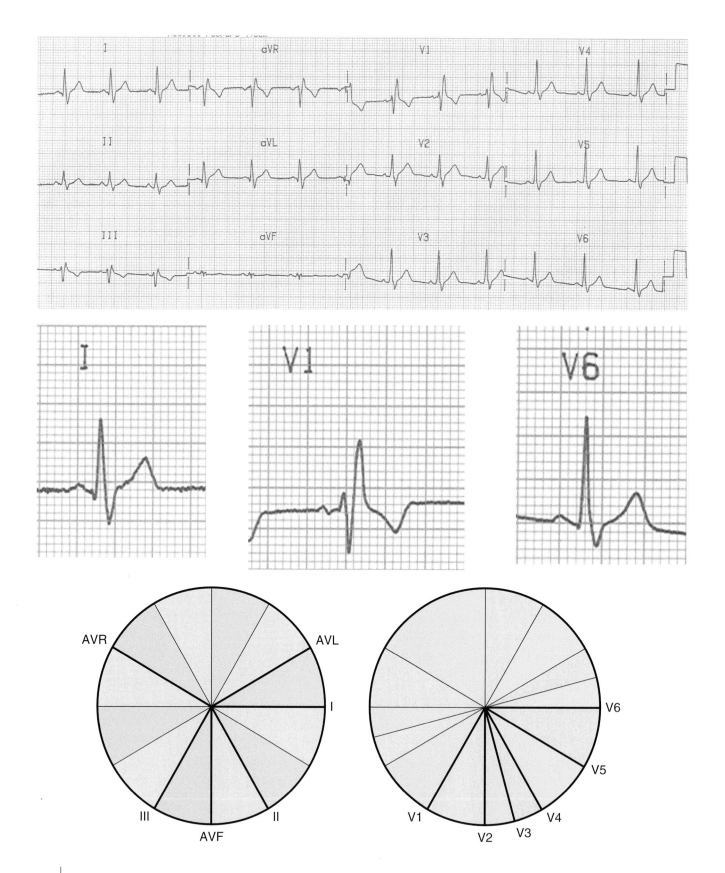

Heart Rate:

Rhythm:

ST Elevation (acute infarction):

II,III,AVF	inferior
I, AVL	lateral
V1, without V2	nonspecific septal
V1 and V2	septal
V3 and V4	anterior
V5 and V6	lateral
V6, without V5.	nonspecific lateral

Intervals (measured in the limb leads)

PR: short (< .12)
        normal (.12 to .20)
        long (>0.20 seconds); this is 1st degree AV
        block

QRS: normal (≤0.09 seconds)
        prolonged (.10 or .11); this is intraventricular
        conduction delay (IVCD)
        Bundle Branch Block (.12 seconds or greater)

QT:

ST Depression (ischemia or infarction):

I,II,III,AVL,AVF	diffuse subendocardial ischemia or infarction
V2,V3,V4,V5	diffuse subendocardial ischemia or infarction

P axis: normal
            rightward
            arm-lead reversal or dextrocardia
            junctional rhythm

QRS axis: normal
            left anterior hemiblock
            left posterior hemiblock
            indeterminate

Q waves (infarction):

II,III,AVF	inferior
I, AVL	lateral
V1, without V2	nonspecific septal
V1 and V2	septal
V3 and V4	anterior
V5 and V6	lateral
V6, without V5	nonspecific lateral

T wave inversion (ischemia or infarction):

II,III,AVF	inferior
I, AVL	lateral
V1, without V2	nonspecific septal
V1 and V2	septal
V3 and V4	anterior
V5 and V6	lateral
V6, without V5	nonspecific lateral

Hypertrophy:

Right atrial: Tall P wave 2.5 mm in II, III, or AVF

Left atrial: Deep negative part of P wave in V1

LVH: R wave in 1 + S wave in III ≥ 25mV
      S wave in V1 + R wave in V5 ≥ 35mV

RVH: Mean QRS either anterior, or rightward

The heart rate is 79 beats per minute. The PR interval measures 0.12 seconds in lead I, and is normal. The QRS interval measures 0.12 seconds in lead I, and indicates bundle branch block (BBB). To determine which bundle is blocked, the last part of the QRS (the last little box or 0.04 seconds) is examined. In the frontal plane, the last part of the QRS (the terminal force of the QRS) is negative in leads I, II, and AVL. It is positive in III, AVR, and AVF. This combination gives an *axis for the last part of the QRS,* of −180°. **This terminal part of the QRS then points rightward, toward the right ventricle. It must be the right bundle that is blocked.** In the horizontal plane, the last part of the QRS (the terminal force of the QRS) is positive in lead V1 but negative in leads V2, V3, V4, V5, and V6. This combination is *an axis for the last part of the QRS* of −165° and points rightward toward the right ventricle. Again it is the right bundle that is blocked. The QT interval is 0.36 seconds. The P axis is normal. The mean QRS axis is positive in I (area under the curve for the Q wave) and the S wave is less than the area under the R wave. The mean QRS is isoelectric in AVF. The mean QRS axis is 0 in the frontal plane. This is normal. The frontal plane ST-T axis is positive in I but isoelectric in lead AVF. This provides an ST-T axis of 0°, which points opposite the terminal QRS axis, as expected. The horizontal plane ST-T axis is negative in lead V1 and positive in leads V2 through V6. This indicates an ST-T axis in the horizontal plane of +15°. This points opposite the terminal QRS and is expected.

Parts of the answer sheets are "grayed out" because these sections have not yet been covered. Answer only the parts that are not highlighted.

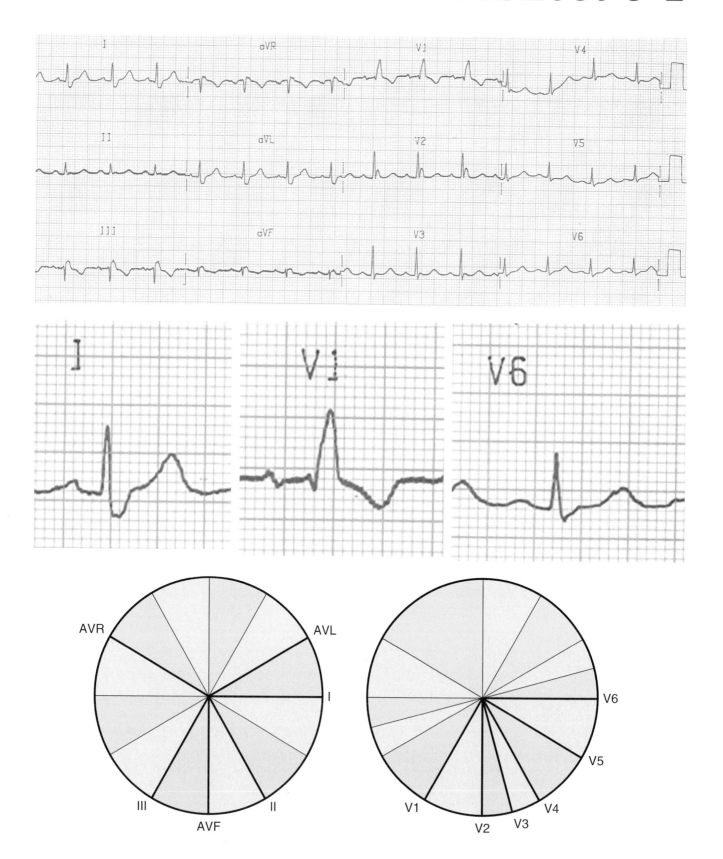

Heart Rate:

Rhythm:

Intervals (measured in the limb leads)

PR: short (< .12)
        normal (.12 to .20)
        long (>0.20 seconds); this is 1st degree AV block

QRS: normal (≤0.09 seconds)
        prolonged (.10 or .11); this is intraventricular conduction delay (IVCD)
        Bundle Branch Block (.12 seconds or greater)

QT:

P axis: normal
                rightward
                arm-lead reversal or dextrocardia
                junctional rhythm

QRS axis: normal
                left anterior hemiblock
                left posterior hemiblock
                indeterminate

T wave inversion (ischemia or infarction):

II,III,AVF	inferior
I, AVL	lateral
V1, without V2	nonspecific septal
V1 and V2	septal
V3 and V4	anterior
V5 and V6	lateral
V6, without V5	nonspecific lateral

ST Elevation (acute infarction):

II,III,AVF	inferior
I, AVL	lateral
V1, without V2	nonspecific septal
V1 and V2	septal
V3 and V4	anterior
V5 and V6	lateral
V6, without V5.	nonspecific lateral

ST Depression (ischemia or infarction):

I,II,III,AVL,AVF	diffuse subendocardial ischemia or infarction
V2,V3,V4,V5	diffuse subendocardial ischemia or infarction

Q waves (infarction):

II,III,AVF	inferior
I, AVL	lateral
V1, without V2	nonspecific septal
V1 and V2	septal
V3 and V4	anterior
V5 and V6	lateral
V6, without V5	nonspecific lateral

Hypertrophy:

Right atrial: Tall P wave 2.5 mm in II, III, or AVF

Left atrial: Deep negative part of P wave in V1

LVH: R wave in 1 + S wave in III ≥ 25mV
      S wave in V1 + R wave in V5 ≥ 35mV

RVH: Mean QRS either anterior, or rightward

The heart rate is 88 beats per minute. The PR interval is 0.2 seconds in lead I, which is normal. The QRS interval is 0.12 seconds, indicating bundle branch block. Because there is bundle branch block, the last part of the QRS must be examined to determine which bundle is blocked. In the frontal plane, the terminal QRS forces are negative in I and AVL. They are positive in III, AVR, and AVF. They are isoelectric in lead II, which is why lead II appears to be only 0.08 seconds wide. The last part of the QRS in II is almost level with the baseline. (You can draw a vertical line from the end of the QRS in lead I to the end of the QRS in lead III. This will help you see the true end of the QRS in lead II.) This combination indicates an axis for the terminal part of the QRS of +150°. This is rightward, towards the right ventricle, and indicates RBBB. The QT interval measures 0.36 in lead III. The P axis (+45) is normal. The mean frontal plane QRS (remember, this measures the axis of the entire QRS complex) is negative in leads I and AVL. It is positive in leads II, III, and AVF. It is probably isoelectric in lead AVR. This combination gives a mean QRS axis of +120° and indicates that left posterior hemiblock is present. The ST-T axis is positive in I, II, and AVL. It is negative in II, AVR, and AVF. This provides an ST-T axis of −15°, which is expected for RBBB.

Parts of the answer sheets are "grayed out" because these sections have not yet been covered. Answer only the parts that are not highlighted.

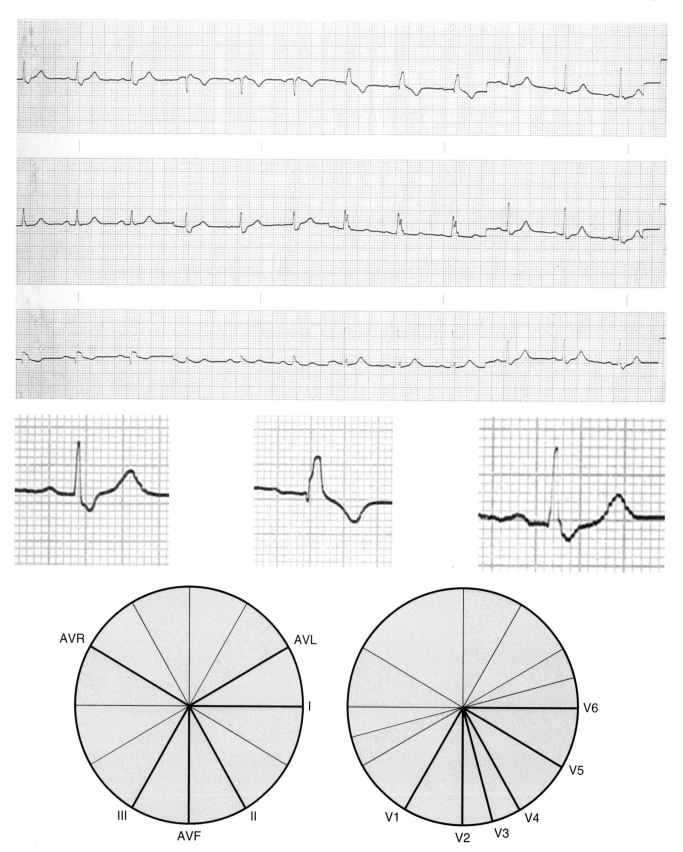

Heart Rate:

Rhythm:

ST Elevation (acute infarction):

II,III,AVF	inferior
I, AVL	lateral
V1, without V2	nonspecific septal
V1 and V2	septal
V3 and V4	anterior
V5 and V6	lateral
V6, without V5.	nonspecific lateral

Intervals (measured in the limb leads)

PR: short (< .12)
normal (.12 to .20)
long (>0.20 seconds); this is 1st degree AV block

QRS: normal (≤0.09 seconds)
prolonged (.10 or .11); this is intraventricular conduction delay (IVCD)
Bundle Branch Block (.12 seconds or greater)

QT:

ST Depression (ischemia or infarction):

I,II,III,AVL,AVF	diffuse subendocardial ischemia or infarction
V2,V3,V4,V5	diffuse subendocardial ischemia or infarction

P axis: normal
rightward
arm-lead reversal or dextrocardia
junctional rhythm

QRS axis: normal
left anterior hemiblock
left posterior hemiblock
indeterminate

Q waves (infarction):

II,III,AVF	inferior
I, AVL	lateral
V1, without V2	nonspecific septal
V1 and V2	septal
V3 and V4	anterior
V5 and V6	lateral
V6, without V5	nonspecific lateral

T wave inversion (ischemia or infarction):

II,III,AVF	inferior
I, AVL	lateral
V1, without V2	nonspecific septal
V1 and V2	septal
V3 and V4	anterior
V5 and V6	lateral
V6, without V5	nonspecific lateral

Hypertrophy:

Right atrial: Tall P wave 2.5 mm in II, III, or AVF

Left atrial: Deep negative part of P wave in V1

LVH: R wave in 1 + S wave in III ≥ 25mV
S wave in V1 + R wave in V5 ≥ 35mV

RVH: Mean QRS either anterior, or rightward

The heart rate is 68 beats per minute. The rhythm is sinus. The PR interval is 0.20 seconds. The QRS interval measures 0.12 seconds and indicates BBB. To determine which bundle branch is blocked, the last part of the QRS must be analyzed. In the frontal plane, the last part of the QRS is negative in I and AVL. It is positive in III, AVR, and AVF. The last part of the QRS is isoelectric in lead II. This combination of forces provides a terminal QRS axis of +150°, which is rightward and indicates RBBB. In the horizontal plane, the terminal part of the QRS complex is positive in leads V1, V2, and V3. It is isoelectric in lead V4 and negative in leads V5 and V6. This combination provides a terminal QRS axis that points to +150°, which is anterior and rightward, toward the right ventricle. This indicates RBBB. The QT interval is 0.40 seconds. The ST-T axis in the frontal plane is positive in leads I, II, AVL, and AVF but negative in leads III and AVR. This indicates a frontal plane ST-T axis of +15°. This points opposite the terminal QRS axis and is as expected.

Parts of the answer sheets are "grayed out" because these sections have not yet been covered. Answer only the parts that are not highlighted.

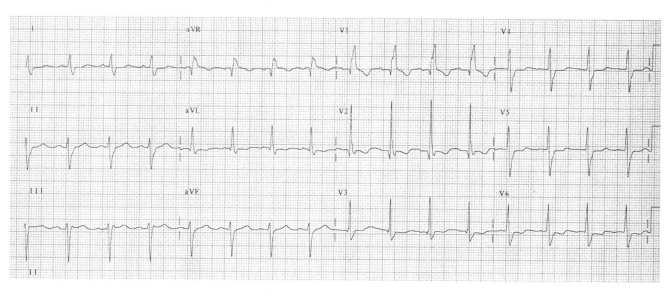

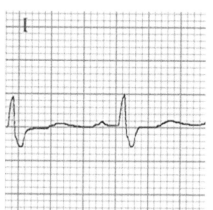

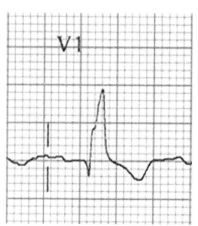

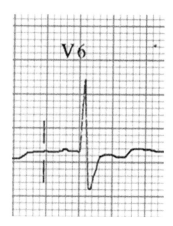

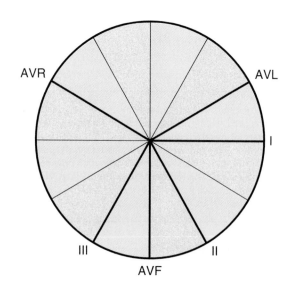

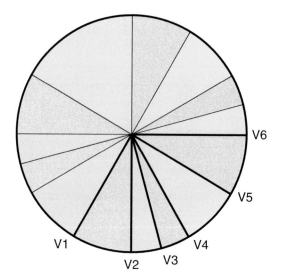

Heart Rate:

Rhythm:

Intervals (measured in the limb leads)

PR: short (< .12)
normal (.12 to .20)
long (>0.20 seconds); this is 1st degree AV block

QRS: normal (≤0.09 seconds)
prolonged (.10 or .11); this is intraventricular conduction delay (IVCD)
Bundle Branch Block (.12 seconds or greater)

QT:

P axis: normal
rightward
arm-lead reversal or dextrocardia
junctional rhythm

QRS axis: normal
left anterior hemiblock
left posterior hemiblock
indeterminate

T wave inversion (ischemia or infarction):

II,III,AVF	inferior
I, AVL	lateral
V1, without V2	nonspecific septal
V1 and V2	septal
V3 and V4	anterior
V5 and V6	lateral
V6, without V5	nonspecific lateral

ST Elevation (acute infarction):

II,III,AVF	inferior
I, AVL	lateral
V1, without V2	nonspecific septal
V1 and V2	septal
V3 and V4	anterior
V5 and V6	lateral
V6, without V5.	nonspecific lateral

ST Depression (ischemia or infarction):

I,II,III,AVL,AVF	diffuse subendocardial ischemia or infarction
V2,V3,V4,V5	diffuse subendocardial ischemia or infarction

Q waves (infarction):

II,III,AVF	inferior
I, AVL	lateral
V1, without V2	nonspecific septal
V1 and V2	septal
V3 and V4	anterior
V5 and V6	lateral
V6, without V5	nonspecific lateral

Hypertrophy:

Right atrial: Tall P wave 2.5 mm in II, III, or AVF

Left atrial: Deep negative part of P wave in V1

LVH: R wave in 1 + S wave in III ≥ 25mV
        S wave in V1 + R wave in V5 ≥ 35mV

RVH: Mean QRS either anterior, or rightward

The heart rate is 93 beats per minute. The PR interval measures 0.18 seconds. The QRS interval measures 0.12 seconds and indicates BBB. To determine which bundle is blocked, analyze the last part of the QRS complex. In the frontal plane, the last part of the QRS is negative in leads I, II, AVL, and AVF. It is positive in leads III and AVR. This combination yields a terminal QRS axis of −165°, which is rightward and indicates RBBB. In the horizontal plane, the terminal part of the QRS is positive in V1 and negative in V2 through V6. This yields an axis (for the last part of the QRS) of −165°. This is rightward, and indicates RBBB. The QT interval measures 0.36 seconds. The P axis is 45°, which is normal. The mean QRS axis in the frontal plane is negative in II, III, and AVF but positive in AVR and AVL. It is isoelectric in lead I. This gives a mean QRS axis in the frontal plane of −90°, which indicates that left anterior hemiblock is present as well. The frontal plane ST-T axis is positive in I, II, III, and AVF. It is negative in AVR and isoelectric in lead AVL. This gives an ST-T axis of +75°. This is not opposite the terminal QRS and is unexpected in RBBB. In the horizontal plane, the ST-T axis is negative in leads V1 through V6, giving an ST-T axis of −120°, which is not opposite the terminal QRS axis. This is unexpected in RBBB as well. Abnormal ST and T axes will be discussed later in Chapters 11 and 12.

Parts of the answer sheets are "grayed out" because these sections have not yet been covered. Answer only the parts that are not highlighted.

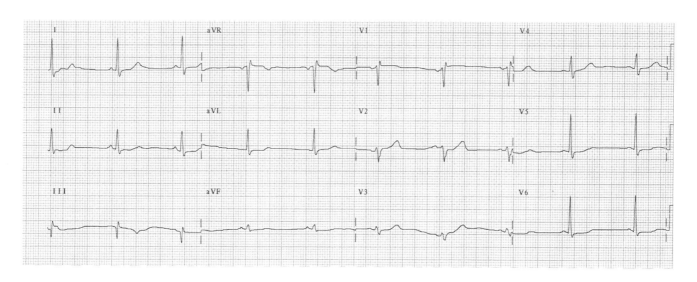

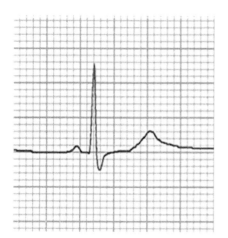
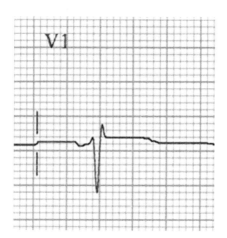
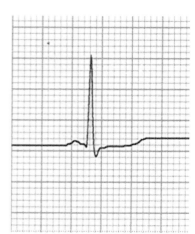

V1

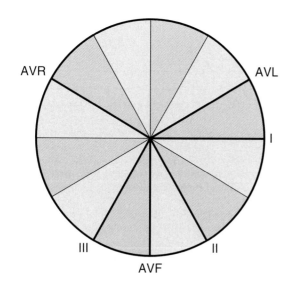
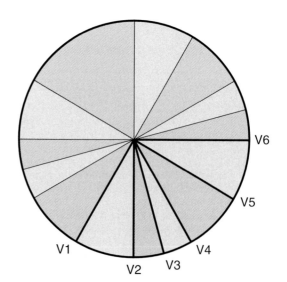

Heart Rate:

Rhythm:

ST Elevation (acute infarction):

II,III,AVF	inferior
I, AVL	lateral
V1, without V2	nonspecific septal
V1 and V2	septal
V3 and V4	anterior
V5 and V6	lateral
V6, without V5.	nonspecific lateral

Intervals (measured in the limb leads)

PR: short (< .12)
      normal (.12 to .20)
      long (>0.20 seconds); this is 1st degree AV
      block

QRS: normal (≤0.09 seconds)
      prolonged (.10 or .11); this is intraventricular
      conduction delay (IVCD)
      Bundle Branch Block (.12 seconds or greater)

QT:

ST Depression (ischemia or infarction):

I,II,III,AVL,AVF	diffuse subendocardial ischemia or infarction
V2,V3,V4,V5	diffuse subendocardial ischemia or infarction

P axis: normal
            rightward
            arm-lead reversal or dextrocardia
            junctional rhythm

QRS axis: normal
            left anterior hemiblock
            left posterior hemiblock
            indeterminate

Q waves (infarction):

II,III,AVF	inferior
I, AVL	lateral
V1, without V2	nonspecific septal
V1 and V2	septal
V3 and V4	anterior
V5 and V6	lateral
V6, without V5	nonspecific lateral

T wave inversion (ischemia or infarction):

II,III,AVF	inferior
I, AVL	lateral
V1, without V2	nonspecific septal
V1 and V2	septal
V3 and V4	anterior
V5 and V6	lateral
V6, without V5	nonspecific lateral

Hypertrophy:

Right atrial: Tall P wave 2.5 mm in II, III, or AVF

Left atrial: Deep negative part of P wave in V1

LVH: R wave in 1 + S wave in III ≥ 25mV
      S wave in V1 + R wave in V5 ≥ 35mV

RVH: Mean QRS either anterior, or rightward

The heart rate is 56 beats per minute. The rhythm is sinus bradycardia. (Causes of sinus bradycardia should be considered, eg, beta blocker therapy.) The PR interval is 0.12 seconds. The QRS interval measures 0.11 seconds in leads II and AVR. This is abnormal and indicates intraventricular conduction delay (IVCD). To determine which bundle is causing the delay, we examine the last part of the QRS complex as though this was BBB. In the frontal plane, the last part of the QRS complex is negative in leads I, II, and AVL. It is positive in leads III and AVR but isoelectric in AVF. This combination gives a terminal QRS axis of +180°. This is rightward and is termed right intraventricular conduction delay (RIVCD). In the past, this was called incomplete right bundle branch block (so much for progress). In the horizontal plane, the last part of the QRS axis is positive in V1 and negative in leads V2 through V6. This combination gives a terminal QRS axis of −165°, which is rightward and also indicates RIVCD. The QT interval is 0.46 seconds. The mean QRS axis in the frontal plane is +15°. The frontal plane ST-T axis is 0°, which is opposite the terminal QRS axis, as expected. The horizontal plane ST-T axis is +135°. This is not opposite the terminal QRS axis and is not expected. The T and ST axes will be discussed in Chapters 10 and 11.

Parts of the answer sheets are "grayed out" because these sections have not yet been covered. Answer only the parts that are not highlighted.

Left Bundle Branch Block

Diseases can impair or destroy the ability of the left bundle to conduct impulses and depolarize the left ventricle. Left intraventricular conduction delay (LIVCD) slows the QRS interval to 0.10 to 0.11 seconds. Left bundle branch block (LBBB) is a more severe form of conduction loss and slows the QRS interval to 0.12 seconds or longer. **A QRS interval of 0.12 seconds or longer defines the presence of bundle branch block.**

Any loss of conduction in either of the bundles slows the process of ventricular depolarization and increases the normal QRS interval of 0.08 to 0.09 seconds.

Disease of the left bundle branch that causes an increase in the **QRS to 0.10 or 0.11 seconds indicates LIVCD.**

Disease of the left bundle branch that causes an increase in the **QRS to 0.12 seconds or more indicates LBBB.**

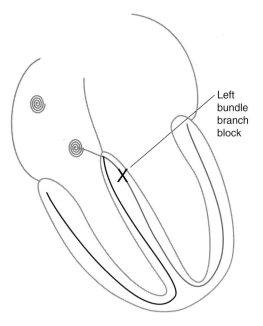

Left bundle branch block

Left Bundle Branch Block: Initial Forces

In Chapter 9 we learned that normal ventricular activation begins with depolarization of the ventricular septum by the left bundle in a direction from left to right. However, if the left bundle is not working, it is unable to depolarize the septum. (From the onset in LBBB, every part of the QRS is formed in an abnormal fashion. In RBBB, the beginning of the QRS is formed normally.)

In LBBB, the ventricular septum is depolarized by the right bundle branch.

This causes the initial force to move leftward.

In the frontal plane, this change in the direction of the force removes the tiny q wave normally seen in lead I and replaces it with a positive deflection.

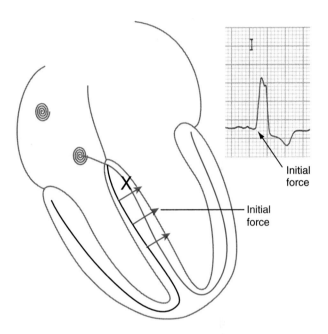

Initial force

Initial force

In the horizontal plane, this change of direction removes the tiny q wave normally seen in V6 and replaces it with a positive deflection.

Also, the first 0.04 seconds (1 little box) of the QRS is negative in lead V1.

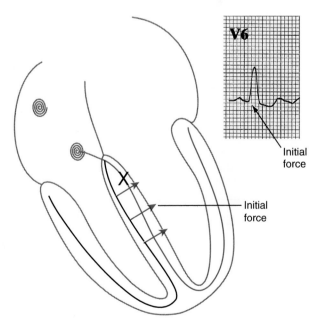

Initial force

Initial force

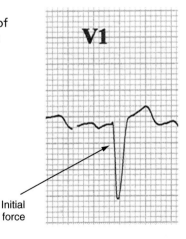

V1

Initial force

Left Bundle Branch Block: Middle Forces

The next event to occur in ventricular depolarization should be activation of the left and right ventricles simultaneously by the right and left bundles. The left bundle is blocked and is unable to depolarize the left ventricle. Because the right bundle is not blocked, it can depolarize the RV normally. **In the frontal plane, this middle part of the QRS represents RV depolarization, which produces a force that points rightward, toward the right ventricle.**

The main force represents the "normally scheduled" right ventricular depolarization.

It produces a force that points rightward, toward the right ventricle. In the frontal plane this produces a downward deflection in the middle of the QRS and is difficult to see.

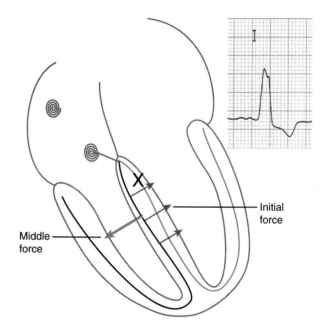

In the horizontal plane, this middle part of the QRS also represents right ventricle depolarization. The middle force points rightward and anterior, toward the right ventricle.

This produces a small downward deflection in V6 (seen here as a notch in the r wave) and an upward deflection (which is typically barely seen) in the middle of the QRS in V1.

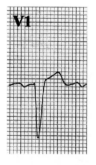

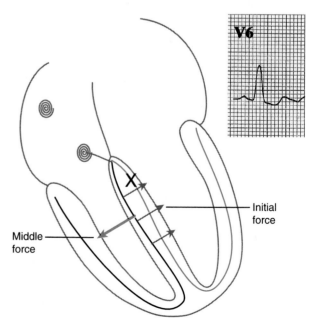

LBBB: Last, Late, or Terminal Forces

Finally, during the last 0.04 seconds of the QRS, the electrical activation spreads from the right bundle branch and depolarizes the left ventricle. In the frontal plane, the late (or terminal) force points leftward toward the left ventricle.

In the frontal plane the late (or terminal) force points leftward toward the left ventricle.

The hallmark of LBBB is that the QRS is delayed to 0.12 seconds and the last part of the QRS points to the left ventricle.

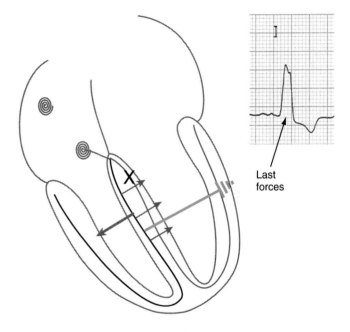

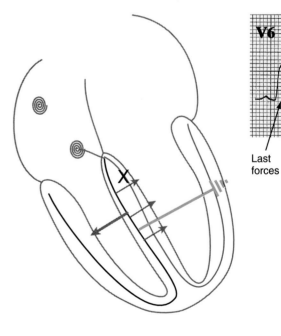

Last forces

Finally, during the last 0.04 seconds of the QRS, the electrical activation spreads to and depolarizes the left ventricle.

In the horizontal plane, the last part of the QRS points leftward and posterior toward the left ventricle.

Last forces

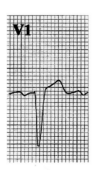

Summary of LBBB: Frontal Plane Concept

LBBB occurs when there is a dysfunction of the left bundle branch that interferes with normal impulse conduction and left ventricular depolarization. This is indicated by a prolonged QRS complex of at least 0.12 seconds. Careful evaluation of the terminal forces of the QRS indicates which bundle branch is blocked. Because the terminal (last 0.04 seconds of the QRS) force points posterior and to the left it must be the left bundle branch that is blocked. In the frontal plane, LBBB produces a terminal R wave in lead I.

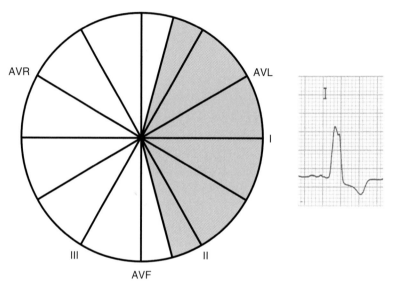

Concept: LBBB causes a wide 0.12-second QRS. The last part of the QRS points to the left ventricle, which is leftward.

Axis: The late or terminal QRS axis in the frontal plane is < +90° and > −90°.

Pattern: The QRS is 0.12 seconds
and
The last part of the QRS in lead I is an R wave.

SUMMARY OF LBBB: HORIZONTAL PLANE CONCEPT

Diseases that affect the left bundle prevent normal impulse conduction and left ventricular depolarization. A QRS interval that is delayed to at least 0.12 seconds indicates bundle branch block. Careful evaluation of the terminal forces of the QRS determines the location of the block. When the terminal (last 0.04 seconds of the QRS) force points posterior and to the left (ie, the left ventricle) it must be the left bundle branch that is blocked. In the horizontal plane in LBBB, the last part of the QRS is positive in lead V6 and negative in lead V1.

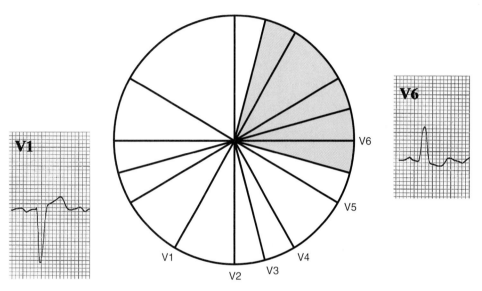

Concept: LBBB causes a wide 0.12-second QRS. The last part of the QRS points to the left ventricle, which is posterior and leftward.

Axis: The late or terminal QRS axis in the frontal plane is > −90° and < +30°.

Pattern: The QRS is 0.12 seconds,
and
The QRS complex ends in an S wave in lead V1, and an R' wave in V6.

SUMMARY OF LBBB: LAST PART OF THE QRS PATTERN

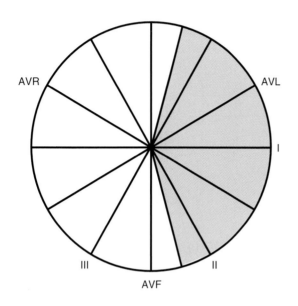

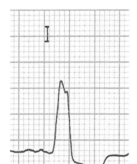

Leads I, V6

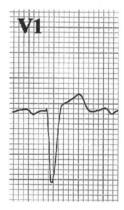

Lead V1

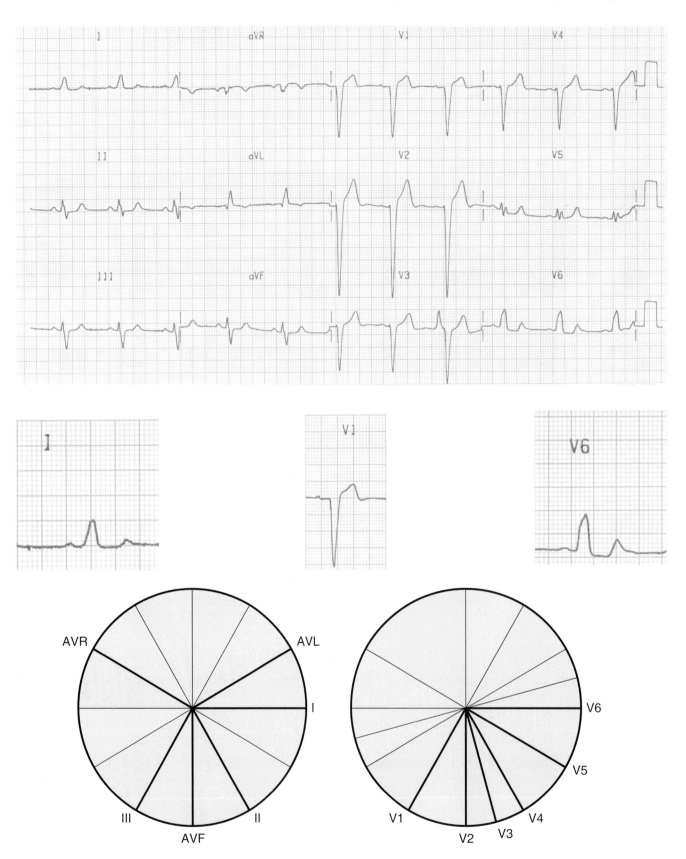

Heart Rate:

Rhythm:

Intervals (measured in the limb leads)

PR: short (< .12)
      normal (.12 to .20)
      long (>0.20 seconds); this is 1st degree AV
      block

QRS: normal (≤0.09 seconds)
      prolonged (.10 or .11); this is intraventricular
      conduction delay (IVCD)
      Bundle Branch Block (.12 seconds or greater)

QT:

P axis: normal
           rightward
           arm-lead reversal or dextrocardia
           junctional rhythm

QRS axis: normal
           left anterior hemiblock
           left posterior hemiblock
           indeterminate

T wave inversion (ischemia or infarction):

II,III,AVF	inferior
I, AVL	lateral
V1, without V2	nonspecific septal
V1 and V2	septal
V3 and V4	anterior
V5 and V6	lateral
V6, without V5	nonspecific lateral

ST Elevation (acute infarction):

II,III,AVF	inferior
I, AVL	lateral
V1, without V2	nonspecific septal
V1 and V2	septal
V3 and V4	anterior
V5 and V6	lateral
V6, without V5.	nonspecific lateral

ST Depression (ischemia or infarction):

I,II,III,AVL,AVF	diffuse subendocardial ischemia or infarction
V2,V3,V4,V5	diffuse subendocardial ischemia or infarction

Q waves (infarction):

II,III,AVF	inferior
I, AVL	lateral
V1, without V2	nonspecific septal
V1 and V2	septal
V3 and V4	anterior
V5 and V6	lateral
V6, without V5	nonspecific lateral

Hypertrophy:

Right atrial: Tall P wave 2.5 mm in II, III, or AVF

Left atrial: Deep negative part of P wave in V1

LVH: R wave in 1 + S wave in III ≥ 25mV
      S wave in V1 + R wave in V5 ≥ 35mV

RVH: Mean QRS either anterior, or rightward

The heart rate is 65 beats per minute. The rhythm is sinus. The PR interval measures 0.12 seconds, which is normal. The QRS interval is 0.14 seconds, which is abnormally long and indicates bundle branch block. The QT interval measures 0.44 seconds, which is long. The P axis is +75° and is normal. The mean QRS axis is −15°. The axis of the last part of the QRS is −60° in the frontal plane, because the last part of the QRS is negative in II and AVF, positive in I and AVL, and isoelectric in AVR. This last part of the QRS points leftward (−60°). The axis of the last part of the QRS is −75° in the horizontal plane, therefore pointing both leftward and posterior. Because the QRS is wide (0.12 seconds) and the last part of the QRS points left and posterior, there is LBBB. LBBB removes the reliability of most criteria that involve the QRS, the ST segment, and the T wave. Thus in LBBB no further analysis should be done.

Parts of the answer sheets are "grayed out" because these sections have not yet been covered. Answer only the parts that are not highlighted.

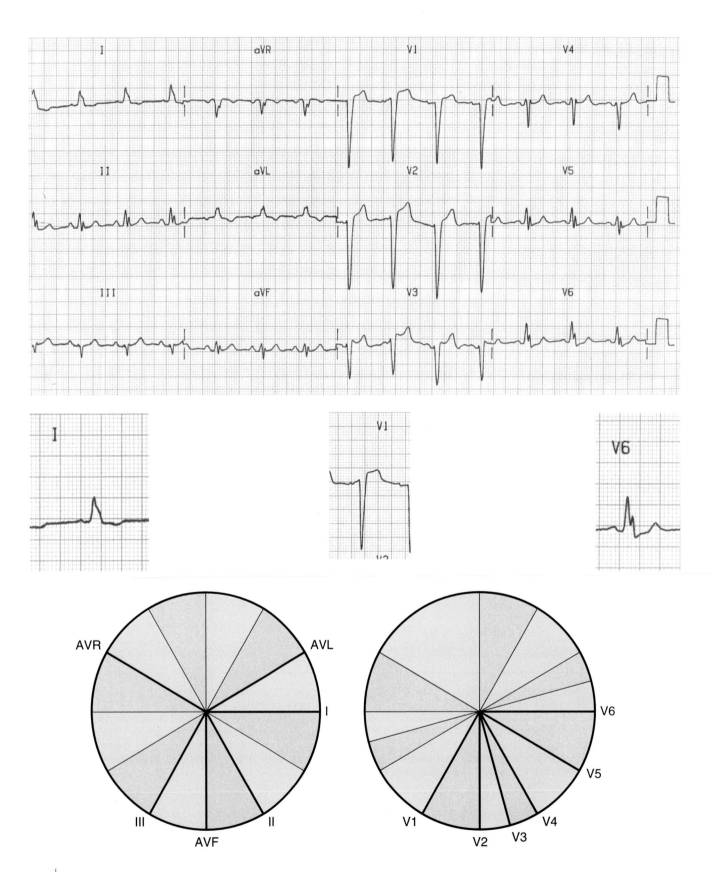

Heart Rate:

Rhythm:

Intervals (measured in the limb leads)

PR: short (< .12)
        normal (.12 to .20)
        long (>0.20 seconds); this is 1st degree AV
        block

QRS: normal (≤0.09 seconds)
        prolonged (.10 or .11); this is intraventricular
        conduction delay (IVCD)
        Bundle Branch Block (.12 seconds or greater)

QT:

P axis: normal
          rightward
          arm-lead reversal or dextrocardia
          junctional rhythm

QRS axis: normal
             left anterior hemiblock
             left posterior hemiblock
             indeterminate

T wave inversion (ischemia or infarction):

II,III,AVF	inferior
I, AVL	lateral
V1, without V2	nonspecific septal
V1 and V2	septal
V3 and V4	anterior
V5 and V6	lateral
V6, without V5	nonspecific lateral

ST Elevation (acute infarction):

II,III,AVF	inferior
I, AVL	lateral
V1, without V2	nonspecific septal
V1 and V2	septal
V3 and V4	anterior
V5 and V6	lateral
V6, without V5.	nonspecific lateral

ST Depression (ischemia or infarction):

I,II,III,AVL,AVF	diffuse subendocardial ischemia or infarction
V2,V3,V4,V5	diffuse subendocardial ischemia or infarction

Q waves (infarction):

II,III,AVF	inferior
I, AVL	lateral
V1, without V2	nonspecific septal
V1 and V2	septal
V3 and V4	anterior
V5 and V6	lateral
V6, without V5	nonspecific lateral

Hypertrophy:

Right atrial: Tall P wave 2.5 mm in II, III, or AVF

Left atrial: Deep negative part of P wave in V1

LVH: R wave in 1 + S wave in III ≥ 25mV
       S wave in V1 + R wave in V5 ≥ 35mV

RVH: Mean QRS either anterior, or rightward

The heart rate is 79 beats per minute. The PR interval is 0.16 seconds and is normal. The QRS interval is 0.12 seconds and indicates BBB. The last part of the QRS must be analyzed to determine which bundle branch is blocked. In the frontal plane, the last part of the QRS is positive in I, II, AVL, and AVF. The last part of the QRS is negative in leads III and AVR. This combination gives a terminal QRS axis of +15°. This is leftward and indicates LBBB. In the horizontal plane, the last part of the QRS is negative in leads V1, V2, and V3. It is positive in leads V4, V5, and V6. This combination gives a terminal QRS axis of −22.5°. This is leftward and posterior and indicates LBBB. The QT interval is 0.36 seconds. The P axis is +75° and is normal. The mean frontal plane QRS axis is +15°. There are no useful criteria for analysis of the frontal plane mean QRS axis in LBBB. Likewise, there are no useful criteria for analysis of the ST or T axis in LBBB.

Parts of the answer sheets are "grayed out" because these sections have not yet been covered. Answer only the parts that are not highlighted.

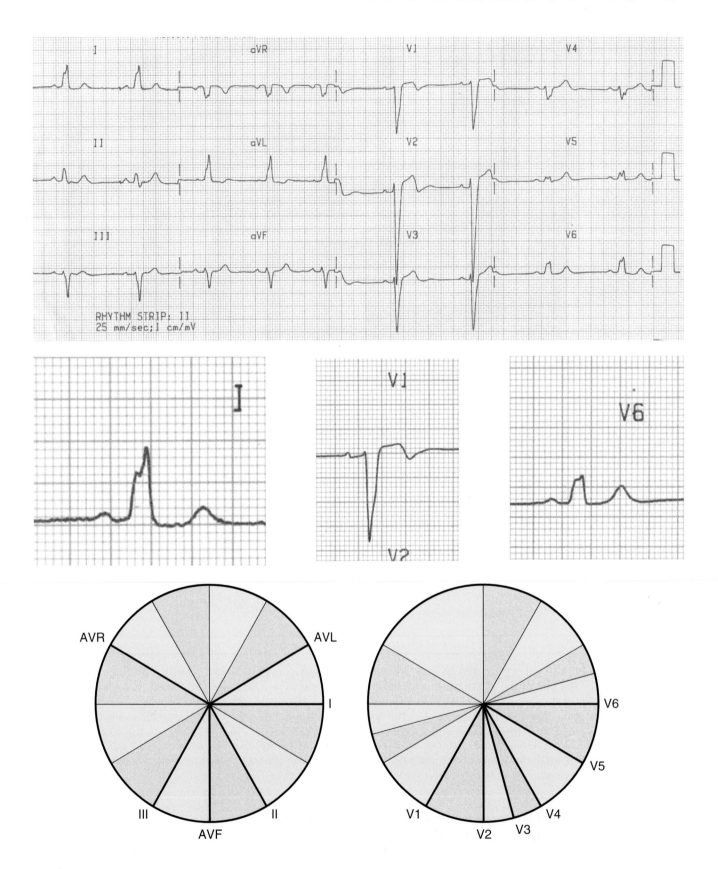

RHYTHM STRIP: II
25 mm/sec; 1 cm/mV

Heart Rate:

Rhythm:

Intervals (measured in the limb leads)

PR: short (< .12)
      normal (.12 to .20)
      long (>0.20 seconds); this is 1st degree AV
      block

QRS: normal (≤0.09 seconds)
      prolonged (.10 or .11); this is intraventricular
      conduction delay (IVCD)
      Bundle Branch Block (.12 seconds or greater)

QT:

P axis: normal
           rightward
           arm-lead reversal or dextrocardia
           junctional rhythm

QRS axis: normal
           left anterior hemiblock
           left posterior hemiblock
           indeterminate

T wave inversion (ischemia or infarction):

II,III,AVF	inferior
I, AVL	lateral
V1, without V2	nonspecific septal
V1 and V2	septal
V3 and V4	anterior
V5 and V6	lateral
V6, without V5	nonspecific lateral

ST Elevation (acute infarction):

II,III,AVF	inferior
I, AVL	lateral
V1, without V2	nonspecific septal
V1 and V2	septal
V3 and V4	anterior
V5 and V6	lateral
V6, without V5.	nonspecific lateral

ST Depression (ischemia or infarction):

I,II,III,AVL,AVF	diffuse subendocardial ischemia or infarction
V2,V3,V4,V5	diffuse subendocardial ischemia or infarction

Q waves (infarction):

II,III,AVF	inferior
I, AVL	lateral
V1, without V2	nonspecific septal
V1 and V2	septal
V3 and V4	anterior
V5 and V6	lateral
V6, without V5	nonspecific lateral

Hypertrophy:

Right atrial: Tall P wave 2.5 mm in II, III, or AVF

Left atrial: Deep negative part of P wave in V1

LVH: R wave in 1 + S wave in III ≥ 25mV
      S wave in V1 + R wave in V5 ≥ 35mV

RVH: Mean QRS either anterior, or rightward

The heart rate is 52 beats per minute. This is sinus bradycardia. Clinical correlation of sinus bradycardia should always be done. Is this patient on beta blockers? The PR interval is 0.16 seconds, which is normal. The QRS interval measures 0.14 seconds, which indicates BBB. Analysis of the terminal part of the QRS again identifies the kind of bundle branch block. To shorten the process, look at lead I. The last part of the QRS is positive, which means the last part of the QRS points leftward, toward the left ventricle. This indicates LBBB. In the horizontal plane, the last part of the QRS is negative in lead VI (posterior) and positive in lead V6 (rightward). This combination points toward the left ventricle and indicates LBBB. Once you have gone through the trouble to calculate the actual axis and understand the location of the terminal QRS force, you really don't need to calculate the axis for the terminal QRS. You can just look at leads I, VI, and V6, and based on these decide whether the last part of the QRS points to the left ventricle or right ventricle. Continuing with the EKG, the QT interval measures 0.44 seconds. The P axis is +60°, which is normal. The mean QRS axis is −15°, but there are no useful criteria for analyzing that. Interestingly, the ST-T axis doesn't point opposite the terminal QRS, as expected. There are no useful criteria for analyzing the ST-T segment in LBBB, so don't.

Parts of the answer sheets are "grayed out" because these sections have not yet been covered. Answer only the parts that are not highlighted.

Worksheet 10-4

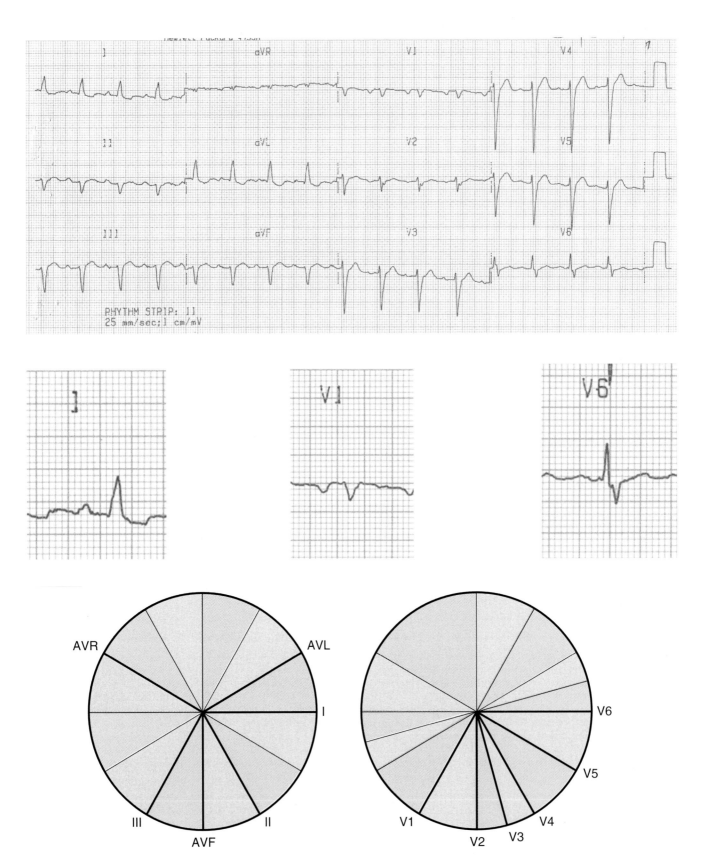

PHYTHM STRIP: II
25 mm/sec;1 cm/mV

Heart Rate:

Rhythm:

Intervals (measured in the limb leads)

PR: short (< .12)
normal (.12 to .20)
long (>0.20 seconds); this is 1st degree AV block

QRS: normal (≤0.09 seconds)
prolonged (.10 or .11); this is intraventricular conduction delay (IVCD)
Bundle Branch Block (.12 seconds or greater)

QT:

P axis: normal
rightward
arm-lead reversal or dextrocardia
junctional rhythm

QRS axis: normal
left anterior hemiblock
left posterior hemiblock
indeterminate

T wave inversion (ischemia or infarction):

II,III,AVF	inferior
I, AVL	lateral
V1, without V2	nonspecific septal
V1 and V2	septal
V3 and V4	anterior
V5 and V6	lateral
V6, without V5	nonspecific lateral

ST Elevation (acute infarction):

II,III,AVF	inferior
I, AVL	lateral
V1, without V2	nonspecific septal
V1 and V2	septal
V3 and V4	anterior
V5 and V6	lateral
V6, without V5.	nonspecific lateral

ST Depression (ischemia or infarction):

I,II,III,AVL,AVF	diffuse subendocardial ischemia or infarction
V2,V3,V4,V5	diffuse subendocardial ischemia or infarction

Q waves (infarction):

II,III,AVF	inferior
I, AVL	lateral
V1, without V2	nonspecific septal
V1 and V2	septal
V3 and V4	anterior
V5 and V6	lateral
V6, without V5	nonspecific lateral

Hypertrophy:

Right atrial: Tall P wave 2.5 mm in II, III, or AVF

Left atrial: Deep negative part of P wave in V1

LVH: R wave in 1 + S wave in III ≥ 25mV
S wave in V1 + R wave in V5 ≥ 35mV

RVH: Mean QRS either anterior, or rightward

The heart rate is 94 beats per minute. The PR interval measures 0.22 seconds. This is long and indicates first degree AV block (1° AV block.) The QRS interval measures 0.11 seconds and indicates intraventricular conduction delay (IVCD). In the frontal plane, the last part of the QRS is positive in lead I, and points leftward toward the left ventricle. This would indicate LIVCD. However, in the horizontal plane, the leads are not consistent with LIVCD. In the horizontal plane, the last part of the QRS is negative in V1 (posterior) but negative in lead V6 as well. Because the last part of the QRS is negative in V6, it is pointing rightward and would typically indicate RIVCD. When the information from the end of the QRS does not all agree with RIVCD or LIVCD, we call the conduction delay atypical. In this EKG, more leads suggest LIVCD than RIVCD. Proper terminology for this EKG would be IVCD (nonspecific) or atypical LIVCD. As in LBBB, LIVCD reduces the useful information obtained from analysis of the QRS, ST, and T axis. The QT interval is 0.32 seconds. The P axis is normal. The mean QRS axis is −60° and indicates left anterior hemiblock.

Parts of the answer sheets are "grayed out" because these sections have not yet been covered. Answer only the parts that are not highlighted.

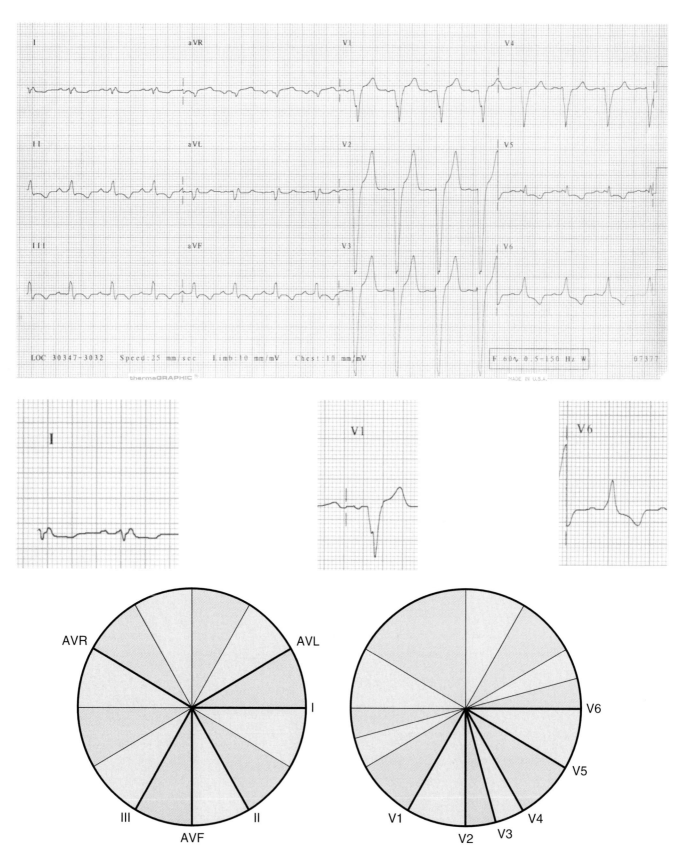

Heart Rate:

Rhythm:

Intervals (measured in the limb leads)

PR: short (< .12)
        normal (.12 to .20)
        long (>0.20 seconds); this is 1st degree AV
        block

QRS: normal (≤0.09 seconds)
        prolonged (.10 or .11); this is intraventricular
        conduction delay (IVCD)
        Bundle Branch Block (.12 seconds or greater)

QT:

P axis: normal
            rightward
            arm-lead reversal or dextrocardia
            junctional rhythm

QRS axis: normal
            left anterior hemiblock
            left posterior hemiblock
            indeterminate

T wave inversion (ischemia or infarction):

II,III,AVF	inferior
I, AVL	lateral
V1, without V2	nonspecific septal
V1 and V2	septal
V3 and V4	anterior
V5 and V6	lateral
V6, without V5	nonspecific lateral

ST Elevation (acute infarction):

II,III,AVF	inferior
I, AVL	lateral
V1, without V2	nonspecific septal
V1 and V2	septal
V3 and V4	anterior
V5 and V6	lateral
V6, without V5.	nonspecific lateral

ST Depression (ischemia or infarction):

I,II,III,AVL,AVF	diffuse subendocardial ischemia or infarction
V2,V3,V4,V5	diffuse subendocardial ischemia or infarction

Q waves (infarction):

II,III,AVF	inferior
I, AVL	lateral
V1, without V2	nonspecific septal
V1 and V2	septal
V3 and V4	anterior
V5 and V6	lateral
V6, without V5	nonspecific lateral

Hypertrophy:

Right atrial: Tall P wave 2.5 mm in II, III, or AVF

Left atrial: Deep negative part of P wave in V1

LVH: R wave in 1 + S wave in III ≥ 25mV
        S wave in V1 + R wave in V5 ≥ 35mV

RVH: Mean QRS either anterior, or rightward

The heart rate is 88 beats per minute in lead I. The PR interval measures 0.18 seconds. The QRS interval measures 0.16 seconds, indicating BBB. In the frontal plane, the last part of the QRS is positive, and therefore, the last part of the QRS points leftward toward the left ventricle. This indicates LBBB. In the horizontal plane, the last part of the QRS is negative in V1 and positive in lead V6. This indicates that the last part of the QRS points leftward and posterior, toward the left ventricle, consistent with LBBB. The QT interval measures 0.36 seconds, which is long. The P axis is +45° and is normal. The mean QRS axis is +90° and is not analyzed in the presence of LBBB. The ST-T axis points rightward (negative in lead I) and anterior (positive in lead VI), which is opposite the last part of the QRS. The ST-T axis is not analyzed further in the presence of LBBB.

Parts of the answer sheets are "grayed out" because these sections have not yet been covered. Answer only the parts that are not highlighted.

The T Axis

The T wave is normally the last deflection in the cardiac cycle and represents electrical activity produced during the rapid ventricular repolarization. The repolarization process allows the depolarized cardiac cells to reset for the next cardiac cycle. The myocardial cells repolarize in the same order as they depolarize. The T axis then normally points toward the left ventricle. much as the QRS does. Ischemia is the most important cause of an altered T wave, and it causes the T wave to point away from the region of ischemia.

The T axis describes the magnitude and direction of the force created during ventricular repolarization.

The T wave axis should point toward all normal areas of myocardium and away from areas of subendocardial ischemia.

Calculating the T wave axis enables a reader to identify the presence or absence of subendocardial ischemia or infarction.

The normal range for the T axis in the frontal plane is between 0° and +60°.

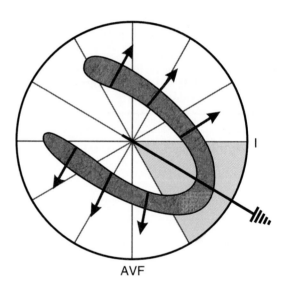

Anatomy of Subendocardial Ischemia

The heart receives oxygen-rich blood via three main arteries commonly called coronary arteries. These arteries are often referred to as epicardial arteries. They lie on the top layer of the heart or the epicardium. When these coronary arteries become diseased with plaque buildup, the heart is deprived of oxygen and nutrients.

Epicardial arteries can become clogged on a chronic basis due to deposition and infiltration by lipid-laden cells.

As the cross-sectional area of the epicardial artery decreases, the supply of blood also decreases.

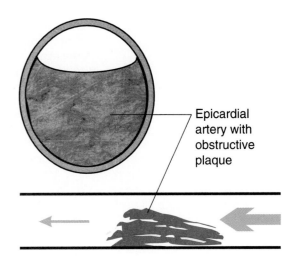

Epicardial artery with obstructive plaque

Anatomy of Subendocardial Ischemia

The part of the myocardium most distant from the arteries is the subendocardial region. The subendocardium is the "last stop" for the arterial supply of oxygen to the heart. This makes the subendocardial region the most sensitive to ischemic conditions, such as increased demand or decreased supply.

Although the subendocardium is the most poorly perfused layer of the heart, its demand for oxygen is high, typically making it the first to become ischemic.

Any increase in demand or decrease in supply of blood at the level of the subendocardium can produce ischemia.

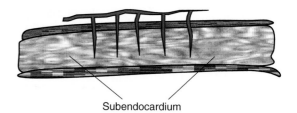

Subendocardium

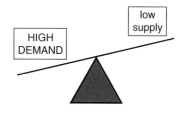

Ischemia

Ischemia occurs when there is an imbalance between the supply of oxygen to the myocardium and the demand for oxygen by the myocardial mitochondria. Any increase in demand or decrease in supply may cause ischemia, which, if it continues, can lead to tissue infarction.

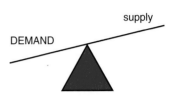

Oxygen demand is increased by:

1. Tachycardia
2. Increased blood pressure
3. Increased heart size (harder to squeeze a basketball than a grape)

Oxygen supply is decreased by:

1. Low hemoglobin
2. Low pO_2
3. Fixed atherosclerotic narrowing
4. A growing atherosclerotic obstruction
5. Coronary artery spasm

Oxygen demand is decreased by:

1. Decreasing a high heart rate
2. Decreasing a high blood pressure
3. Decreasing a dilated heart size

Oxygen supply is increased by:

1. Increasing a low hemoglobin
2. Increasing a low pO^2
3. Reducing thrombotic narrowing
4. Dilating or bypassing a fixed lesion
5. Decreasing coronary artery spasm, if present

The Normal T Wave

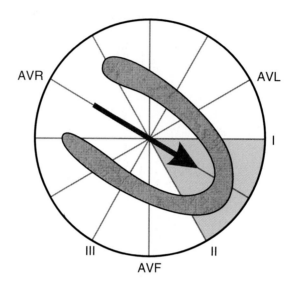

Concept: On the normal EKG, the T axis points toward all the normal areas of myocardium.

Axis: This provides a T axis of 0° to + 60°.

Pattern: The T waves are upright in leads I, II, and AVF. The T wave can be isoelectric in AVF or AVL but not negative.

Inferior Wall Ischemia

The T wave points away from an area of subendocardial ischemia. By localizing the area that the T axis points away from, the reader can determine the area of subendocardial ischemia. In subendocardial ischemia of the inferior wall, the T axis points away from the inferior wall.

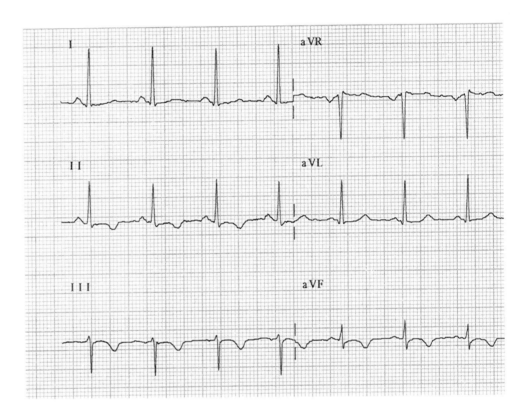

Frontal plane T axis = −75°.

Concept: The T axis points away from the inferior wall, indicating subendocardial ischemia of the inferior wall.

Axis: In inferior wall ischemia, the T axis points from −45° to −90° in the frontal plane.

Pattern: The T axis points away from leads, II, III, and AVF, giving an inverted T wave in these leads.

Lateral Wall Ischemia

The T wave points away from an area of subendocardial ischemia. By localizing the area that the T axis points away from, the reader can determine the area of subendocardial ischemia. In subendocardial ischemia of the lateral wall, the T axis points away from the lateral wall.

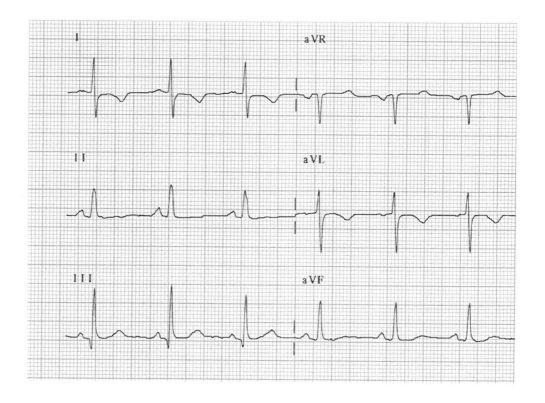

Frontal plane T axis = +150°.

Concept: The T axis points away from the lateral wall, indicating subendocardial ischemia of the lateral wall.

Axis: In ischemia of the lateral wall, the T axis points from +105° to +180° in the frontal plane.

Pattern: The T axis points away from leads I and AVL, giving an inverted T wave in these leads.

Apical Wall Ischemia

The T wave points away from an area of subendocardial ischemia. By localizing the area that the T axis points away from, the reader can determine the area of subendocardial ischemia. In subendocardial ischemia of the apical wall, the T axis points away from the apex.

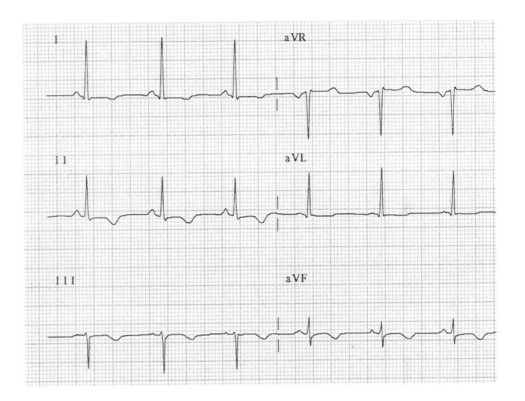

Frontal plane T axis = −135°.

Concept: The T axis points away from the apex, indicating subendocardial ischemia of the apical wall.

Axis: In apical wall ischemia, the T axis points from −105° to −165° in the frontal plane.

Pattern: The T axis points away from leads I, II, and AVF (and may point away from AVL and/or III as well), giving an inverted T wave in these leads.

Septal and Anterior Wall Ischemia

The T wave points away from an area of subendocardial ischemia. In subendocardial ischemia of the anterior wall, the T axis points away from the anterior wall.

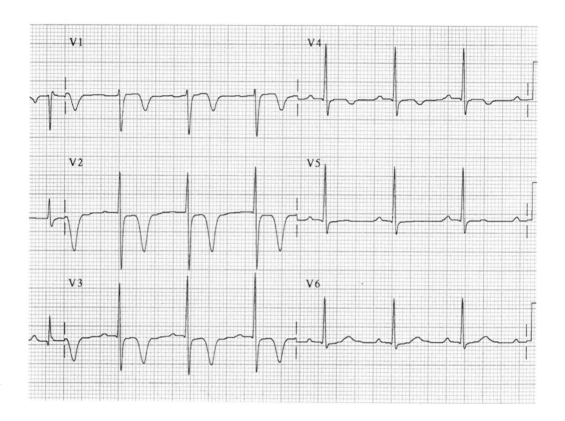

Horizontal plane T axis = −60°.

Concept: The T axis points away from the septum and anterior walls, indicating subendocardial ischemia of the septal and anterior walls.

Axis: In septal and anterior wall ischemia, the T axis points from −22.5° to −60° in the horizontal plane.

Pattern: The T axis points away from leads V1, V2, and V3 (and may point away from V4 as well), giving an inverted T wave in these leads.

SUMMARY OF FRONTAL PLANE T AXIS

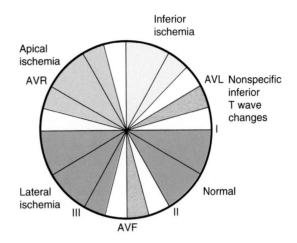

Location of Subendocardial Ischemia	Concept to Understand	T Axis to Translate the Concept (Don't Memorize This)	Inverted T Wave Pattern (memorize)
Inferior	T axis points away from the inferior wall	−45 to −90	II, III, AVF
Lateral	T axis points away from lateral wall	+105 to +180	I, AVL
Apical	T axis points away from apex	−105 to −165	I, II, AVF
Nonspecific inferior T wave changes	T axis borderline superior	−15 to −30	III, AVF, but not II
Nonspecific lateral T wave changes	T axis borderline rightward	+75 to +90	L, but not I
Normal T axis	T axis points toward the apex	0 to +60	If any, only III

SUMMARY OF HORIZONTAL PLANE T AXIS

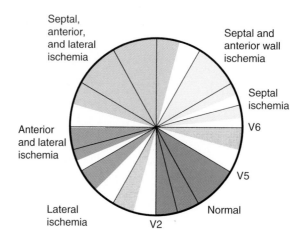

Location of Subendocardial Ischemia	Concept to Understand	T Axis to Translate the Concept (Don't Memorize This)	Inverted T Wave Pattern (Memorize!)
Nonspecific septal T wave changes	T axis points borderline away from the septum	0 to +15	V1 only
Septal	T axis points away from septum	−7.5 to −15	V1 and V2
Septal and anterior	T axis points away from septum and anterior wall	−22.5 to −60	V2 and V3 (+/− V1, +/− V4)
Septal anterior and lateral	T axis points away from septum, anterior and lateral walls	−75 to −165	V2, V3, V4, V5 (+/− V1, +/− V6)
Anterior and lateral	T axis points away from anterior and lateral walls	+162.5 to +180	V4 and V5 (+/− V3, +/− V6)
Lateral	T axis points away from the lateral wall	+135 to +150	V5 and V6
Nonspecific lateral T wave changes	T axis points borderline away from the lateral wall	+105 to +120	V6 only
Normal	T axis points toward the apex	+30 to +75	No T wave inversion

SUMMARY CHART OF T WAVE INVERSIONS

Patterns of T Wave Inversions	Locations of Ischemia
II, III, AVF	Inferior
I, AVL	Lateral
I, II, AVF	Apical
V1, V2	Septal
V3, V4	Anterior
V5, V6	Lateral

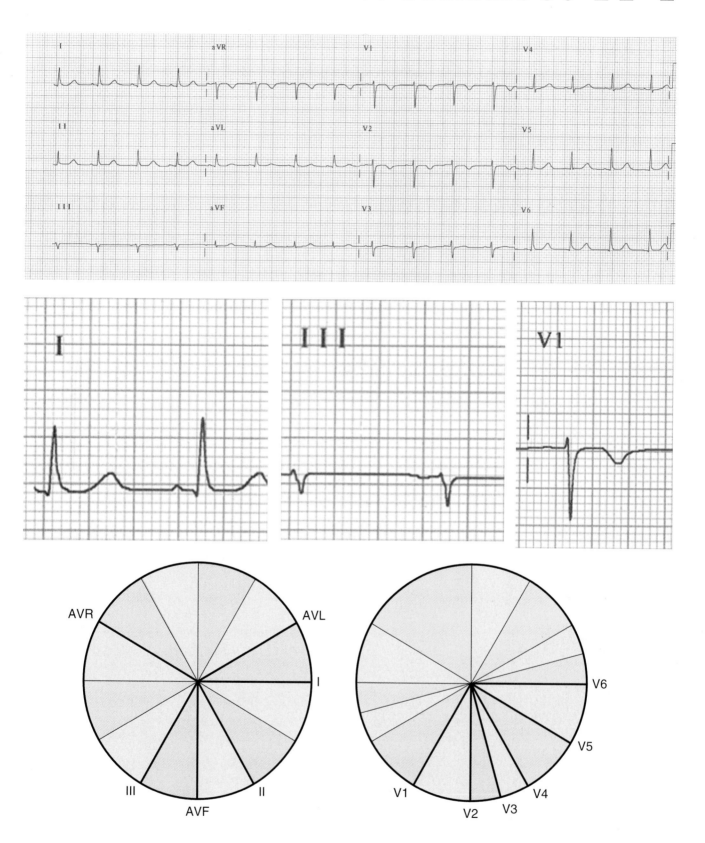

Heart Rate:

Rhythm:

Intervals (measured in the limb leads)

PR: short (< .12)
       normal (.12 to .20)
       long (>0.20 seconds); this is 1st degree AV
       block

QRS: normal (≤0.09 seconds)
       prolonged (.10 or .11); this is intraventricular
       conduction delay (IVCD)
       Bundle Branch Block (.12 seconds or greater)

QT:

P axis: normal
           rightward
           arm-lead reversal or dextrocardia
           junctional rhythm

QRS axis: normal
           left anterior hemiblock
           left posterior hemiblock
           indeterminate

T wave inversion (ischemia or infarction):

II,III,AVF	inferior
I, AVL	lateral
V1, without V2	nonspecific septal
V1 and V2	septal
V3 and V4	anterior
V5 and V6	lateral
V6, without V5	nonspecific lateral

ST Elevation (acute infarction):

II,III,AVF	inferior
I, AVL	lateral
V1, without V2	nonspecific septal
V1 and V2	septal
V3 and V4	anterior
V5 and V6	lateral
V6, without V5.	nonspecific lateral

ST Depression (ischemia or infarction):

I,II,III,AVL,AVF	diffuse subendocardial ischemia or infarction
V2,V3,V4,V5	diffuse subendocardial ischemia or infarction

Q waves (infarction):

II,III,AVF	inferior
I, AVL	lateral
V1, without V2	nonspecific septal
V1 and V2	septal
V3 and V4	anterior
V5 and V6	lateral
V6, without V5	nonspecific lateral

Hypertrophy:

Right atrial: Tall P wave 2.5 mm in II, III, or AVF

Left atrial: Deep negative part of P wave in V1

LVH: R wave in 1 + S wave in III ≥ 25mV
      S wave in V1 + R wave in V5 ≥ 35mV

RVH: Mean QRS either anterior, or rightward

The heart rate is 94 beats per minute. The PR interval is 0.12 seconds, which is normal. The QRS interval measures 0.08 seconds, which is normal. The QT interval is 0.34 seconds. The P axis is 0°. The mean QRS axis is +15°, which is normal. The frontal plane T axis is +30°, which is normal. The horizontal plane T axis is −15° and is pointing away from the septum. This is consistent with subendocardial ischemia or infarction of the septum. Infarction cannot be diagnosed with confidence on a single EKG by looking at the ST segment or the T wave. If the T wave changes reverse on the next EKG, then ischemia was present. If the T wave changes persist in the appropriate clinical setting (such as pain and diagnostic cardiac enzymes), then infarction is present.

Importantly, when the T wave is inverted in V1 and V2, there is another possible clinical explanation. This T axis in the horizontal plane points away from both the septum and the free wall of the right ventricle. It is clinically possible for these T wave changes to reflect strain of the free wall of the right ventricle, as in acute pulmonary embolism. History is always key. Is the patient obese, young, with risk factors for thromboembolism? Or is the patient an elderly patient with risk factors for coronary disease?

Parts of the answer sheets are "grayed out" because these sections have not yet been covered. Answer only the parts that are not highlighted.

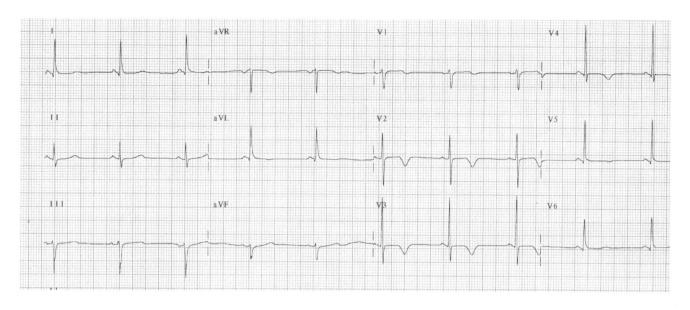

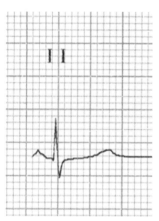

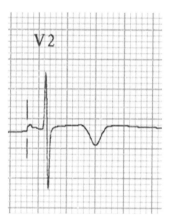

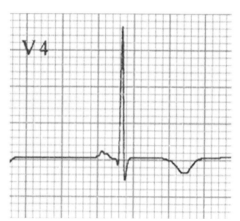

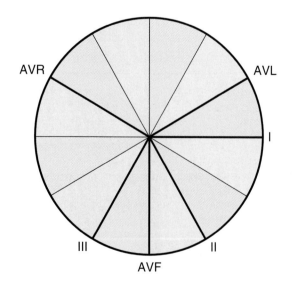

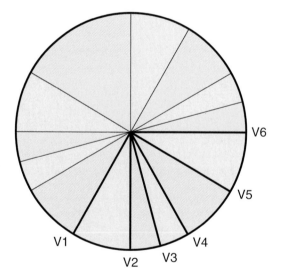

Heart Rate:

Rhythm:

Intervals (measured in the limb leads)

PR: short (< .12)
normal (.12 to .20)
long (>0.20 seconds); this is 1st degree AV block

QRS: normal (≤0.09 seconds)
prolonged (.10 or .11); this is intraventricular conduction delay (IVCD)
Bundle Branch Block (.12 seconds or greater)

QT:

P axis:	normal
	rightward
	arm-lead reversal or dextrocardia
	junctional rhythm
QRS Axis:	normal
	Left anterior hemiblock
	Left posterior hemiblock
	Indeterminate

T wave inversion (ischemia or infarction):

II,III,AVF	inferior
I, AVL	lateral
V1, without V2	nonspecific septal
V1 and V2	septal
V3 and V4	anterior
V5 and V6	lateral
V6, without V5.	nonspecific lateral

ST Elevation (acute infarction):

II,III,AVF	inferior
I, AVL	lateral
V1, without V2	nonspecific septal
V1 and V2	septal
V3 and V4	anterior
V5 and V6	lateral
V6, without V5.	nonspecific lateral

ST Depression (ischemia or infarction):

I,II,III,AVL,AVF	diffuse subendocardial ischemia or infarction
V2,V3,V4,V5	diffuse subendocardial ischemia or infarction

Q waves (infarction):

II,III,AVF	inferior
I, AVL	lateral
V1, without V2	nonspecific septal
V1 and V2	septal
V3 and V4	anterior
V5 and V6	lateral
V6, without V5.	nonspecific lateral

Hypertrophy:

Right atrial: Tall P wave 2.5 mm in II, III, or AVF

Left atrial: Deep negative part of P wave in V1

LVH: R wave in 1 + S wave in III ≥ 25mV
S wave in V1 + R wave in V5 ≥ 35mV

RVH: Mean QRS either anterior, or rightward

The heart rate is 60 beats per minute. The PR interval is 0.12 seconds. The QRS interval measures 0.09 seconds. The QT interval measures 0.40 seconds. The P axis is +45°, which is normal. The mean QRS axis is −15°, which is normal. The frontal plane T axis is +75°, which is normal. The horizontal T axis is −60°. This points away from the septum and anterior wall. It indicates subendocardial ischemia or infarction of the septum and anterior walls.

Parts of the answer sheets are "grayed out" because these sections have not yet been covered. Answer only the parts that are not highlighted.

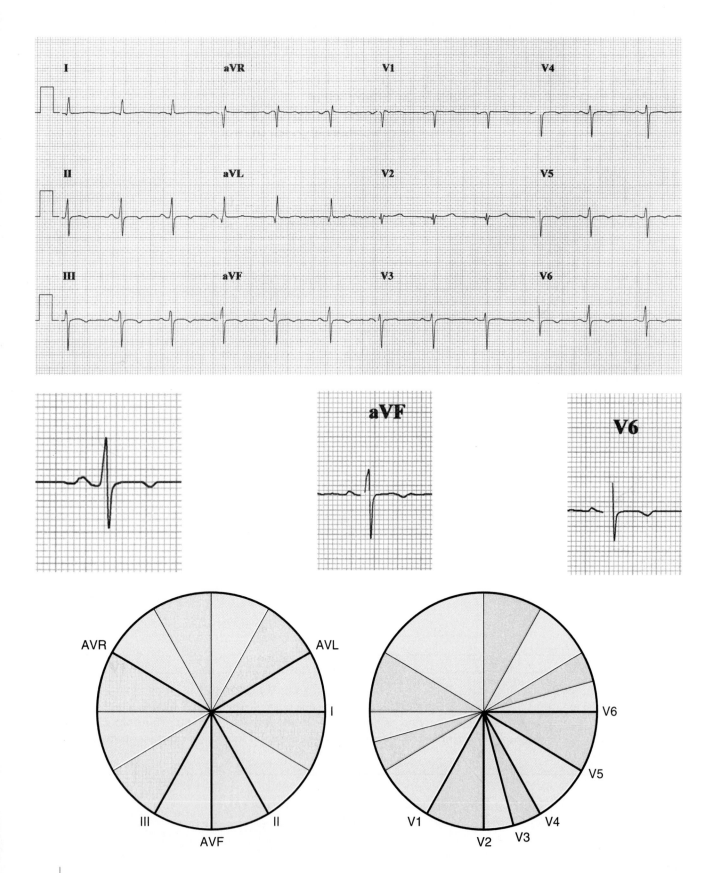

Heart Rate:

Rhythm:

Intervals (measured in the limb leads)

PR: short (< .12)
     normal (.12 to .20)
     long (>0.20 seconds); this is 1st degree AV block

QRS: normal (≤0.09 seconds)
      prolonged (.10 or .11); this is intraventricular conduction delay (IVCD)
      Bundle Branch Block (.12 seconds or greater)

QT:

P axis: normal
         rightward
         arm-lead reversal or dextrocardia
         junctional rhythm

QRS axis: normal
           left anterior hemiblock
           left posterior hemiblock
           indeterminate

T wave inversion (ischemia or infarction):

II,III,AVF	inferior
I, AVL	lateral
V1, without V2	nonspecific septal
V1 and V2	septal
V3 and V4	anterior
V5 and V6	lateral
V6, without V5	nonspecific lateral

ST Elevation (acute infarction):

II,III,AVF	inferior
I, AVL	lateral
V1, without V2	nonspecific septal
V1 and V2	septal
V3 and V4	anterior
V5 and V6	lateral
V6, without V5.	nonspecific lateral

ST Depression (ischemia or infarction):

I,II,III,AVL,AVF	diffuse subendocardial ischemia or infarction
V2,V3,V4,V5	diffuse subendocardial ischemia or infarction

Q waves (infarction):

II,III,AVF	inferior
I, AVL	lateral
V1, without V2	nonspecific septal
V1 and V2	septal
V3 and V4	anterior
V5 and V6	lateral
V6, without V5	nonspecific lateral

Hypertrophy:

Right atrial: Tall P wave 2.5 mm in II, III, or AVF

Left atrial: Deep negative part of P wave in V1

LVH: R wave in 1 + S wave in III ≥ 25mV
      S wave in V1 + R wave in V5 ≥ 35mV

RVH: Mean QRS either anterior, or rightward

The heart rate is 74 beats per minute. The PR interval is 0.16 seconds. The QRS interval measures 0.09 seconds. The QT interval measures 0.40 seconds, which is long. It is difficult to measure the QT interval in this EKG, because it is difficult to find tall enough T waves to measure. *When the T waves are very small, it suggests hypokalemia. Clinically, the patient's history (vomiting? nasogastric tube? diuretics?) should be evaluated, as well as the serum potassium level.* The frontal plane T axis is −90°, pointing away from the inferior wall. The T waves, like all forces, have magnitude and direction. To be significant, a T wave abnormality should have abnormal direction and magnitude. The inverted T waves should be at least 1 mm deep. If the T waves are abnormally directed (as in this EKG) away from the inferior wall, but of low amplitude, then the specificity of the diagnosis is reduced. These T waves (abnormally directed away from the inferior wall, but of minimal amplitude) are termed **nonspecific inferior T wave changes.** Significantly, *hypokalemia (as discussed in Chapter 19) causes T wave and ST segment changes.* Thus, this EKG clinically suggests hypokalemia or inferior ischemia or infarction. The horizontal T axis points away from the lateral wall but is also of very low amplitude, making it nonspecific as well. The horizontal T axis indicates nonspecific lateral T wave changes consistent with hypokalemia or ischemia or infarction.

Parts of the answer sheets are "grayed out" because these sections have not yet been covered. Answer only the parts that are not highlighted.

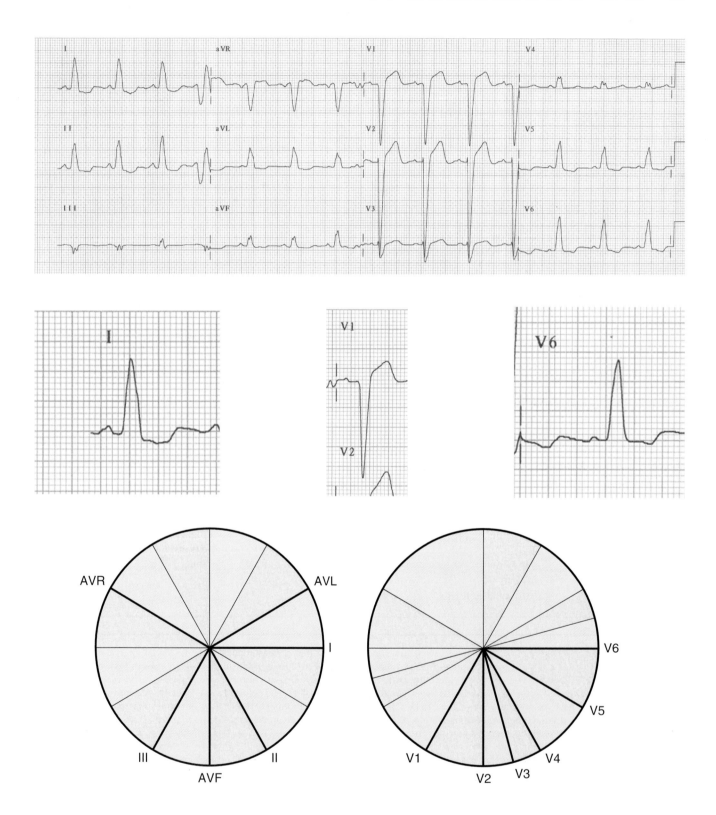

Heart Rate:

Rhythm:

Intervals (measured in the limb leads)

PR: short (< .12)
     normal (.12 to .20)
     long (>0.20 seconds); this is 1st degree AV block

QRS: normal (≤0.09 seconds)
     prolonged (.10 or .11); this is intraventricular conduction delay (IVCD)
     Bundle Branch Block (.12 seconds or greater)

QT:

P axis:	normal
	rightward
	arm-lead reversal or dextrocardia
	junctional rhythm
QRS axis:	normal
	left anterior hemiblock
	left posterior hemiblock
	indeterminate

T wave inversion (ischemia or infarction):

II,III,AVF	inferior
I, AVL	lateral
V1, without V2	nonspecific septal
V1 and V2	septal
V3 and V4	anterior
V5 and V6	lateral
V6, without V5	nonspecific lateral

ST Elevation (acute infarction):

II,III,AVF	inferior
I, AVL	lateral
V1, without V2	nonspecific septal
V1 and V2	septal
V3 and V4	anterior
V5 and V6	lateral
V6, without V5.	nonspecific lateral

ST Depression (ischemia or infarction):

| I,II,III,AVL,AVF | diffuse subendocardial ischemia or infarction |
| V2,V3,V4,V5 | diffuse subendocardial ischemia or infarction |

Q waves (infarction):

II,III,AVF	inferior
I, AVL	lateral
V1, without V2	nonspecific septal
V1 and V2	septal
V3 and V4	anterior
V5 and V6	lateral
V6, without V5	nonspecific lateral

Hypertrophy:

Right atrial: Tall P wave 2.5 mm in II, III, or AVF

Left atrial: Deep negative part of P wave in V1

LVH: R wave in 1 + S wave in III ≥ 25mV
      S wave in V1 + R wave in V5 ≥ 35mV

RVH: Mean QRS either anterior, or rightward

The heart rate is 83 beats per minute. The PR interval is 0.16 seconds. The QRS interval measures 0.14 seconds. This indicates BBB. In the frontal plane, the last part of the QRS points leftward and indicates LBBB. In the horizontal plane, the last part of the QRS points posterior and leftward, and also indicates LBBB. The QT interval measures 0.40 seconds. The P axis is +30°, which is normal. The mean QRS axis is −15°. (Remember, in LBBB the mean QRS axis is noted but not analyzed.) The ST-T axis is opposite the last part of the QRS as expected. There are no useful criteria for analyzing the ST-T axis in LBBB. Do not diagnose T wave abnormalities in this setting.

Parts of the answer sheets are "grayed out" because these sections have not yet been covered. Answer only the parts that are not highlighted.

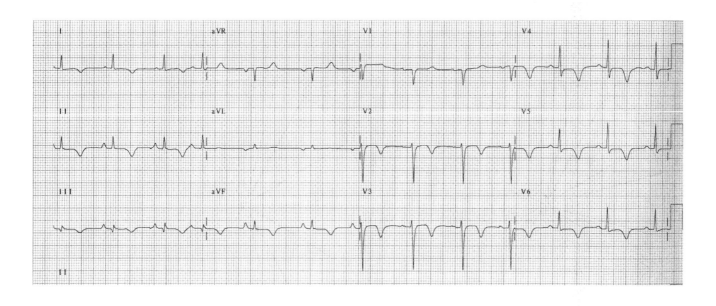

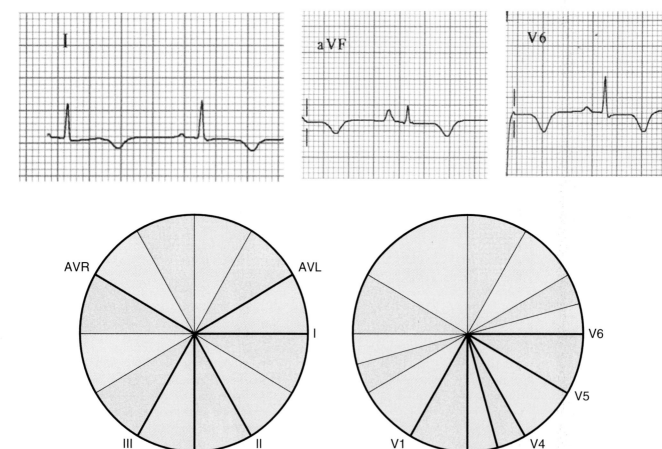

Heart Rate:

Rhythm:

Intervals (measured in the limb leads)

PR: short (< .12)
normal (.12 to .20)
long (>0.20 seconds); this is 1st degree AV block

QRS: normal (≤0.09 seconds)
prolonged (.10 or .11); this is intraventricular conduction delay (IVCD)
Bundle Branch Block (.12 seconds or greater)

QT:

P axis: normal
rightward
arm-lead reversal or dextrocardia
junctional rhythm

QRS axis: normal
left anterior hemiblock
left posterior hemiblock
indeterminate

T wave inversion (ischemia or infarction):

II,III,AVF	inferior
I, AVL	lateral
V1, without V2	nonspecific septal
V1 and V2	septal
V3 and V4	anterior
V5 and V6	lateral
V6, without V5	nonspecific lateral

ST Elevation (acute infarction):

II,III,AVF	inferior
I, AVL	lateral
V1, without V2	nonspecific septal
V1 and V2	septal
V3 and V4	anterior
V5 and V6	lateral
V6, without V5.	nonspecific lateral

ST Depression (ischemia or infarction):

I,II,III,AVL,AVF	diffuse subendocardial ischemia or infarction
V2,V3,V4,V5	diffuse subendocardial ischemia or infarction

Q waves (infarction):

II,III,AVF	inferior
I, AVL	lateral
V1, without V2	nonspecific septal
V1 and V2	septal
V3 and V4	anterior
V5 and V6	lateral
V6, without V5	nonspecific lateral

Hypertrophy:

Right atrial: Tall P wave 2.5 mm in II, III, or AVF

Left atrial: Deep negative part of P wave in V1

LVH: R wave in 1 + S wave in III ≥ 25mV
S wave in V1 + R wave in V5 ≥ 35mV

RVH: Mean QRS either anterior, or rightward

The heart rate is 71 beats per minute. The PR interval measures 0.16 second. The QRS interval is 0.08 seconds. The QT interval measures 0.40 seconds. The P axis is +75°, which is normal. The mean QRS axis is +30°, which is normal. The T wave is abnormal. In the frontal plane, the T axis is −120° and indicates apical subendocardial ischemia or infarction. In the horizontal plane, the T axis is −165° and points away from the septum, anterior, and lateral walls, consistent with subendocardial ischemia or infarction. When the T waves are abnormal throughout the EKG, it can be read as diffuse T wave changes and suggests global ischemia or infarction. To get such diffuse ischemic changes, a large supply and demand mismatch would be expected. This can sometimes follow a cardiac arrest or other sustained hypotensive episode, which would affect the entire myocardium.

Parts of the answer sheets are "grayed out" because these sections have not yet been covered. Answer only the parts that are not highlighted.

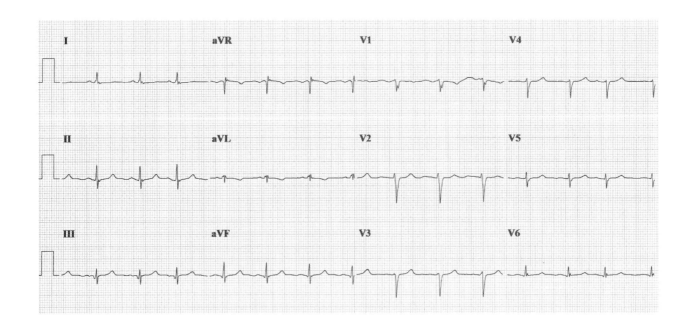

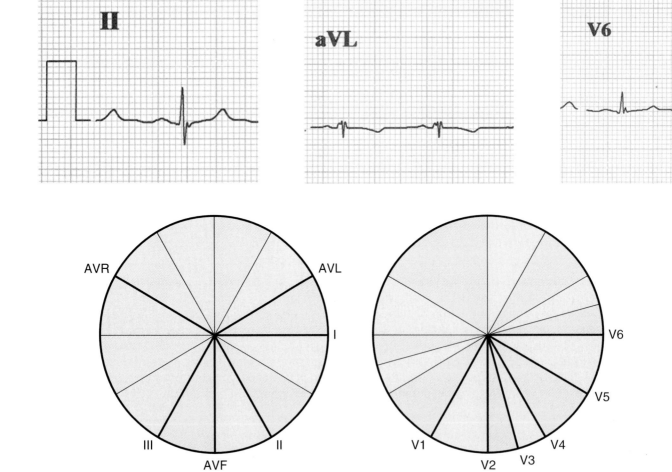

Heart Rate:

Rhythm:

Intervals (measured in the limb leads)

PR: short (< .12)
normal (.12 to .20)
long (>0.20 seconds); this is 1st degree AV block

QRS: normal (≤0.09 seconds)
prolonged (.10 or .11); this is intraventricular conduction delay (IVCD)
Bundle Branch Block (.12 seconds or greater)

QT:

P axis: normal
rightward
arm-lead reversal or dextrocardia
junctional rhythm

QRS axis: normal
left anterior hemiblock
left posterior hemiblock
indeterminate

T wave inversion (ischemia or infarction):

II,III,AVF	inferior
I, AVL	lateral
V1, without V2	nonspecific septal
V1 and V2	septal
V3 and V4	anterior
V5 and V6	lateral
V6, without V5	nonspecific lateral

ST Elevation (acute infarction):

II,III,AVF	inferior
I, AVL	lateral
V1, without V2	nonspecific septal
V1 and V2	septal
V3 and V4	anterior
V5 and V6	lateral
V6, without V5.	nonspecific lateral

ST Depression (ischemia or infarction):

I,II,III,AVL,AVF	diffuse subendocardial ischemia or infarction
V2,V3,V4,V5	diffuse subendocardial ischemia or infarction

Q waves (infarction):

II,III,AVF	inferior
I, AVL	lateral
V1, without V2	nonspecific septal
V1 and V2	septal
V3 and V4	anterior
V5 and V6	lateral
V6, without V5	nonspecific lateral

Hypertrophy:

Right atrial: Tall P wave 2.5 mm in II, III, or AVF

Left atrial: Deep negative part of P wave in V1

LVH: R wave in 1 + S wave in III ≥ 25mV
S wave in V1 + R wave in V5 ≥ 35mV

RVH: Mean QRS either anterior, or rightward

The heart rate is 83. The PR interval measures 0.18 seconds. The QRS interval measures 0.08 seconds. The QT interval is 0.38 seconds. The P axis is +45° and is normal. The mean QRS axis is +75°. The T waves are of low amplitude. The frontal plane T axis is +90°, which indicates nonspecific lateral T wave changes. This may be caused by ischemia or infarction as well as other diseases, hence the description nonspecific. Among other causes of nonspecific T wave changes are drug and electrolyte effects, hypertrophy, pericarditis, myocarditis, and no clinically detectable disease. If the EKG was taken to rule in ischemic disease, and this is the first EKG, a second EKG 20 minutes later may show more diagnostic EKG changes.

Parts of the answer sheets are "grayed out" because these sections have not yet been covered. Answer only the parts that are not highlighted.

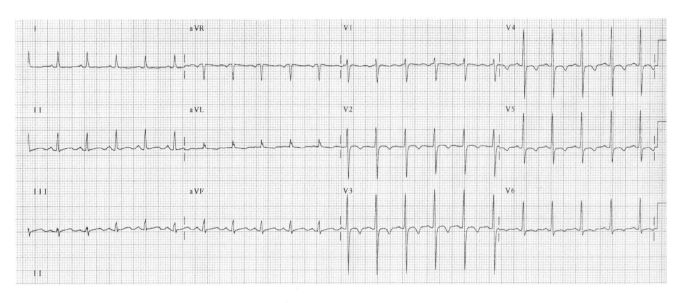

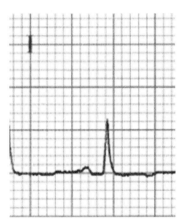
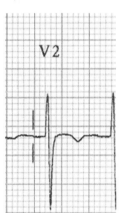
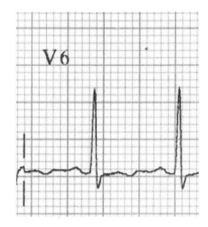

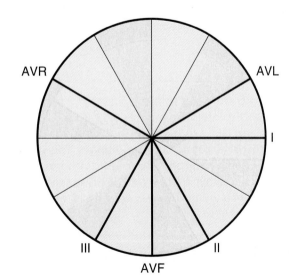
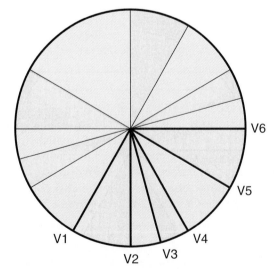

Heart Rate:

Rhythm:

Intervals (measured in the limb leads)

PR: short (< .12)
normal (.12 to .20)
long (>0.20 seconds); this is 1st degree AV block

QRS: normal (≤0.09 seconds)
prolonged (.10 or .11); this is intraventricular conduction delay (IVCD)
Bundle Branch Block (.12 seconds or greater)

QT:

P axis: normal
rightward
arm-lead reversal or dextrocardia
junctional rhythm

QRS axis: normal
left anterior hemiblock
left posterior hemiblock
indeterminate

T wave inversion (ischemia or infarction):

II,III,AVF	inferior
I, AVL	lateral
V1, without V2	nonspecific septal
V1 and V2	septal
V3 and V4	anterior
V5 and V6	lateral
V6, without V5	nonspecific lateral

ST Elevation (acute infarction):

II,III,AVF	inferior
I, AVL	lateral
V1, without V2	nonspecific septal
V1 and V2	septal
V3 and V4	anterior
V5 and V6	lateral
V6, without V5.	nonspecific lateral

ST Depression (ischemia or infarction):

I,II,III,AVL,AVF	diffuse subendocardial ischemia or infarction
V2,V3,V4,V5	diffuse subendocardial ischemia or infarction

Q waves (infarction):

II,III,AVF	inferior
I, AVL	lateral
V1, without V2	nonspecific septal
V1 and V2	septal
V3 and V4	anterior
V5 and V6	lateral
V6, without V5	nonspecific lateral

Hypertrophy:

Right atrial: Tall P wave 2.5 mm in II, III, or AVF

Left atrial: Deep negative part of P wave in V1

LVH: R wave in 1 + S wave in III ≥ 25mV
S wave in V1 + R wave in V5 ≥ 35mV

RVH: Mean QRS either anterior, or rightward

The heart rate is 125. This is sinus tachycardia. Clinical determination of the cause of sinus tachycardia should always be attempted. Causes such as hypovolemia, sepsis, congestive failure, shock, anxiety, pain and pulmonary embolus, should be considered as clinically appropriate from the history and physical examination. The PR interval measures 0.14 seconds. The QRS interval measures 0.08 seconds. The QT interval measures 0.30 seconds, and low-amplitude T waves are noted. This QT interval is long for the heart rate and may be due to hypokalemia. The P axis is +60° and is normal. The mean QRS axis is +30° and is normal. The frontal plane T wave is of low amplitude. Its direction or axis is +90°, which indicates nonspecific lateral T wave changes. The horizontal plane T axis is −150°, and indicates septal, anterior, and lateral wall subendocardial ischemia or infarction. Because of the lower amplitude of the horizontal T waves, the specificity of this finding is less than if the T waves were of more amplitude.

Clinically, the patient may have been overdiuresed, producing hypovolemia (sinus tachycardia) and hypokalemia (low-amplitude T waves, diffuse T wave inversion). Ischemia is another possibility.

Parts of the answer sheets are "grayed out" because these sections have not yet been covered. Answer only the parts that are not highlighted.

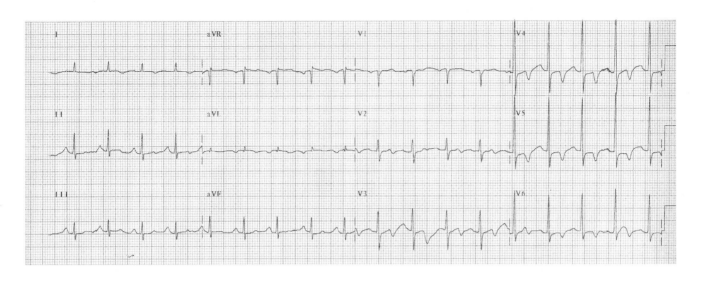

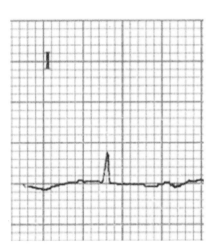

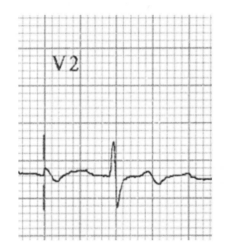

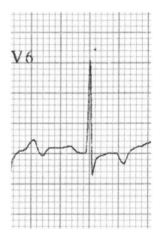

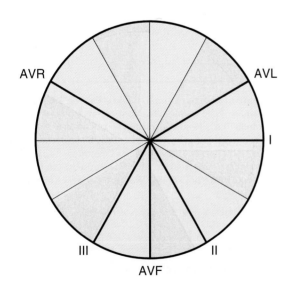

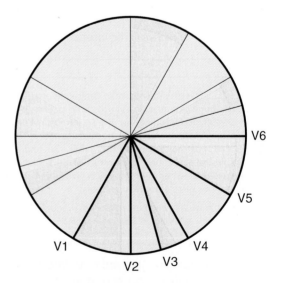

Heart Rate:

Rhythm:

Intervals (measured in the limb leads)

PR: short (< .12)
      normal (.12 to .20)
      long (>0.20 seconds); this is 1st degree AV
      block

QRS: normal (≤0.09 seconds)
      prolonged (.10 or .11); this is intraventricular
      conduction delay (IVCD)
      Bundle Branch Block (.12 seconds or greater)

QT:

P axis: normal
           rightward
           arm-lead reversal or dextrocardia
           junctional rhythm

QRS axis: normal
           left anterior hemiblock
           left posterior hemiblock
           indeterminate

T wave inversion (ischemia or infarction):

II,III,AVF	inferior
I, AVL	lateral
V1, without V2	nonspecific septal
V1 and V2	septal
V3 and V4	anterior
V5 and V6	lateral
V6, without V5	nonspecific lateral

ST Elevation (acute infarction):

II,III,AVF	inferior
I, AVL	lateral
V1, without V2	nonspecific septal
V1 and V2	septal
V3 and V4	anterior
V5 and V6	lateral
V6, without V5.	nonspecific lateral

ST Depression (ischemia or infarction):

I,II,III,AVL,AVF	diffuse subendocardial ischemia or infarction
V2,V3,V4,V5	diffuse subendocardial ischemia or infarction

Q waves (infarction):

II,III,AVF	inferior
I, AVL	lateral
V1, without V2	nonspecific septal
V1 and V2	septal
V3 and V4	anterior
V5 and V6	lateral
V6, without V5	nonspecific lateral

Hypertrophy:

Right atrial: Tall P wave 2.5 mm in II, III, or AVF

Left atrial: Deep negative part of P wave in V1

LVH: R wave in 1 + S wave in III ≥ 25mV
      S wave in V1 + R wave in V5 ≥ 35mV

RVH: Mean QRS either anterior, or rightward

The heart rate is 107 beats per minute. The PR interval measures 0.16 seconds. The QRS interval measures 0.06 seconds. The QT interval measures 0.26 seconds. The P axis is +75° and is normal. The mean QRS axis is +60°, which is normal. The frontal plane T wave is low amplitude and points at 120° away from the lateral wall. It is consistent with lateral subendocardial ischemia, but at this low amplitude is really a nonspecific finding (nonspecific lateral T wave changes). In the horizontal plane, the T axis is of greater amplitude, so the abnormal T axis is more specific for ischemia or infarction. The horizontal T axis is +180° and points away from the anterior and lateral walls, consistent with ischemia or infarction.

Parts of the answer sheets are "grayed out" because these sections have not yet been covered. Answer only the parts that are not highlighted.

ST Segment Depression

The baseline of the EKG is defined as a line that runs through the end of the T wave to the beginning of the following P wave. The ST segment is the region that begins at the end of the QRS and ends at beginning of the T wave. In the normal EKG, the ST segment appears flat and lies on the baseline. **Any elevation or depression of the ST segment 1 mm above or below the baseline represents an abnormality.** When the ST segment is above or below the baseline, it represents an electrical force that has magnitude and direction. Calculation of the ST axis allows characterization of this force.

Bundle branch block (Chapters 9 and 10) can cause ST segment depression and elevation. Right and left ventricular hypertrophy can as well (Chapters 17 and 18). **The most important cause of ST segment depression is subendocardial ischemia. In subendocardial ischemia, the ST segment can become abnormal and points away from regions of subendocardial ischemia. It is a more specific finding of subendocardial ischemia than T-wave inversion.**

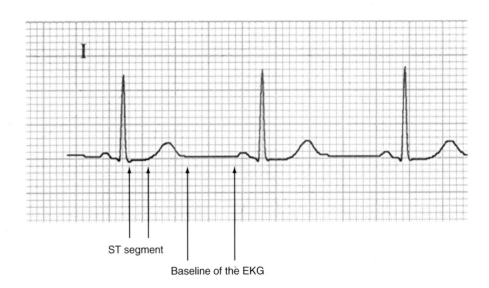

ST segment

Baseline of the EKG

ST Segment Depression: Induced by Exercise

ST segment depression indicates subendocardial ischemia. ST segment depression can be either spontaneous or provoked. In the following example each EKG lead has two complexes. The first of the pair was taken at rest. The second of the pair was taken at the peak stress of an exercise test. The increased demand of the stress test provoked subendocardial ischemia in this patient. A significant obstructive lesion in an epicardial artery is likely present.

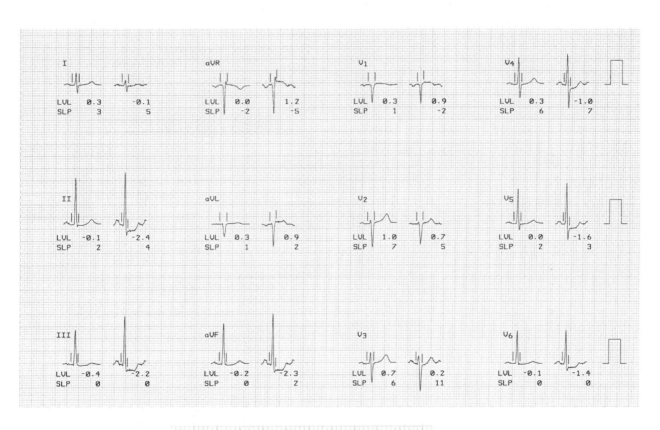

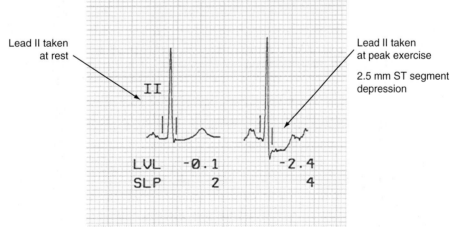

Lead II taken at rest

Lead II taken at peak exercise

2.5 mm ST segment depression

Frontal Plane: ST Depression

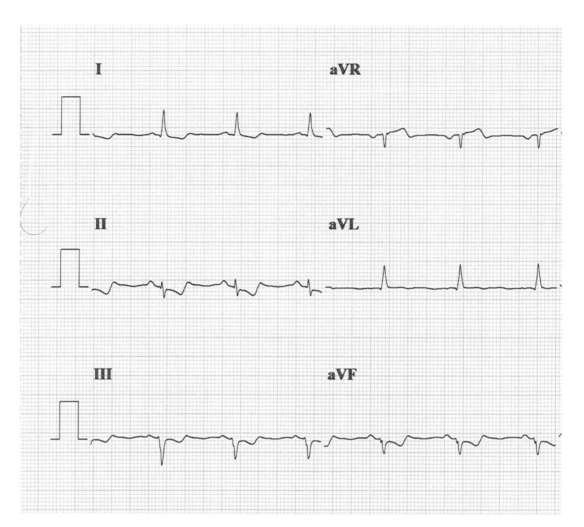

Frontal plane ST axis: −120°.

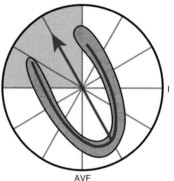

Concept: The ST segment points away from subendocardial inferior, apical, and lateral wall ischemia.

Axis: The ST axis points at −90° to −180° in the frontal plane.

Pattern: ST depression is present in lead II. Leads I and AVF must be isoelectric or have ST depression.

Horizontal Plane: ST Depression

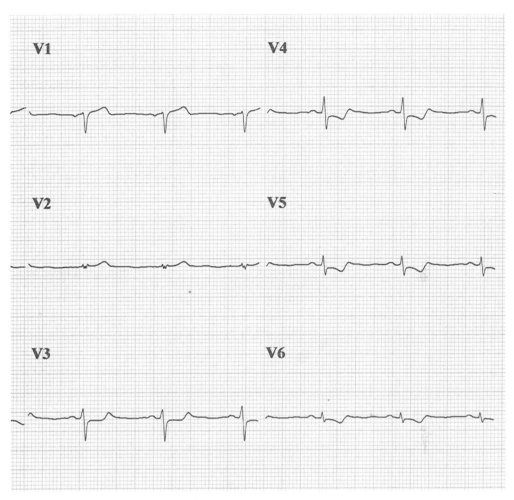

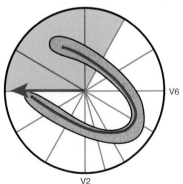

Horizontal plane ST axis: −180°.

Concept: The ST segment points away from subendocardial septal, anterior, and lateral wall ischemia.

Axis: The ST axis points at −60° to −180° in the horizontal plane.

Pattern: ST depression is present in V3 and V4. Leads V2 and V5 can be isoelectric or depressed but never elevated.

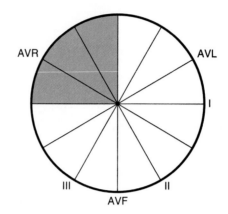

Location of Subendocardial Ischemia	Concept to Understand	ST Axis to Translate the Concept	ST Segment Depression Pattern
Inferior, apical, and lateral	ST axis points away from inferior, apical, and lateral walls	−90° to −180°	ST depression is present in lead II. Leads I and AVF must be isoelectric or have ST depression

SUMMARY OF HORIZONTAL PLANE ST SEGMENT

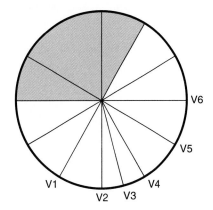

Location of Subendocardial Ischemia	Concept to Understand	ST Axis to Translate the Concept	ST Segment Depression Pattern
Septal, anterior, and lateral	ST axis points away from septum, anterior, and lateral walls	−60° to −180°	ST depression is present in V3 and V4. Leads V2 and V5 can be isoelectric or depressed but never elevated.

SUMMARY CHART OF ST SEGMENT DEPRESSION

Patterns of ST Segment Depression	Locations of Ischemia
II is depressed. I and AVF are not elevated.	Inferior, apical, and lateral subendocardial ischemia or infarction
V3 and V4 are depressed. V2 and V5 are not elevated.	Septal, anterior, and lateral subendocardial ischemia or infarction

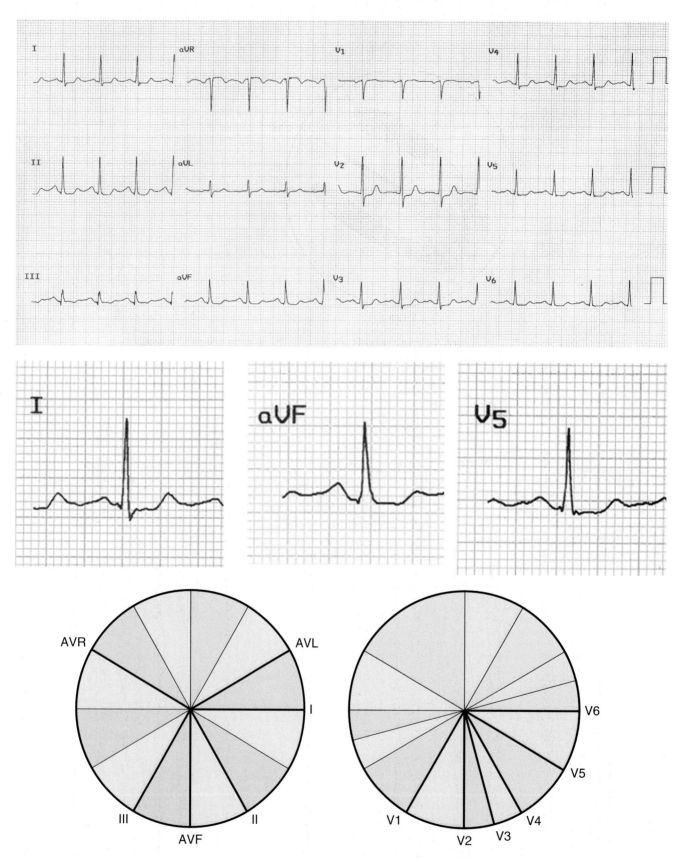

Heart Rate:

Rhythm:

Intervals (measured in the limb leads)

PR: short (< .12)
         normal (.12 to .20)
         long (>0.20 seconds); this is 1st degree AV
         block

QRS: normal (≤0.09 seconds)
         prolonged (.10 or .11); this is intraventricular
         conduction delay (IVCD)
         Bundle Branch Block (.12 seconds or greater)

QT:

P axis: normal
             rightward
             arm-lead reversal or dextrocardia
             junctional rhythm

QRS axis: normal
             left anterior hemiblock
             left posterior hemiblock
             indeterminate

T wave inversion (ischemia or infarction):

II,III,AVF	inferior
I, AVL	lateral
V1, without V2	nonspecific septal
V1 and V2	septal
V3 and V4	anterior
V5 and V6	lateral
V6, without V5	nonspecific lateral

ST Elevation (acute infarction):

II,III,AVF	inferior
I, AVL	lateral
V1, without V2	nonspecific septal
V1 and V2	septal
V3 and V4	anterior
V5 and V6	lateral
V6, without V5.	nonspecific lateral

ST Depression (ischemia or infarction):

I,II,III,AVL,AVF	diffuse subendocardial ischemia or infarction
V2,V3,V4,V5	diffuse subendocardial ischemia or infarction

Q waves (infarction):

II,III,AVF	inferior
I, AVL	lateral
V1, without V2	nonspecific septal
V1 and V2	septal
V3 and V4	anterior
V5 and V6	lateral
V6, without V5	nonspecific lateral

Hypertrophy:

Right atrial: Tall P wave 2.5 mm in II, III, or AVF

Left atrial: Deep negative part of P wave in V1

LVH: R wave in 1 + S wave in III ≥ 25mV
       S wave in V1 + R wave in V5 ≥ 35mV

RVH: Mean QRS either anterior, or rightward

The heart rate is 100 beats per minute. The PR interval is 0.16 seconds, which is normal. The QRS interval measures 0.09 seconds, which is normal. The QT interval measures 0.36 seconds. The P axis is +75°, which is normal. In the frontal plane, the mean QRS axis is +45°. In the horizontal plane, the mean QRS axis is +15°. In the frontal plane, the ST segment is negative in leads I, II, III, and AVF. It is positive in AVR and isoelectric in lead AVL. This combination gives an ST axis of −120°. This is consistent with diffuse subendocardial ischemia or infarction. *ST changes are more specific than T wave changes for the diagnosis of ischemia.* In the horizontal plane, the ST axis is negative in leads V2 through V6 but isoelectric in lead V1. This gives an ST axis in the horizontal plane of −150°, which also indicates diffuse subendocardial ischemia or infarction. *The pathophysiology of ST segment depression is a severe mismatch of supply and demand for oxygen at the mitochondrial level of the myocardium. A total obstruction to flow is not present, or there would be ST segment elevation present.*

Bundle branch block can cause ST depression, but the QRS interval is normal on this EKG, so BBB is not present.

Parts of the answer sheets are "grayed out" because these sections have not yet been covered. Answer only the parts that are not highlighted.

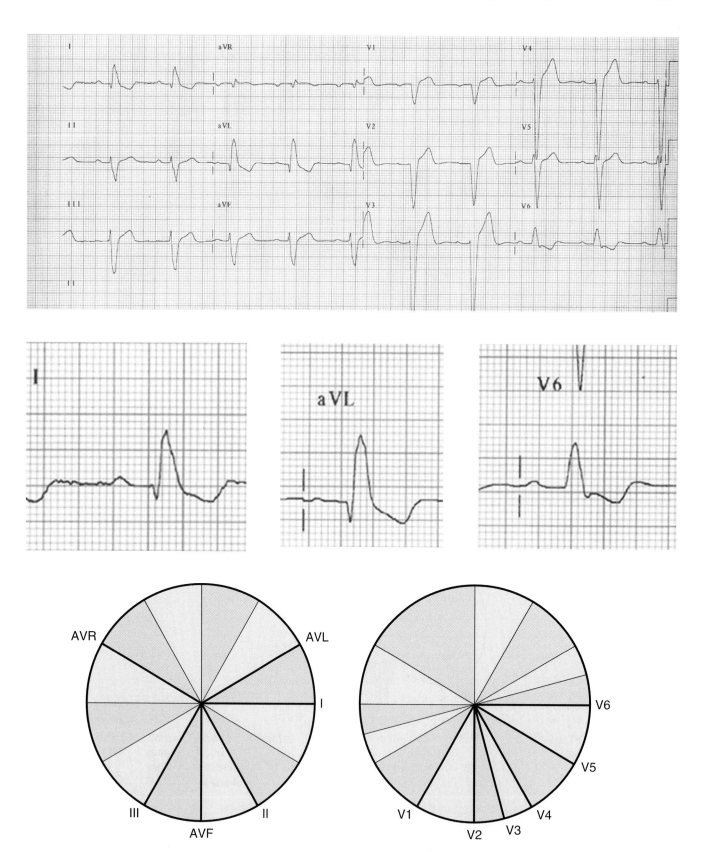

Heart Rate:

Rhythm:

Intervals (measured in the limb leads)

PR: short (< .12)
      normal (.12 to .20)
      long (>0.20 seconds); this is 1st degree AV block

QRS: normal (≤0.09 seconds)
      prolonged (.10 or .11); this is intraventricular conduction delay (IVCD)
      Bundle Branch Block (.12 seconds or greater)

QT:

ST Elevation (acute infarction):

II,III,AVF	inferior
I, AVL	lateral
V1, without V2	nonspecific septal
V1 and V2	septal
V3 and V4	anterior
V5 and V6	lateral
V6, without V5.	nonspecific lateral

ST Depression (ischemia or infarction):

I,II,III,AVL,AVF	diffuse subendocardial ischemia or infarction
V2,V3,V4,V5	diffuse subendocardial ischemia or infarction

P axis: normal
              rightward
              arm-lead reversal or dextrocardia
              junctional rhythm

QRS axis: normal
              left anterior hemiblock
              left posterior hemiblock
              indeterminate

Q waves (infarction):

II,III,AVF	inferior
I, AVL	lateral
V1, without V2	nonspecific septal
V1 and V2	septal
V3 and V4	anterior
V5 and V6	lateral
V6, without V5	nonspecific lateral

T wave inversion (ischemia or infarction):

II,III,AVF	inferior
I, AVL	lateral
V1, without V2	nonspecific septal
V1 and V2	septal
V3 and V4	anterior
V5 and V6	lateral
V6, without V5	nonspecific lateral

Hypertrophy:

Right atrial: Tall P wave 2.5 mm in II, III, or AVF

Left atrial: Deep negative part of P wave in V1

LVH: R wave in 1 + S wave in III ≥ 25mV
      S wave in V1 + R wave in V5 ≥ 35mV

RVH: Mean QRS either anterior, or rightward

The heart rate is 60 beats per minute. The PR interval measures 0.22 seconds, which is prolonged, and indicates 1° AV block. The QRS interval measures 0.16 seconds, which indicates BBB. In the frontal plane, the last part of the QRS points leftward and indicates LBBB. In the horizontal plane, the last part of the QRS is negative in V1 and V2 and points posterior to the left ventricle. This also indicates LBBB. Because the last part of the QRS in V6 is not leftward, this is called LBBB, atypical BBB, or atypical LBBB. These are similar clinically and have the same differential diagnoses as LBBB. The QT interval measures 0.44 seconds. The P axis is +30°. The mean QRS axis is −60°. *In the setting of LBBB (or atypical BBB or atypical LBBB) there are no useful criteria for interpreting the mean QRS axis, so do not interpret hemiblock in this setting.* The ST and T axis will not be analyzed further because of the presence of atypical LBBB. **Do not analyze the ST or T segment as subendocardial ischemia in this setting!**

Parts of the answer sheets are "grayed out" because these sections have not yet been covered. Answer only the parts that are not highlighted.

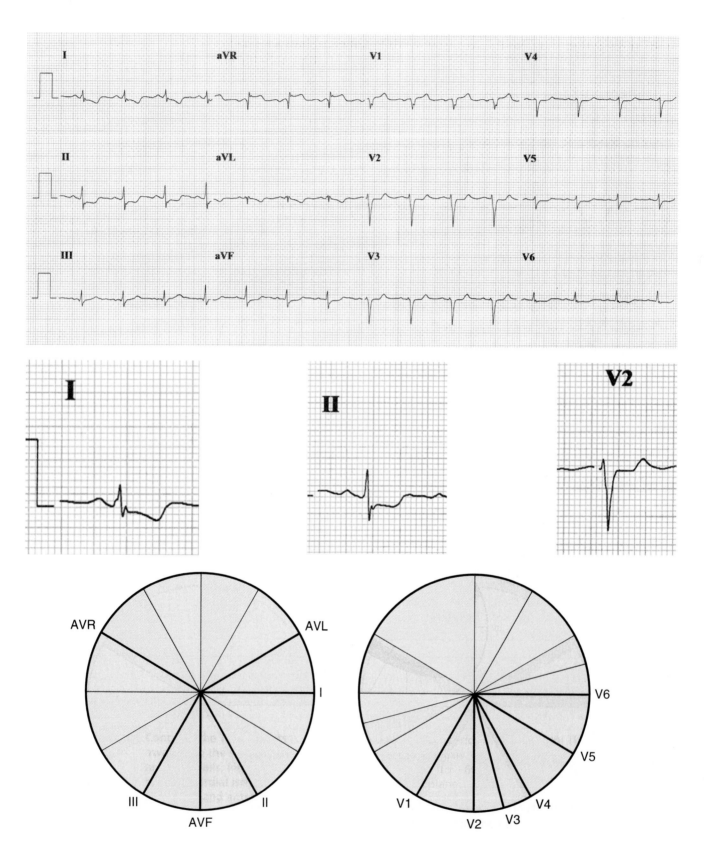

Heart Rate:

Rhythm:

ST Elevation (acute infarction):

II,III,AVF	inferior
I, AVL	lateral
V1, without V2	nonspecific septal
V1 and V2	septal
V3 and V4	anterior
V5 and V6	lateral
V6, without V5.	nonspecific lateral

Intervals (measured in the limb leads)

PR: short (< .12)
normal (.12 to .20)
long (>0.20 seconds); this is 1st degree AV
block

QRS: normal (≤0.09 seconds)
prolonged (.10 or .11); this is intraventricular
conduction delay (IVCD)
Bundle Branch Block (.12 seconds or greater)

QT:

ST Depression (ischemia or infarction):

I,II,III,AVL,AVF	diffuse subendocardial ischemia or infarction
V2,V3,V4,V5	diffuse subendocardial ischemia or infarction

P axis: normal
rightward
arm-lead reversal or dextrocardia
junctional rhythm

QRS axis: normal
left anterior hemiblock
left posterior hemiblock
indeterminate

Q waves (infarction):

II,III,AVF	inferior
I, AVL	lateral
V1, without V2	nonspecific septal
V1 and V2	septal
V3 and V4	anterior
V5 and V6	lateral
V6, without V5	nonspecific lateral

T wave inversion (ischemia or infarction):

II,III,AVF	inferior
I, AVL	lateral
V1, without V2	nonspecific septal
V1 and V2	septal
V3 and V4	anterior
V5 and V6	lateral
V6, without V5	nonspecific lateral

Hypertrophy:

Right atrial: Tall P wave 2.5 mm in II, III, or AVF

Left atrial: Deep negative part of P wave in V1

LVH: R wave in 1 + S wave in III ≥ 25mV
S wave in V1 + R wave in V5 ≥ 35mV

RVH: Mean QRS either anterior, or rightward

The heart rate is 88 beats per minute. The PR interval measures 0.16 seconds. The QRS interval measures 0.08 seconds. The QT interval measures 0.32 seconds. The P axis is +30. The frontal plane QRS axis is +75°. The horizontal plane QRS axis is −75°. In the frontal plane, the ST axis is −150°. In the horizontal plane, the ST axis is −150°. This indicates diffuse subendocardial ischemia or infarction. *ST changes are more specific than T wave changes for the diagnosis of ischemia.*

As with T wave changes, ischemia cannot be differentiated from infarction based solely on one EKG. If the next EKG on the above patient was normal, then this EKG would represent ischemia. If the previous EKG was normal, and the EKG a week from now demonstrated no change from above, then infarction would be present. The T wave and ST segment on a single EKG are part of the answer, but don't answer all the questions.

Parts of the answer sheets are "grayed out" because these sections have not yet been covered. Answer only the parts that are not highlighted.

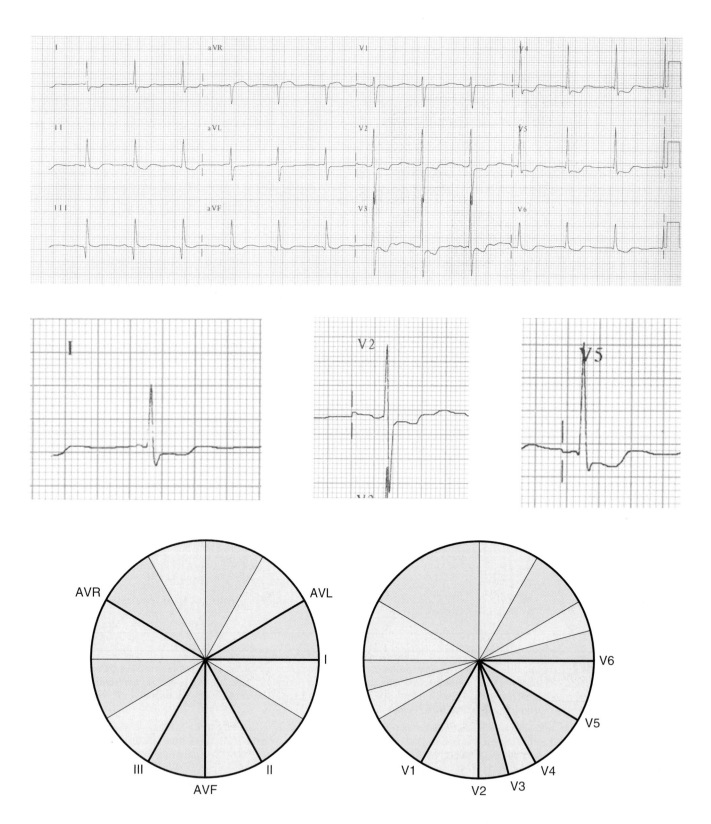

Heart Rate:

Rhythm:

Intervals (measured in the limb leads)

PR: short (< .12)
        normal (.12 to .20)
        long (>0.20 seconds); this is 1st degree AV
        block

QRS: normal (≤0.09 seconds)
        prolonged (.10 or .11); this is intraventricular
        conduction delay (IVCD)
        Bundle Branch Block (.12 seconds or greater)

QT:

P axis: normal
            rightward
            arm-lead reversal or dextrocardia
            junctional rhythm

QRS axis: normal
            left anterior hemiblock
            left posterior hemiblock
            indeterminate

T wave inversion (ischemia or infarction):

II,III,AVF	inferior
I, AVL	lateral
V1, without V2	nonspecific septal
V1 and V2	septal
V3 and V4	anterior
V5 and V6	lateral
V6, without V5	nonspecific lateral

ST Elevation (acute infarction):

II,III,AVF	inferior
I, AVL	lateral
V1, without V2	nonspecific septal
V1 and V2	septal
V3 and V4	anterior
V5 and V6	lateral
V6, without V5.	nonspecific lateral

ST Depression (ischemia or infarction):

I,II,III,AVL,AVF	diffuse subendocardial ischemia or infarction
V2,V3,V4,V5	diffuse subendocardial ischemia or infarction

Q waves (infarction):

II,III,AVF	inferior
I, AVL	lateral
V1, without V2	nonspecific septal
V1 and V2	septal
V3 and V4	anterior
V5 and V6	lateral
V6, without V5	nonspecific lateral

Hypertrophy:

Right atrial: Tall P wave 2.5 mm in II, III, or AVF

Left atrial: Deep negative part of P wave in V1

LVH: R wave in 1 + S wave in III ≥ 25mV
      S wave in V1 + R wave in V5 ≥ 35mV

RVH: Mean QRS either anterior, or rightward

The heart rate is 75 beats per minute. The PR interval measures 0.16 seconds. The QRS interval measures 0.11 seconds. This indicates intraventricular conduction delay (IVCD). In the frontal plane, the last part of the QRS points rightward. In the horizontal plane, the last part of the QRS points posterior. These are not consistent with either RIVCD or LIVCD, so the conduction delay is considered nonspecific (nonspecific IVCD). The P axis is +90°, which is rightward. In the frontal plane, the mean QRS axis is +45°. In the horizontal plane, the mean QRS is +15°. Continuing in the frontal plane, the ST axis is negative in leads I, II, AVL, and AVF. It is positive in AVR but isoelectric in lead III. This combination points to −150°. This indicates diffuse subendocardial ischemia or infarction. In the horizontal plane, the ST segment is negative in leads V2 through V6. It is isoelectric in lead V1. This indicates diffuse subendocardial ischemia or infarction as well.

Parts of the answer sheets are "grayed out" because these sections have not yet been covered. Answer only the parts that are not highlighted.

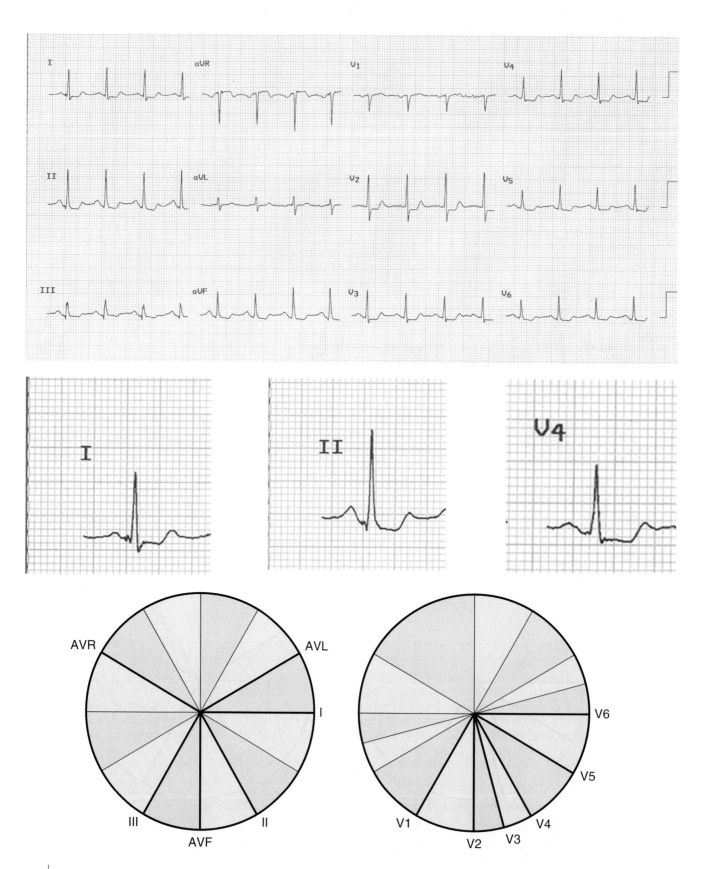

Heart Rate:

Rhythm:

Intervals (measured in the limb leads)

PR: short (< .12)
normal (.12 to .20)
long (>0.20 seconds); this is 1st degree AV block

QRS: normal (≤0.09 seconds)
prolonged (.10 or .11); this is intraventricular conduction delay (IVCD)
Bundle Branch Block (.12 seconds or greater)

QT:

P axis: normal
rightward
arm-lead reversal or dextrocardia
junctional rhythm

QRS axis: normal
left anterior hemiblock
left posterior hemiblock
indeterminate

T wave inversion (ischemia or infarction):

II,III,AVF	inferior
I, AVL	lateral
V1, without V2	nonspecific septal
V1 and V2	septal
V3 and V4	anterior
V5 and V6	lateral
V6, without V5	nonspecific lateral

ST Elevation (acute infarction):

II,III,AVF	inferior
I, AVL	lateral
V1, without V2	nonspecific septal
V1 and V2	septal
V3 and V4	anterior
V5 and V6	lateral
V6, without V5.	nonspecific lateral

ST Depression (ischemia or infarction):

I,II,III,AVL,AVF	diffuse subendocardial ischemia or infarction
V2,V3,V4,V5	diffuse subendocardial ischemia or infarction

Q waves (infarction):

II,III,AVF	inferior
I, AVL	lateral
V1, without V2	nonspecific septal
V1 and V2	septal
V3 and V4	anterior
V5 and V6	lateral
V6, without V5	nonspecific lateral

Hypertrophy:

Right atrial: Tall P wave 2.5 mm in II, III, or AVF

Left atrial: Deep negative part of P wave in V1

LVH: R wave in 1 + S wave in III ≥ 25mV
S wave in V1 + R wave in V5 ≥ 35mV

RVH: Mean QRS either anterior, or rightward

The heart rate is 100 beats per minute. The PR interval measures 0.16 seconds. The QRS interval measures 0.09 seconds. The QT interval measures 0.32 seconds. The P axis is +75°, which is normal. In the frontal plane, the mean QRS axis is +60°. In the horizontal plane, the mean QRS axis is +15°. In the frontal plane, the ST is negative in leads I, II, AVL, and AVF. It is positive in lead AVR but isoelectric in lead III. This combination gives an ST axis of −150°, which points away from the entire subendocardium and indicates diffuse subendocardial ischemia or infarction. In the horizontal plane, the ST is isoelectric in lead V1 and negative in leads V2 through V6. This combination gives an ST axis of −150°, which points away from the entire subendocardium as well.

In the setting of ST changes, the heart rate of 100 should be carefully examined clinically. Increased heart rate is a major determinant of increased demand for oxygen. This would only make the ischemic burden worse. Is the patient having chest pain, anxiety, congestive failure, bleeding with hypovolemia? Any of these would cause sinus tachycardia and could be worsening the degree of ischemia.

Parts of the answer sheets are "grayed out" because these sections have not yet been covered. Answer only the parts that are not highlighted.

Worksheet 12-6

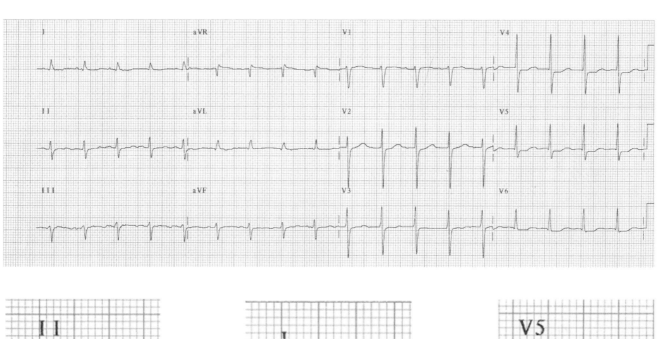

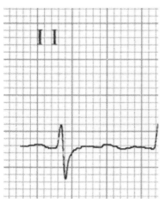

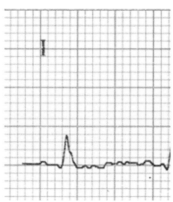

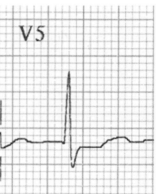

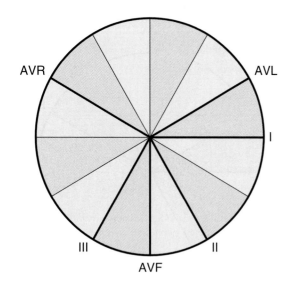

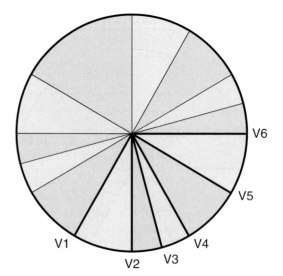

Heart Rate:

Rhythm:

ST Elevation (acute infarction):

II,III,AVF	inferior
I, AVL	lateral
V1, without V2	nonspecific septal
V1 and V2	septal
V3 and V4	anterior
V5 and V6	lateral
V6, without V5.	nonspecific lateral

Intervals (measured in the limb leads)

PR: short (< .12)
normal (.12 to .20)
long (>0.20 seconds); this is 1st degree AV block

QRS: normal (≤0.09 seconds)
prolonged (.10 or .11); this is intraventricular conduction delay (IVCD)
Bundle Branch Block (.12 seconds or greater)

QT:

ST Depression (ischemia or infarction):

I,II,III,AVL,AVF	diffuse subendocardial ischemia or infarction
V2,V3,V4,V5	diffuse subendocardial ischemia or infarction

P axis: normal
rightward
arm-lead reversal or dextrocardia
junctional rhythm

QRS axis: normal
left anterior hemiblock
left posterior hemiblock
indeterminate

Q waves (infarction):

II,III,AVF	inferior
I, AVL	lateral
V1, without V2	nonspecific septal
V1 and V2	septal
V3 and V4	anterior
V5 and V6	lateral
V6, without V5	nonspecific lateral

T wave inversion (ischemia or infarction):

II,III,AVF	inferior
I, AVL	lateral
V1, without V2	nonspecific septal
V1 and V2	septal
V3 and V4	anterior
V5 and V6	lateral
V6, without V5	nonspecific lateral

Hypertrophy:

Right atrial: Tall P wave 2.5 mm in II, III, or AVF

Left atrial: Deep negative part of P wave in V1

LVH: R wave in 1 + S wave in III ≥ 25mV
S wave in V1 + R wave in V5 ≥ 35mV

RVH: Mean QRS either anterior, or rightward

The heart rate is 107 beats per minute. The PR interval is indeterminate and cannot be clearly seen with confidence. Baseline electrical artifact is present, and a repeat tracing should be obtained. The QRS interval measures 0.08 seconds. The QT interval cannot be clearly measured, due to low-amplitude T waves. It should be considered indeterminate as well. The P axis cannot be measured and is indeterminate. In the frontal plane, the mean QRS axis is −30°. In the horizontal plane, the mean QRS axis is −22.5°. In the frontal plane, there are not ST deviations greater than ½ box deep. These ST changes are nonspecific, meaning the ST segment is displaced finitely below the baseline, but not in a clear direction, and of low amplitude. In the horizontal plane, the ST segment is slightly negative in lead V2 and is negative in leads V3 through V6. The magnitude of the deflection reaches 1 little box in lead V5 and becomes more specific. This is a borderline case and frequently is read as nonspecific ST changes. When the ST segment depression reaches 1 little box as in lead V5, it should probably be termed subendocardial ischemia or infarction.

Parts of the answer sheets are "grayed out" because these sections have not yet been covered. Answer only the parts that are not highlighted.

ST Segment Elevation

There should be no **ST segment elevation (STE)** on the EKG. ST segment elevation, which measures **less than 1mm (1 little box)**, is a nonspecific finding. STE should be **considered an indication of 100% occlusion of an** epicardial artery. STE **that is bulging upward is also more specific than** STE that is sagging.

This "bulging upward" STE is always specific for transmural ischemia or infarction.

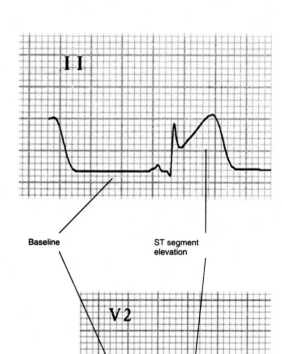

This "sway back" STE is not specific for transmural ischemia or infarction.

More clinical information is required.

If the 74-year-old patient has hypertension, hypercholesterolemia, diabetes, and chest pain and smokes, then this elevation is more likely due to ischemia.

Transmural Ischemia: Pathophysiology

STE should be considered an indication of 100% occlusion of an epicardial artery. The occlusion is the result of chronic disease with an acute superimposed thrombus.

The chronic event requires an atherosclerotic plaque that builds up slowly along the inside of the epicardial artery. At this point, the lesion does not obstruct blood flow either at rest or with increased demand.

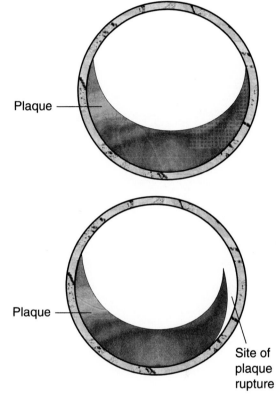

Plaque

The acute event begins with a separation or rupture of the atherosclerotic plaque.

This separation uncovers new surface that immediately attracts the attention of the coagulation system.

Plaque

Site of plaque rupture

The acute event continues with a thrombus formation at the site of the ruptured plaque.

When this occludes 100% of the lumen, the myocardium distal receives no blood flow and suffers ischemia across the entire thickness of myocardium. This is called transmural ischemia.

The ST segment is attracted to the part of the ventricle supplied by the blocked artery.

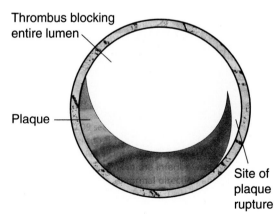

Thrombus blocking entire lumen

Plaque

Site of plaque rupture

Transmural Ischemia: Pathophysiology

The complete occlusion of the epicardial artery results in transmural ischemia in the area of the heart supplied by the involved artery.

Complete occlusion of an epicardial artery represents a severe case of supply and demand mismatch.

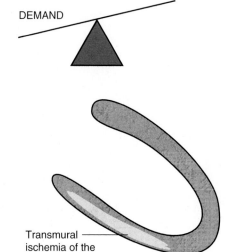

The region of ischemia involves not only the subendocardium but also the entire thickness of myocardium.

Therefore, it is called "transmural" ischemia. After 6 to 12 hours of transmural ischemia, the myocardial cells die, causing permanent cell death, which is known as myocardial infarction.

Transmural ischemia of the inferior wall

Transmural Ischemia: Inferior Wall

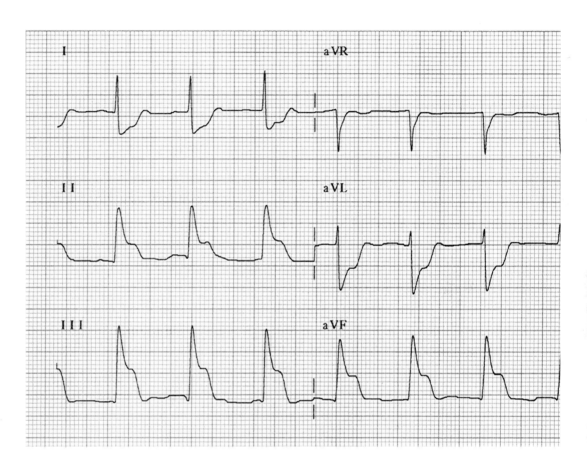

Frontal plane ST axis: +120°.

Concept: ST segment points toward inferior wall transmural ischemia or infarction.

Axis: ST axis points from +90° to +165°.

Pattern: ST elevation in leads III and AVF. Lead II can be elevated, depressed, or isoelectric.

Transmural Inferior Ischemia: Reciprocal Changes

Transmural ischemia of the inferior wall attracts the ST segment toward the inferior wall. This produces STE in the inferior leads III and AVF and usually II as well. The observers or leads on the other side of the heart also see the transmural process, but they see it as going away from them. Therefore, leads I and AVL show ST segment depression. This ST segment depression does not represent additional subendocardial ischemia of the lateral wall. There is no way for the ST segment to point toward the inferior wall without also pointing away from the lateral lead observers. This geometric fact of life is called reciprocal changes. It occurs in lateral transmural ischemia and anterior transmural ischemia as well.

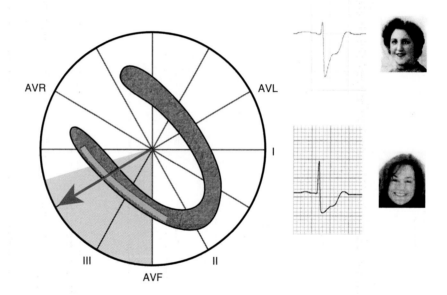

Transmural Inferior Ischemia: Posterior Extension

Transmural ischemia of the inferior wall attracts the ST segment toward the inferior wall. This produces STE in the inferior leads III and AVF, and usually II as well. The ST depression in leads I and AVL are due to reciprocal changes from the inferior process. The anterior leads in inferior transmural ischemia sometimes demonstrate ST segment depression. Following is a side view of the heart from a hypothetical lateral view (from the patient's left side) that shows inferior transmural ischemia. The observer in lead V2 sees this process as going away from him, and this can explain the ST segment depression in lead V2. **The transmural ischemia in this example is not only inferior but also posterior.** (There is also a chance that the ST segment in V2 is pointing away from subendocardial ischemia of the anterior wall, but this adds another disease. "No one test answers all the questions.")

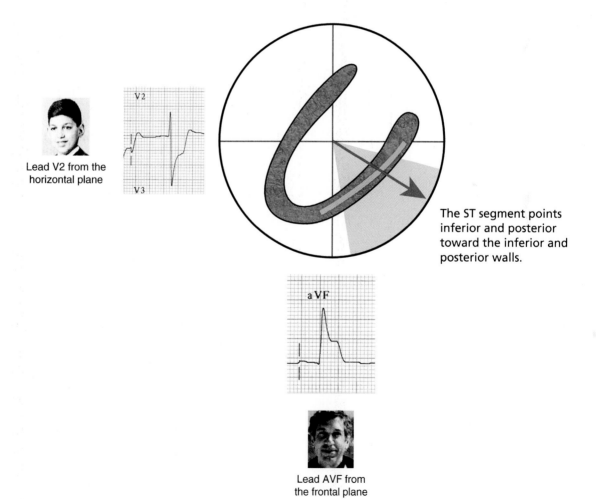

Lead V2 from the
horizontal plane

The ST segment points
inferior and posterior
toward the inferior and
posterior walls.

Lead AVF from
the frontal plane

Transmural Ischemia: Lateral and Apical

Concept: The ST segment points toward apical wall transmural ischemia or infarction.

Axis: The ST axis points from +15° to +75°.

Pattern: There is ST elevation in leads I, II, and AVF. Lead AVL or lead III may show ST elevation as well.

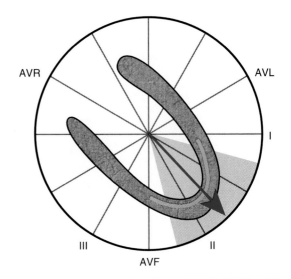

Concept: The ST segment points toward lateral wall transmural ischemia or infarction.

Axis: The ST axis points from 0° to −75°.

Pattern: There is ST elevation in leads I and AVL.

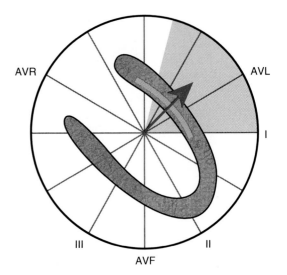

Transmural Ischemia: Septum and Anterior Walls

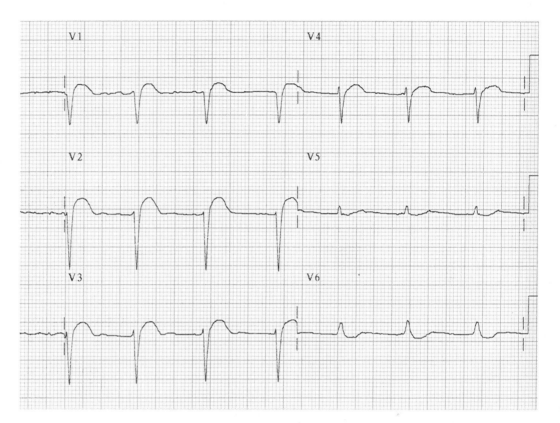

Horizontal plane ST axis: +120°.

Concept: The ST segment points toward the septal and anterior wall transmural ischemia.

Axis: The horizontal plane ST axis points from +120° to +157.5°.

Pattern: ST elevation in leads V1, V2, and V3. V4 may have ST elevation as well.

SUMMARY OF ST AXIS: FRONTAL PLANE

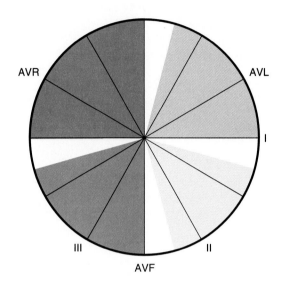

Location of Subendocardial Ischemia	Concept to Understand	ST Axis to Translate the Concept (Don't Memorize)	Pattern of ST Depression (Memorize)
Inferior, apical, lateral	*ST points away from subendocardial ischemia*	−90° to −180°	ST depression in II; leads I and AVF must be isoelectric or depressed

Location of Transmural Ischemia	Concept to Understand	ST Axis to Translate the Concept (Don't Memorize)	Pattern of ST Segment Elevation (Memorize)
Inferior wall	*ST points toward the inferior wall*	+90° to +165°	ST elevation in III, and AVF; lead II may show ST elevation
Apical wall	*ST points toward the apex*	+15° to +75°	ST elevation in I, II, and AVF
Lateral wall	*ST points toward the lateral wall*	0° to −75°	ST elevation in I and AVL

SUMMARY OF ST AXIS: HORIZONTAL PLANE

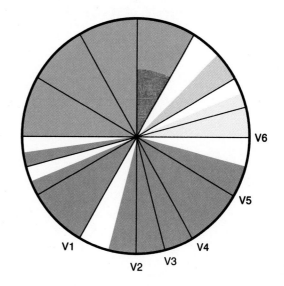

Location of Transmural Ischemia	Concept to Understand	ST Axis to Translate the Concept (Don't' Memorize)	ST Wave Elevation Pattern (Memorize)
Septal	ST axis points toward the septum	+165° to +172.5°	V1 and V2
Septal and anterior	ST axis points toward septum and anterior wall	+120° to +157.5°	V1, V2, V3 (+/− V4)
Septal anterior and lateral	ST axis points toward septum and anterior and lateral walls	+15° to +105°	V2, V3, V4, V5 (+/− V1, +/− V6)
Anterior and lateral	ST axis points toward anterior and lateral walls	+0° to −22.5°	V4, V5, V6 (+/− V3)
Lateral	ST axis points toward the lateral wall	−30° to −45°	V5 and V6
Posterior (only read with an inferior transmural process)	ST axis points toward the posterior wall	−60° to −90°	ST depression in V1 to V5 along with ST elevation in II, II, and AVF
Subendocardial ischemia	ST axis points away from the septum and anterior and lateral walls	−60° to −180°	ST depression in leads V3 and V4. Leads V2 and V5 can be isoelectric or depressed, but **never** elevated

SUMMARY OF ST SEGMENT PATTERNS

Patterns of ST Wave Elevations	Locations of Ischemia
III, AVF (+/− II)	Inferior
I, AVL	Lateral
I, II, AVF	Apical
V1, V2	Septal
V3, V4	Anterior
V5, V6	Lateral

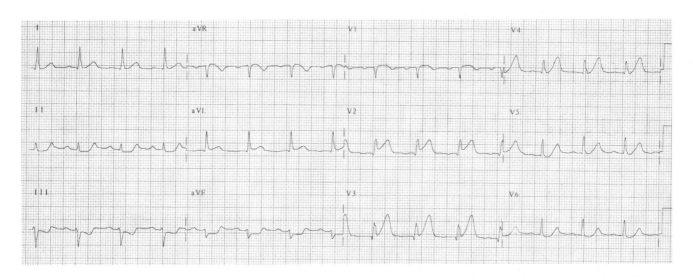

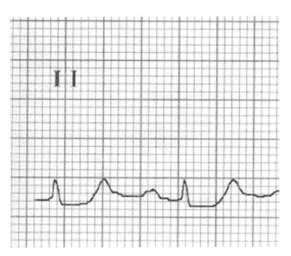

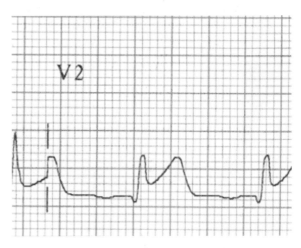

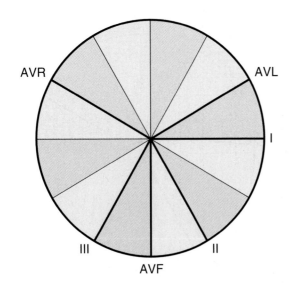

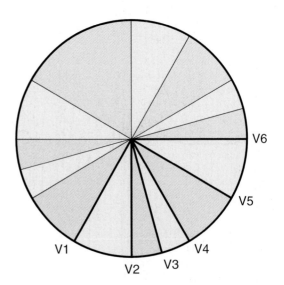

Heart Rate:

Rhythm:

ST Elevation (acute infarction):

II, III, AVF	inferior
I, AVL	lateral
V1, without V2	nonspecific septal
V1 and V2	septal
V3 and V4	anterior
V5 and V6	lateral
V6, without V5	nonspecific lateral

Intervals (measured in the limb leads)

PR: short (< .12)
      normal (.12 to .20)
      long (>0.20 seconds); this is 1st degree AV
      block

QRS: normal (≤0.09 seconds)
      prolonged (.10 or .11); this is intraventricular
      conduction delay (IVCD)
      Bundle Branch Block (.12 seconds or greater)

QT:

ST Depression (ischemia or infarction):

I, II, III, AVL, AVF	diffuse subendocardial ischemia or infarction
V2, V3, V4, V5	diffuse subendocardial ischemia or infarction

P axis: normal
           rightward
           arm-lead reversal or dextrocardia
           junctional rhythm

QRS axis: normal
           left anterior hemiblock
           left posterior hemiblock
           indeterminate

Q waves (infarction):

II, III, AVF	inferior
I, AVL	lateral
V1, without V2	nonspecific septal
V1 and V2	septal
V3 and V4	anterior
V5 and V6	lateral
V6, without V5	nonspecific lateral

T wave inversion (ischemia or infarction):

II, III, AVF	inferior
I, AVL	lateral
V1, without V2	nonspecific septal
V1 and V2	septal
V3 and V4	anterior
V5 and V6	lateral
V6, without V5	nonspecific lateral

Hypertrophy:

Right atrial: Tall P wave 2.5 mm in II, III, or AVF

Left atrial: Deep negative part of P wave in V1

LVH: R wave in 1 + S wave in III ≥ 25mV
     S wave in V1 + R wave in V5 ≥ 35mV

RVH: Mean QRS either anterior, or rightward

The heart rate is 88; the rhythm is sinus. The PR interval measures 0.22 seconds; this indicates 1° AV block. The QRS interval measures 0.08 seconds and is normal. The QT interval measures 0.34 seconds. The P axis is normal at +60°. The mean QRS axis is −15° in the frontal plane and +15° in the horizontal plane. The ST axis in the horizontal plane is +150° and points toward the septum and anterior walls, consistent with transmural ischemia or infarction. *(The EKG results from rupture of an atherosclerotic plaque with a superimposed 100% occlusive thrombus. The ST axis in the frontal plane is −90°. This may represent subendocardial ischemia or reciprocal changes from the anterior process (Because the anterior wall is also superior). Regardless, ST elevation always takes precedence over ST depression or T wave changes, because the transmural process requires immediate therapy. This EKG will progress to myocardial infarction (Chapter 15) of the septum and anterior walls if the 100% occlusion lesion is not relieved quickly.*

Localizing exactly where the transmural process is occurring is not as rock solid as it sounds. Remember this is a 100-year-old test done by having a patient put his or her hands and feet in pickle brine, and then connecting wires to a galvanometer. *The key finding is that the ST segment points toward an area of myocardium. This means transmural ischemia and a 100% occluded artery, which requires intervention to eliminate the obstruction.*

Parts of the answer sheets are "grayed out" because these sections have not yet been covered. Answer only the parts that are not highlighted.

Worksheet 13-2

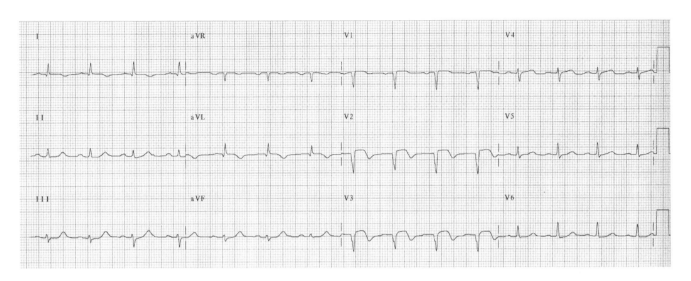

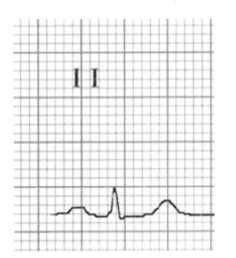

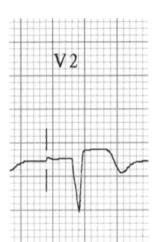

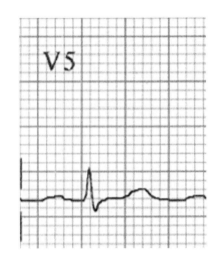

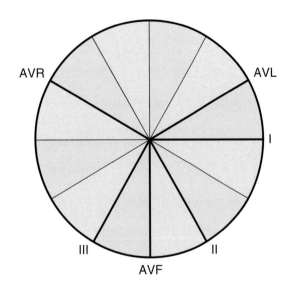

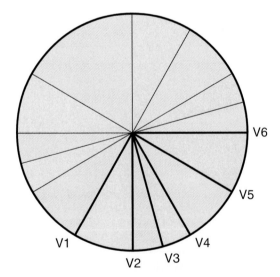

Heart Rate:

Rhythm:

Intervals (measured in the limb leads)

PR: short (< .12)
        normal (.12 to .20)
        long (>0.20 seconds); this is 1st degree AV block

QRS: normal (≤0.09 seconds)
        prolonged (.10 or .11); this is intraventricular conduction delay (IVCD)
        Bundle Branch Block (.12 seconds or greater)

QT:

P axis: normal
         rightward
         arm-lead reversal or dextrocardia
         junctional rhythm

QRS axis: normal
           left anterior hemiblock
           left posterior hemiblock
           indeterminate

T wave inversion (ischemia or infarction):

II,III,AVF	inferior
I, AVL	lateral
V1, without V2	nonspecific septal
V1 and V2	septal
V3 and V4	anterior
V5 and V6	lateral
V6, without V5	nonspecific lateral

ST Elevation (acute infarction):

II,III,AVF	inferior
I, AVL	lateral
V1, without V2	nonspecific septal
V1 and V2	septal
V3 and V4	anterior
V5 and V6	lateral
V6, without V5	nonspecific lateral

ST Depression (ischemia or infarction):

I,II,III,AVL,AVF	diffuse subendocardial ischemia or infarction
V2,V3,V4,V5	diffuse subendocardial ischemia or infarction

Q waves (infarction):

II,III,AVF	inferior
I, AVL	lateral
V1, without V2	nonspecific septal
V1 and V2	septal
V3 and V4	anterior
V5 and V6	lateral
V6, without V5	nonspecific lateral

Hypertrophy:

Right atrial: Tall P wave 2.5 mm in II, III, or AVF

Left atrial: Deep negative part of P wave in V1

LVH: R wave in 1 + S wave in III ≥ 25mV
       S wave in V1 + R wave in V5 ≥ 35mV

RVH: Mean QRS either anterior, or rightward

The heart rate is 83 beats per minute. The PR interval measures 0.18 seconds. The QRS interval measures 0.08 seconds. The QT interval measures 0.36 seconds. (There is low voltage on this EKG. This is discussed in Chapter 17.) The P axis is +60°. The mean QRS axis is 0° in the frontal plane and −45° in the horizontal plane. The frontal plane T axis is +105°, which points away from the lateral wall, indicating subendocardial or ischemia. In the horizontal plane, the ST axis is +120°, indicating septal and anterior wall transmural ischemia or infarction. Again, this patient should be immediately evaluated to determine the clinical appropriateness of clot removing therapy. The ST depression in lead V6 may represent its reciprocal view of the ST segment moving toward the septum.

Parts of the answer sheets are "grayed out" because these sections have not yet been covered. Answer only the parts that are not highlighted.

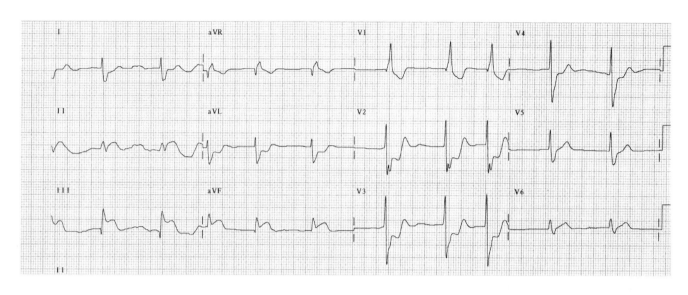

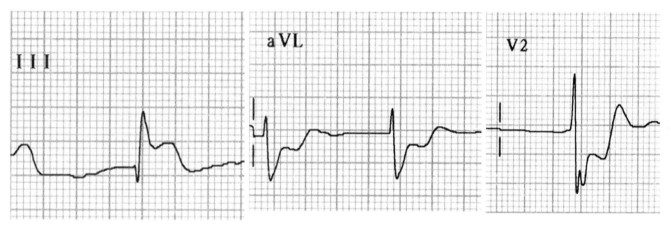

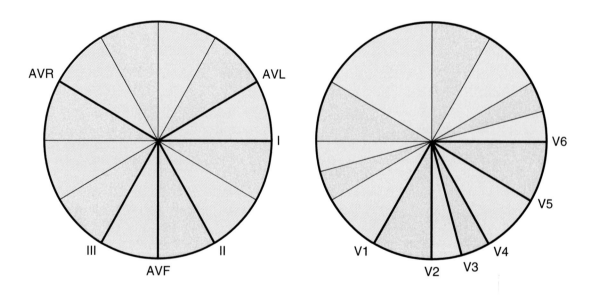

Heart Rate:

Rhythm:

Intervals (measured in the limb leads)

PR: short (< .12)
normal (.12 to .20)
long (>0.20 seconds); this is 1st degree AV block

QRS: normal (≤0.09 seconds)
prolonged (.10 or .11); this is intraventricular conduction delay (IVCD)
Bundle Branch Block (.12 seconds or greater)

QT:

P axis: normal
rightward
arm-lead reversal or dextrocardia
junctional rhythm

QRS axis: normal
left anterior hemiblock
left posterior hemiblock
indeterminate

T wave inversion (ischemia or infarction):

II,III,AVF	inferior
I, AVL	lateral
V1, without V2	nonspecific septal
V1 and V2	septal
V3 and V4	anterior
V5 and V6	lateral
V6, without V5	nonspecific lateral

ST Elevation (acute infarction):

II,III,AVF	inferior
I, AVL	lateral
V1, without V2	nonspecific septal
V1 and V2	septal
V3 and V4	anterior
V5 and V6	lateral
V6, without V5	nonspecific lateral

ST Depression (ischemia or infarction):

I,II,III,AVL,AVF	diffuse subendocardial ischemia or infarction
V2,V3,V4,V5	diffuse subendocardial ischemia or infarction

Q waves (infarction):

II,III,AVF	inferior
I, AVL	lateral
V1, without V2	nonspecific septal
V1 and V2	septal
V3 and V4	anterior
V5 and V6	lateral
V6, without V5	nonspecific lateral

Hypertrophy:

Right atrial: Tall P wave 2.5 mm in II, III, or AVF

Left atrial: Deep negative part of P wave in V1

LVH: R wave in 1 + S wave in III ≥ 25mV
S wave in V1 + R wave in V5 ≥ 35mV

RVH: Mean QRS either anterior, or rightward

The rhythm is irregularly irregular, which indicates atrial fibrillation. The rate is determined by counting the number of QRS complexes between the 6-second markers on the EKG. These each mark a 3-second interval. There are six QRS complexes between the markers, which makes the ventricular rate 60 per minute. The PR interval is then undefined. The QRS interval measures 0.12 seconds, indicating BBB. The last part of the QRS points rightward in lead I in the frontal plane and rightward in the horizontal plane in V6. The last part of the QRS is positive in lead V1, pointing toward the right ventricle, indicating RBBB. The QT interval is 0.36. The P axis is undefined in atrial fibrillation. The mean QRS axis in the frontal plane is +150°, indicating left posterior hemiblock. The ST axis in the frontal plane is +120° pointing at the inferior wall and indicating transmural ischemia or infarction. Leads I and AVL show reciprocal ST depression, because they watch the ST pointing toward the inferior wall and away from them. In the horizontal plane, the ST axis is −60°, and is pointing toward the posterior wall, indicating transmural ischemia or infarction of the posterior wall. When the ST segment is pointing toward the posterior wall, it shows up on the EKG as going backward, away from lead V2, and showing ST depression in lead V2. When there is ST elevation in the inferior leads, the ST axis of −60° to −90° in the horizontal plane probably represents posterior transmural ischemia or infarction.

Parts of the answer sheets are "grayed out" because these sections have not yet been covered. Answer only the parts that are not highlighted.

Worksheet 13-4

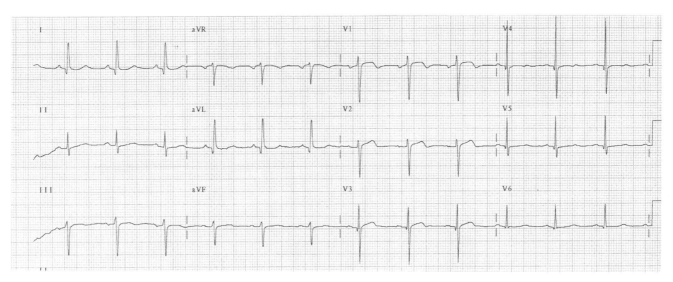

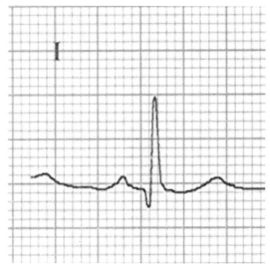

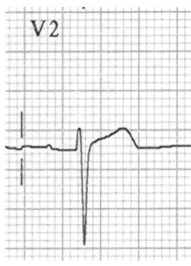

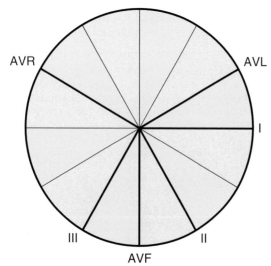

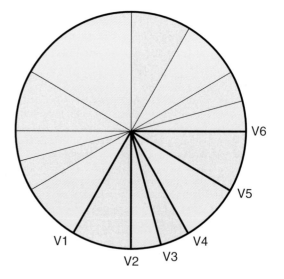

Heart Rate:

Rhythm:

Intervals (measured in the limb leads)

PR: short (< .12)
            normal (.12 to .20)
            long (>0.20 seconds); this is 1st degree AV
            block

QRS: normal (≤0.09 seconds)
            prolonged (.10 or .11); this is intraventricular
            conduction delay (IVCD)
            Bundle Branch Block (.12 seconds or greater)

QT:

P axis / QRS axis

P axis: normal
              rightward
              arm-lead reversal or dextrocardia
              junctional rhythm

QRS axis: normal
              left anterior hemiblock
              left posterior hemiblock
              indeterminate

T wave inversion (ischemia or infarction):

II,III,AVF	inferior
I, AVL	lateral
V1, without V2	nonspecific septal
V1 and V2	septal
V3 and V4	anterior
V5 and V6	lateral
V6, without V5	nonspecific lateral

ST Elevation (acute infarction):

II,III,AVF	inferior
I, AVL	lateral
V1, without V2	nonspecific septal
V1 and V2	septal
V3 and V4	anterior
V5 and V6	lateral
V6, without V5	nonspecific lateral

ST Depression (ischemia or infarction):

I,II,III,AVL,AVF	diffuse subendocardial ischemia or infarction
V2,V3,V4,V5	diffuse subendocardial ischemia or infarction

Q waves (infarction):

II,III,AVF	inferior
I, AVL	lateral
V1, without V2	nonspecific septal
V1 and V2	septal
V3 and V4	anterior
V5 and V6	lateral
V6, without V5	nonspecific lateral

Hypertrophy:

Right atrial: Tall P wave 2.5 mm in II, III, or AVF

Left atrial: Deep negative part of P wave in V1

LVH: R wave in 1 + S wave in III ≥ 25mV
        S wave in V1 + R wave in V5 ≥ 35mV

RVH: Mean QRS either anterior, or rightward

The heart rate is 75 per minute and represents sinus rhythm. The PR interval measures 0.16 seconds. The QRS interval measures 0.09 seconds and is normal. The QT interval measures 0.40 seconds and is long. The P axis is normal at +15°. The mean QRS axis is −15° in the frontal plane and −22.5° in the horizontal plane. The T axis in the frontal plane is +30° and is normal. The frontal plane ST axis is normal. There is ST segment elevation in V1, V2, and V3. The ST axis in the horizontal plane is +150°, indicating septal and anterior wall transmural ischemia or infarction.

ST segment elevation indicates a 100% occlusion of an epicardial artery. The pathophysiology is a ruptured atherosclerotic plaque, with a superimposed thrombus. The patient should be evaluated as soon as possible. Immediate therapy would be directed at opening the artery. The location of the defect should be in the left anterior descending artery because that supplies the septum and anterior wall. Some complications include bundle branch block, congestive heart failure, pulmonary edema, and shock.

Parts of the answer sheets are "grayed out" because these sections have not yet been covered. Answer only the parts that are not highlighted.

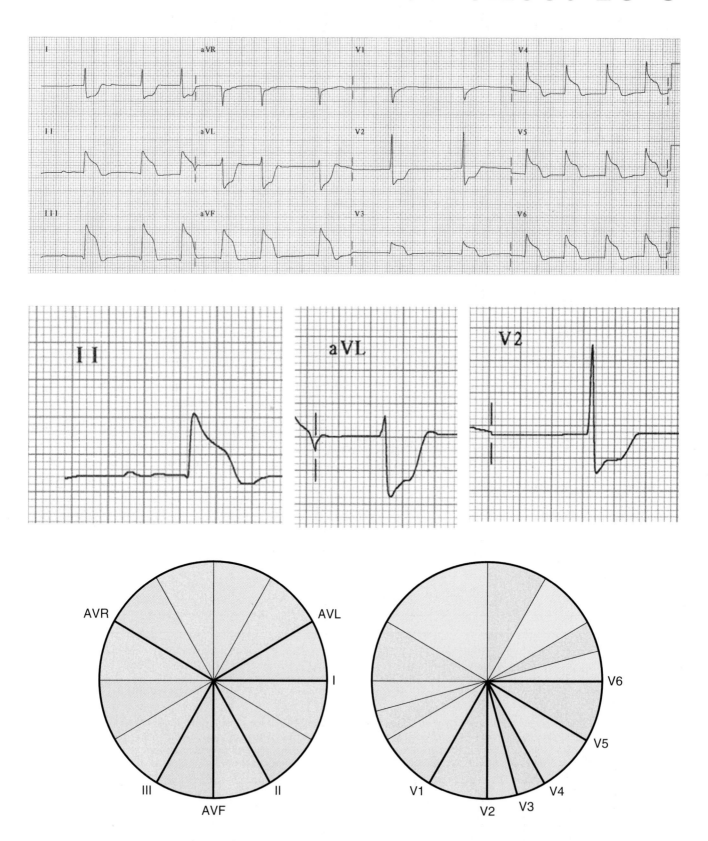

Heart Rate:

Rhythm:

Intervals (measured in the limb leads)

PR: short (< .12)
     normal (.12 to .20)
     long (>0.20 seconds); this is 1st degree AV
     block

QRS: normal (≤0.09 seconds)
      prolonged (.10 or .11); this is intraventricular
      conduction delay (IVCD)
      Bundle Branch Block (.12 seconds or greater)

QT:

P axis: normal
           rightward
           arm-lead reversal or dextrocardia
           junctional rhythm

QRS axis: normal
           left anterior hemiblock
           left posterior hemiblock
           indeterminate

T wave inversion (ischemia or infarction):

II,III,AVF	inferior
I, AVL	lateral
V1, without V2	nonspecific septal
V1 and V2	septal
V3 and V4	anterior
V5 and V6	lateral
V6, without V5	nonspecific lateral

ST Elevation (acute infarction):

II,III,AVF	inferior
I, AVL	lateral
V1, without V2	nonspecific septal
V1 and V2	septal
V3 and V4	anterior
V5 and V6	lateral
V6, without V5	nonspecific lateral

ST Depression (ischemia or infarction):

I,II,III,AVL,AVF	diffuse subendocardial ischemia or infarction
V2,V3,V4,V5	diffuse subendocardial ischemia or infarction

Q waves (infarction):

II,III,AVF	inferior
I, AVL	lateral
V1, without V2	nonspecific septal
V1 and V2	septal
V3 and V4	anterior
V5 and V6	lateral
V6, without V5	nonspecific lateral

Hypertrophy:

Right atrial: Tall P wave 2.5 mm in II, III, or AVF

Left atrial: Deep negative part of P wave in V1

LVH: R wave in 1 + S wave in III ≥ 25mV
      S wave in V1 + R wave in V5 ≥ 35mV

RVH: Mean QRS either anterior, or rightward

The rhythm is irregularly irregular, therefore it is atrial fibrillation. To calculate the ventricular rate, measure the number of QRS complexes between the marked 6-second intervals, which are present of most EKGs. On this EKG, there are six QRS complexes, which makes the ventricular rate 60 per minute. The PR interval is undefined, because in atrial fibrillation there is no P wave activity. The QRS interval measures 0.08 seconds and can only be seen reliably in lead AVR. The QT interval measures 0.32 seconds. The P axis is undefined. The mean QRS axis in the frontal plane is +90° and in the horizontal plane is +15°. The ST axis in the frontal plane is +105°. It is pointing at the inferior wall and indicates transmural ischemia or infarction of the inferior wall. This EKG is caused by a ruptured atherosclerotic plaque in a coronary artery, with a 100% occlusion by a superimposed thrombus. Note the ST depression in leads I and AVL. These are called reciprocal changes and reflect the ST segment pointing toward the inferior wall and away from them. There is no way for the ST to point toward the inferior wall at +105° without leads I and AVL having the ST show up as negative. In the horizontal plane, the ST axis is +15° and indicates transmural ischemia of the anterior and lateral walls as well. The ST segment in the horizontal plane, by pointing at the anterior and lateral walls, shows up in lead V1 and V2 as negative. These are probably reciprocal changes as well.

Parts of the answer sheets are "grayed out" because these sections have not yet been covered. Answer only the parts that are not highlighted.

Inferior Q Waves (Initial QRS Axis)

The QRS complex represents ventricular depolarization. The initial part of the complex, called the QRS init 0.04, can be evaluated separately from the rest of the QRS complex. This initial part of the QRS provides information on transmural infarction.

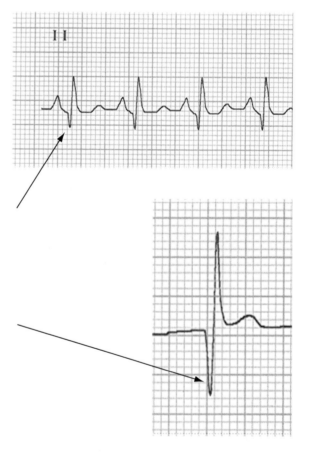

The initial part of the QRS is considered the first little box or 0.04 seconds of the complex.

In these examples, the initial part of the QRS is negative.

The Normal Initial Part of the QRS

The normal initial part (defined as the first 0.04 seconds of the QRS) of the QRS in the frontal plane results from normal initial depolarization of all segments of the left ventricle. A tiny q wave in leads I and V6 is normal and expected (Chapter 9), because it represents septal depolarization. However, **these q waves must be less than 0.04 seconds wide to be normal.**

When each part is added together, the resultant force points inferior and to the left.

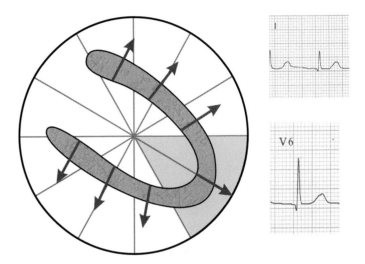

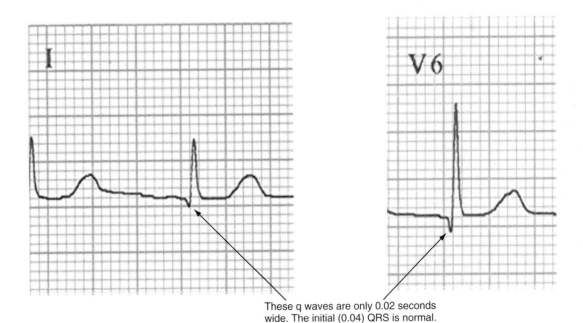

These q waves are only 0.02 seconds wide. The initial (0.04) QRS is normal.

Transmural Infarction

Complete occlusion of an epicardial artery by a ruptured plaque and superimposed thrombus causes transmural ischemia (Chapter 13). When the obstruction is not relieved, transmural infarction results. **The hallmark of transmural infarction on the EKG is an abnormality of the initial part of the QRS, which points away from the infarcted area.** Since the initial part (0.04 seconds) of the QRS points away from the infarct, it produces a negative part of the QRS in the leads that look directly at the affected region. This negative part is called a Q wave, although a very narrow and short r wave, with a wide S wave would be equivalent.

After a transmural infarction the damaged segment of the myocardium can no longer depolarize normally.

The infarcted area is unable to contribute its share to the QRS initial forces.

This changes the axis, pointing it away from the infarcted area.

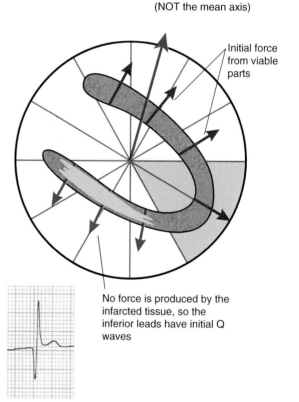

The initial 0.04 seconds of the QRS (NOT the mean axis)

Initial force from viable parts

No force is produced by the infarcted tissue, so the inferior leads have initial Q waves

Transmural Inferior Infarction

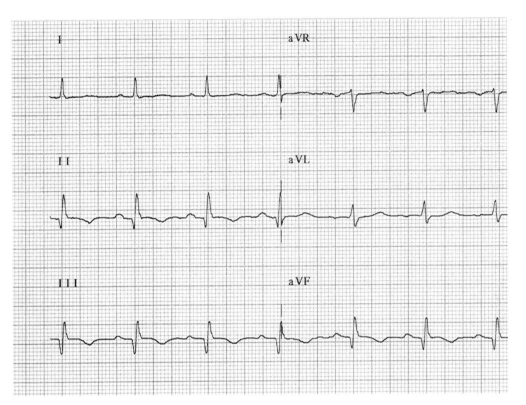

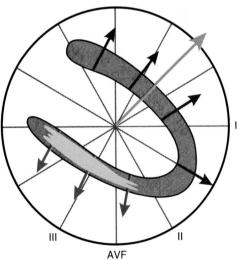

Frontal plane initial QRS axis: −45°.

Concept: The initial part of the QRS points away from inferior transmural infarction.

Axis: The initial part of the QRS points at −45° to −90° in the frontal plane.

Pattern: There are initial significant Q waves in leads II, III, and AVF.

Concept: The QRSinit.04 axis points away from lateral transmural infarction.

Axis: The points at +105° to +180° in the frontal plane.

Pattern: There are initial 0.04 second Q waves in leads I and AVL.

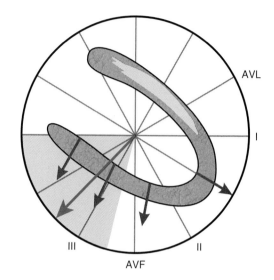

Concept: The QRSinit.04 axis points away from apical transmural infarction.

Axis: The points at −105° to −165° in the frontal plane.

Pattern: There are initial Q waves in leads I, II, and AVF.

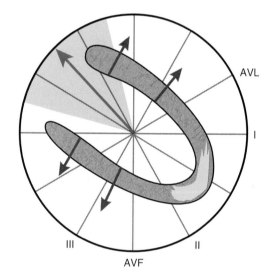

Transmural Infarction: Less Specific Criteria

The following EKG shows a common pattern, where the initial QRS falls in a gray area, between clearly normal and clearly abnormal. The initial QRS points slightly away from the apex but not definitely away from the inferior wall. **This pattern is sometimes called "nonspecific inferior Q waves."** It is less specific than the standard criteria for inferior infarction. Roughly half of the patients with this pattern have other evidence of inferior infarction.

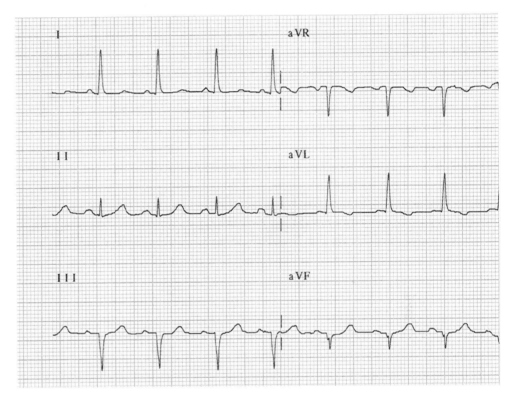

Frontal plane initial QRS axis: −15°.

Concept: The initial QRS isn't clearly normal but is not clearly abnormal either. It doesn't point comfortably toward the apex but doesn't point definitely away from the inferior wall.

Axis: Points at −15° to −30° in the frontal plane.

Pattern: There are Q waves in leads III and AVF, but NOT in lead II.

SUMMARY OF INITIAL QRS AXIS: FRONTAL PLANE

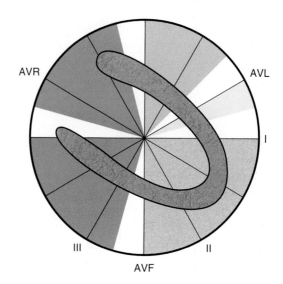

Location of Transmural Infarction	Concept to Understand	Initial QRS Axis to Translate the Concept (Don't Memorize)	Q Wave Pattern (Memorize)
Inferior	$QRS_{init.\ 04}$ axis points away from inferior wall	−45° to −90°	II, III, AVF
Lateral	$QRS_{init.\ 04}$ axis points away from lateral wall	+105° to +180°	I, AVL
Apical	$QRS_{init.\ 04}$ axis points away from apex	−105° to −165°	I, II, AVF
Nonspecific inferior	$QRS_{init.\ 04}$ axis borderline superior	−15° to −30°	III, AVF, but not II
Normal $QRS_{init.\ 04}$ axis	$QRS_{init.\ 04}$ axis points toward the apex	0° to +60°	If any, only III or AVL

SUMMARY OF INITIAL QRS: FRONTAL PLANE PATTERN

Patterns of Q Waves	Locations of Infarct
II, III, AVF	Inferior
I, AVL	Lateral
I, II, AVF	Apical

Worksheet 14-1

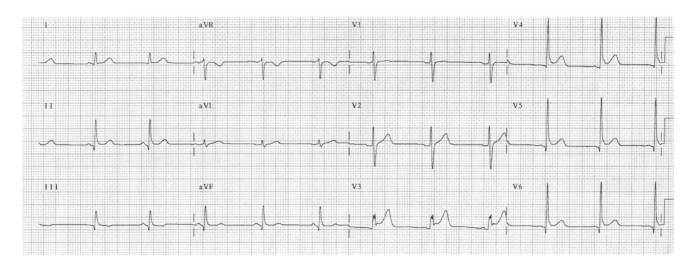

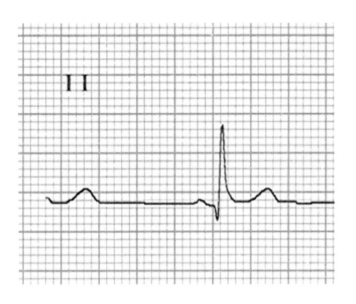

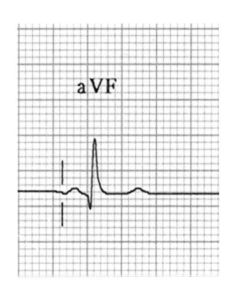

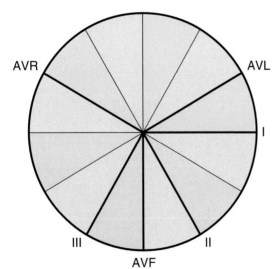

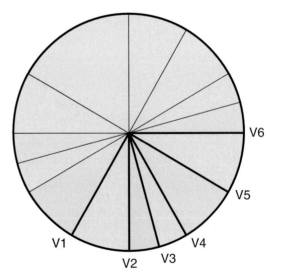

Heart Rate:

Rhythm:

Intervals (measured in the limb leads)

PR: short (< .12)
        normal (.12 to .20)
        long (>0.20 seconds); this is 1st degree AV
        block

QRS: normal (≤0.09 seconds)
        prolonged (.10 or .11); this is intraventricular
        conduction delay (IVCD)
        Bundle Branch Block (.12 seconds or greater)

QT:

P axis: normal
          rightward
          arm-lead reversal or dextrocardia
          junctional rhythm

QRS axis: normal
          left anterior hemiblock
          left posterior hemiblock
          indeterminate

T wave inversion (ischemia or infarction):

II,III,AVF	inferior
I, AVL	lateral
V1, without V2	nonspecific septal
V1 and V2	septal
V3 and V4	anterior
V5 and V6	lateral
V6, without V5	nonspecific lateral

ST Elevation (acute infarction):

II,III,AVF	inferior
I, AVL	lateral
V1, without V2	nonspecific septal
V1 and V2	septal
V3 and V4	anterior
V5 and V6	lateral
V6, without V5.	nonspecific lateral

ST Depression (ischemia or infarction):

I,II,III,AVL,AVF	diffuse subendocardial ischemia or infarction
V2,V3,V4,V5	diffuse subendocardial ischemia or infarction

Q waves (infarction):

II,III,AVF	inferior
I, AVL	lateral
V1, without V2	nonspecific septal
V1 and V2	septal
V3 and V4	anterior
V5 and V6	lateral
V6, without V5	nonspecific lateral

Hypertrophy:

Right atrial: Tall P wave 2.5 mm in II, III, or AVF

Left atrial: Deep negative part of P wave in V1

LVH: R wave in 1 + S wave in III ≥ 25mV
        S wave in V1 + R wave in V5 ≥ 35mV

RVH: Mean QRS either anterior, or rightward

The heart rate is 68 beats per minute. The PR interval is 0.12 seconds. The QRS interval is 0.08 seconds (measured best in leads I and AVL). The QT interval measures 0.36 seconds. The P axis is $+60°$. The mean QRS axis is $+60°$ in the frontal plane and $-7.5°$ in the horizontal plane. The axis for the initial part of the QRS is negative in leads II, III, AVF, and AVR. It is positive in leads I and AVL. This combination gives an axis of $-45°$, which points away from the inferior wall and indicates transmural infarction. An estimate of the time the infarction occurred can be given based on the T wave and ST segments in the plane of the infarction. If the T and ST are normal, the time is considered "age indeterminate, or old." If the T waves or ST segment are abnormal in the plane, then the infarction is considered "recent or possibly acute." In the horizontal plane, the initial part of the QRS points to $+90°$. This points away from the posterior wall and indicates that the inferior infarction has extended to the posterior wall as well (remember the right coronary artery typically supplies both walls). In the horizontal plane, the ST segment points to $+30°$, this points toward the septum and anterior and lateral walls, indicating transmural ischemia or infarction. When any degree of ST elevation or depression is present on the first EKG, a second EKG taken 20 minutes later may show evolution of changes and be more specific and helpful in the diagnostic process.

Parts of the answer sheets are "grayed out" because these sections have not yet been covered. Answer only the parts that are not highlighted.

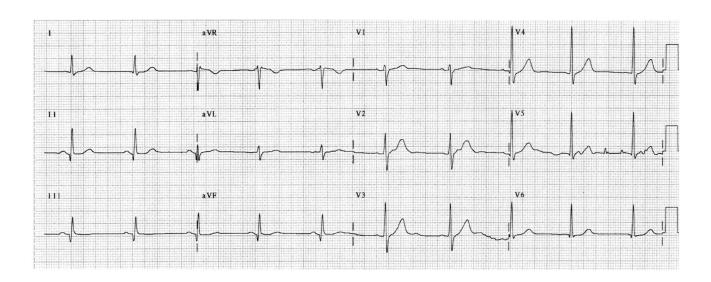

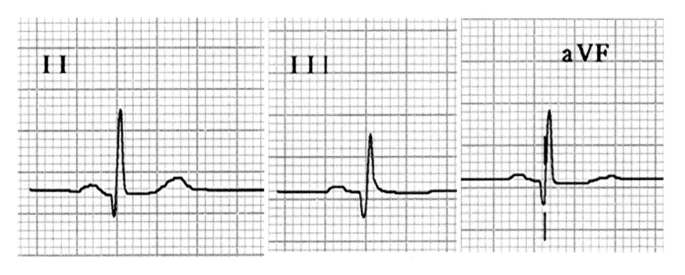

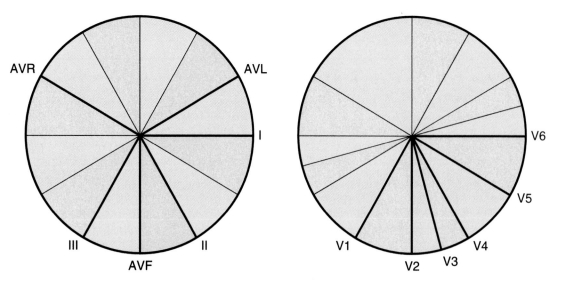

Heart Rate:

Rhythm:

Intervals (measured in the limb leads)

PR: short (< .12)
       normal (.12 to .20)
       long (>0.20 seconds); this is 1st degree AV
       block

QRS: normal (≤0.09 seconds)
       prolonged (.10 or .11); this is intraventricular
       conduction delay (IVCD)
       Bundle Branch Block (.12 seconds or greater)

QT:

P axis: normal
               rightward
               arm-lead reversal or dextrocardia
               junctional rhythm

QRS axis: normal
               left anterior hemiblock
               left posterior hemiblock
               indeterminate

T wave inversion (ischemia or infarction):

II,III,AVF	inferior
I, AVL	lateral
V1, without V2	nonspecific septal
V1 and V2	septal
V3 and V4	anterior
V5 and V6	lateral
V6, without V5	nonspecific lateral

ST Elevation (acute infarction):

II,III,AVF	inferior
I, AVL	lateral
V1, without V2	nonspecific septal
V1 and V2	septal
V3 and V4	anterior
V5 and V6	lateral
V6, without V5.	nonspecific lateral

ST Depression (ischemia or infarction):

I,II,III,AVL,AVF	diffuse subendocardial ischemia or infarction
V2,V3,V4,V5	diffuse subendocardial ischemia or infarction

Q waves (infarction):

II,III,AVF	inferior
I, AVL	lateral
V1, without V2	nonspecific septal
V1 and V2	septal
V3 and V4	anterior
V5 and V6	lateral
V6, without V5	nonspecific lateral

Hypertrophy:

Right atrial: Tall P wave 2.5 mm in II, III, or AVF

Left atrial: Deep negative part of P wave in V1

LVH: R wave in 1 + S wave in III ≥ 25mV
      S wave in V1 + R wave in V5 ≥ 35mV

RVH: Mean QRS either anterior, or rightward

The heart rate is 58 beats per minute. The PR interval 0.16 seconds. The QRS interval is 0.08 seconds. The QT interval is 0.40 seconds. The P axis is +75°. The mean QRS axis is +60° in the frontal plane and +15° in the horizontal plane. In the frontal plane, the axis of the initial part of the QRS is −45°, pointing away from the inferior wall and indicating infarction of the inferior wall. In the horizontal plane, the axis for the initial part of the QRS is +90°, which indicates infarction of the posterior wall as well. The T waves and ST segments in the frontal plane are normal. In the horizontal plane, the T waves and ST segments have nonspecific changes only. There, the infarction diagnosed by the initial parts of the QRS (inferior and posterior) is considered age indeterminate, or old.

Parts of the answer sheets are "grayed out" because these sections have not yet been covered. Answer only the parts that are not highlighted.

Worksheet 14-3

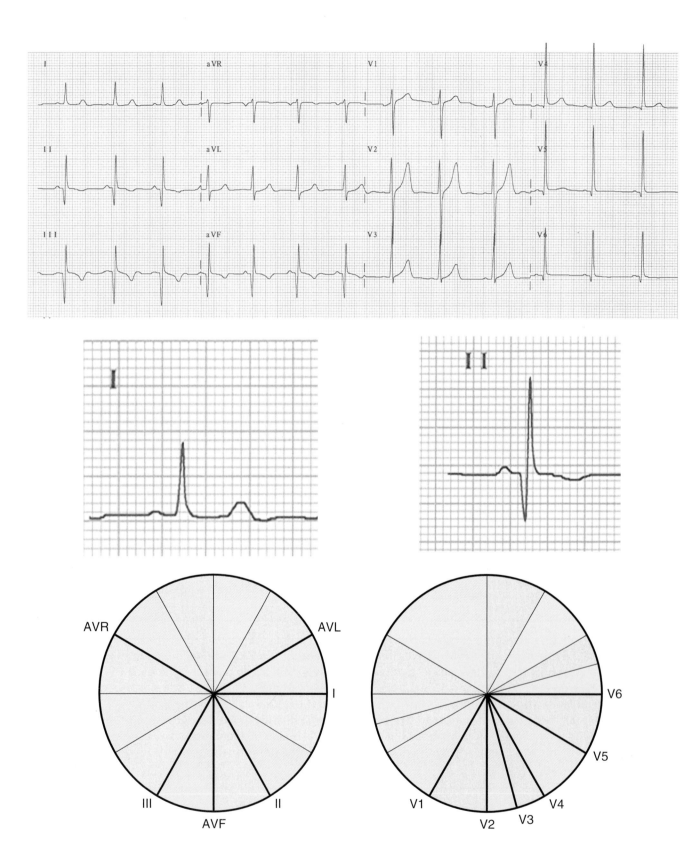

Heart Rate:

Rhythm:

ST Elevation (acute infarction):

II,III,AVF	inferior
I, AVL	lateral
V1, without V2	nonspecific septal
V1 and V2	septal
V3 and V4	anterior
V5 and V6	lateral
V6, without V5.	nonspecific lateral

Intervals (measured in the limb leads)

PR: short (< .12)
        normal (.12 to .20)
        long (>0.20 seconds); this is 1st degree AV
        block

QRS: normal (≤0.09 seconds)
        prolonged (.10 or .11); this is intraventricular
        conduction delay (IVCD)
        Bundle Branch Block (.12 seconds or greater)

QT:

ST Depression (ischemia or infarction):

I,II,III,AVL,AVF	diffuse subendocardial ischemia or infarction
V2,V3,V4,V5	diffuse subendocardial ischemia or infarction

P axis: normal
            rightward
            arm-lead reversal or dextrocardia
            junctional rhythm

QRS axis: normal
            left anterior hemiblock
            left posterior hemiblock
            indeterminate

Q waves (infarction):

II,III,AVF	inferior
I, AVL	lateral
V1, without V2	nonspecific septal
V1 and V2	septal
V3 and V4	anterior
V5 and V6	lateral
V6, without V5	nonspecific lateral

T wave inversion (ischemia or infarction):

II,III,AVF	inferior
I, AVL	lateral
V1, without V2	nonspecific septal
V1 and V2	septal
V3 and V4	anterior
V5 and V6	lateral
V6, without V5	nonspecific lateral

Hypertrophy:

Right atrial: Tall P wave 2.5 mm in II, III, or AVF

Left atrial: Deep negative part of P wave in V1

LVH: R wave in 1 + S wave in III ≥ 25mV
      S wave in V1 + R wave in V5 ≥ 35mV

RVH: Mean QRS either anterior, or rightward

The heart rate is 79 beats per minute. This is sinus rhythm. The PR interval measures 0.12 seconds. The QRS interval measures 0.09 seconds. The QT interval measures 0.38 seconds, which is long. The P axis is normal (+60°). The mean QRS axis is 0° in the frontal plane and −7.5° in the horizontal plane. The initial QRS axis is abnormal in the frontal plane (pattern: Q waves in II, III, and AVF or axis: initial part of QRS is −45°, indicating transmural infarction of the inferior wall. There is no ST elevation, so it does not appear that the transmural ischemia, which caused this infarction is still present. When ST elevation is associated with Q waves, it suggests that the infarction is acute. When the ST segments and T waves are not totally normal, it is still useful to consider the infarction as possibly acute or recent, so that appropriate clinical caution is taken. (Reading the T wave axis in the frontal plane, the T is −60°, consistent with inferior ischemia or infarction.) When Q waves are present, the most useful reading of the ST segments and T waves is an estimation of the time infarction occurred. In the horizontal plane, the initial QRS is abnormal as well. (Tall wide R wave in lead V2, Q waves in leads V5 and V6.) The initial part of the QRS is +120°. This is borderline but suggests infarction of the posterior and lateral walls. The ST axis in the horizontal plane is nonspecific.

Parts of the answer sheets are "grayed out" because these sections have not yet been covered. Answer only the parts that are not highlighted.

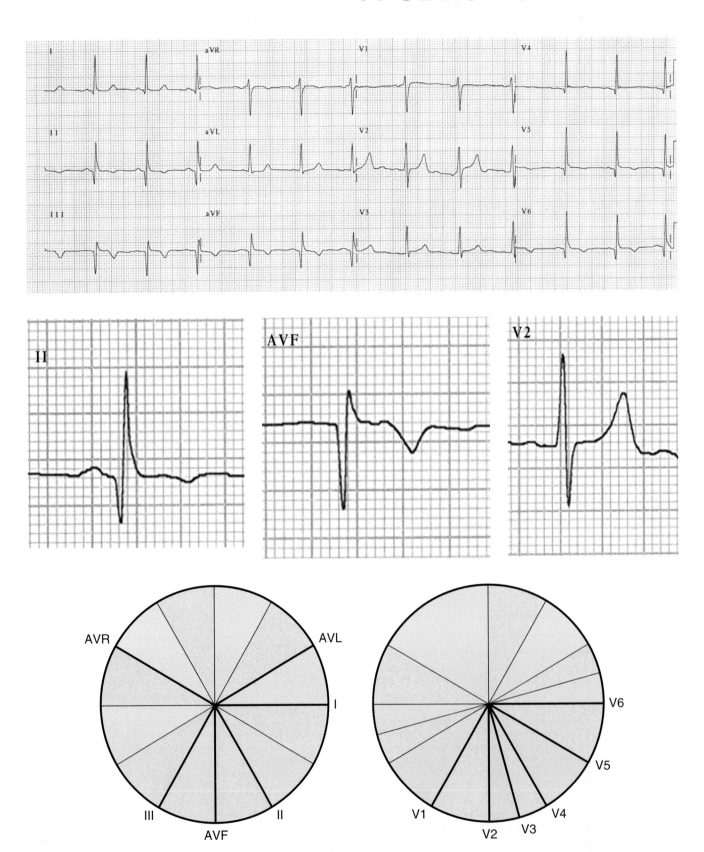

Heart Rate:

Rhythm:

ST Elevation (acute infarction):

II,III,AVF	inferior
I, AVL	lateral
V1, without V2	nonspecific septal
V1 and V2	septal
V3 and V4	anterior
V5 and V6	lateral
V6, without V5.	nonspecific lateral

Intervals (measured in the limb leads)

PR: short (< .12)
normal (.12 to .20)
long (>0.20 seconds); this is 1st degree AV block

QRS: normal (≤0.09 seconds)
prolonged (.10 or .11); this is intraventricular conduction delay (IVCD)
Bundle Branch Block (.12 seconds or greater)

QT:

ST Depression (ischemia or infarction):

I,II,III,AVL,AVF	diffuse subendocardial ischemia or infarction
V2,V3,V4,V5	diffuse subendocardial ischemia or infarction

P axis: normal
rightward
arm-lead reversal or dextrocardia
junctional rhythm

QRS axis: normal
left anterior hemiblock
left posterior hemiblock
indeterminate

Q waves (infarction):

II,III,AVF	inferior
I, AVL	lateral
V1, without V2	nonspecific septal
V1 and V2	septal
V3 and V4	anterior
V5 and V6	lateral
V6, without V5	nonspecific lateral

T wave inversion (ischemia or infarction):

II,III,AVF	inferior
I, AVL	lateral
V1, without V2	nonspecific septal
V1 and V2	septal
V3 and V4	anterior
V5 and V6	lateral
V6, without V5	nonspecific lateral

Hypertrophy:

Right atrial: Tall P wave 2.5 mm in II, III, or AVF

Left atrial: Deep negative part of P wave in V1

LVH: R wave in 1 + S wave in III ≥ 25mV
S wave in V1 + R wave in V5 ≥ 35mV

RVH: Mean QRS either anterior, or rightward

The heart rate is 71 beats per minute. The PR interval is 0.16 seconds. The QRS interval is 0.10 seconds (LIVCD); the QT interval is 0.40 seconds. The P axis is +30°. The mean QRS axis is 0° in the frontal plane and +15° in the horizontal plane. In the frontal plane, the initial part of the QRS is abnormal *(pattern: Q waves in II, III, and AVF or axis: −45°)*, indicating transmural infarction of the inferior wall. In the frontal plane, the T axis is abnormal *(pattern: inverted in leads II, III, and AVF, or axis: −45°)*, indicating that the inferior infarction is recent or possibly acute. In the horizontal plane, the initial part of the QRS is abnormal (pattern: tall wide initial R wave in leads V1 and V2 or axis: +120°), indicating posterior infarction.

Parts of the answer sheets are "grayed out" because these sections have not yet been covered. Answer only the parts that are not highlighted.

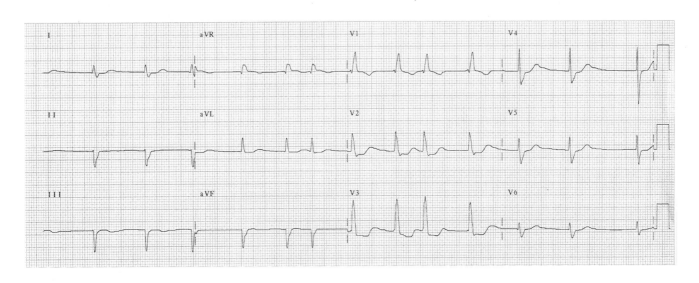

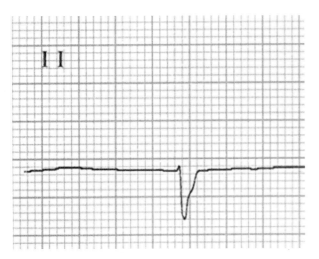

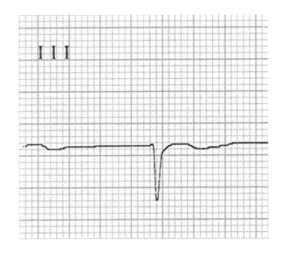

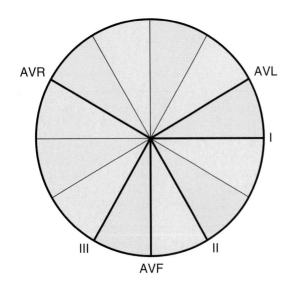

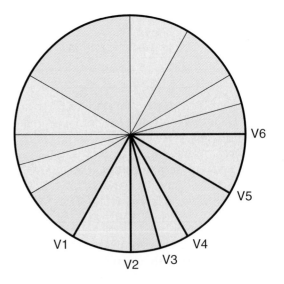

Heart Rate:

Rhythm:

Intervals (measured in the limb leads)

PR: short (< .12)
          normal (.12 to .20)
          long (>0.20 seconds); this is 1st degree AV block

QRS: normal (≤0.09 seconds)
          prolonged (.10 or .11); this is intraventricular conduction delay (IVCD)
          Bundle Branch Block (.12 seconds or greater)

QT:

P axis: normal
            rightward
            arm-lead reversal or dextrocardia
            junctional rhythm

QRS axis: normal
            left anterior hemiblock
            left posterior hemiblock
            indeterminate

T wave inversion (ischemia or infarction):

II,III,AVF	inferior
I, AVL	lateral
V1, without V2	nonspecific septal
V1 and V2	septal
V3 and V4	anterior
V5 and V6	lateral
V6, without V5	nonspecific lateral

ST Elevation (acute infarction):

II,III,AVF	inferior
I, AVL	lateral
V1, without V2	nonspecific septal
V1 and V2	septal
V3 and V4	anterior
V5 and V6	lateral
V6, without V5.	nonspecific lateral

ST Depression (ischemia or infarction):

I,II,III,AVL,AVF	diffuse subendocardial ischemia or infarction
V2,V3,V4,V5	diffuse subendocardial ischemia or infarction

Q waves (infarction):

II,III,AVF	inferior
I, AVL	lateral
V1, without V2	nonspecific septal
V1 and V2	septal
V3 and V4	anterior
V5 and V6	lateral
V6, without V5	nonspecific lateral

Hypertrophy:

Right atrial: Tall P wave 2.5 mm in II, III, or AVF

Left atrial: Deep negative part of P wave in V1

LVH: R wave in 1 + S wave in III ≥ 25mV
       S wave in V1 + R wave in V5 ≥ 35mV

RVH: Mean QRS either anterior, or rightward

The rhythm is irregularly irregular, which indicates atrial fibrillation. The ventricular rate is 80 beats per minute. The PR interval is undefined. The QRS interval measures 0.12 seconds in lead I. This is bundle branch block. The last part of the QRS points to the right (in leads I and V6) and anterior (in VI), indicating RBBB. The QT interval varies but is hard to see and measure, suggesting low-amplitude T waves and possible hypokalemia. The mean QRS axis is −90° in the frontal plane, indicating LAHB. (This mean QRS axis may be due to the inferior infarction, but it's useful to read hemiblock as well, especially in the face of RBBB.) The mean QRS axis is +157.5° in the horizontal plane. Since this is RBBB, both the mean QRS axis (to determine the presence of hemiblock) and the initial QRS axis (to determine the presence of infarction) should be calculated. The initial QRS axis is abnormal in the frontal plane (pattern: Q waves in II, III, and AVF or axis: initial part of QRS is −75°), indicating transmural infarction of the inferior wall. There is no ST elevation, depression, or T wave change in the frontal plane, so the inferior infarction is considered old, or "age indeterminate."

Parts of the answer sheets are "grayed out" because these sections have not yet been covered. Answer only the parts that are not highlighted.

Anterior Q Waves (Initial QRS Axis)

Transmural infarction of the septum and anterior and lateral walls of the myocardium is the result of a complete occlusion of the left anterior descending (LAD) branch of the left coronary artery.

The LAD artery is a branch of the left coronary artery.

It has branches that supply the septum, as well as branches that supply the anterior and lateral walls of the left ventricle.

The distal portion of the LAD artery frequently wraps around and supplies the apex.

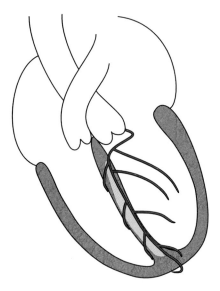

Cardiac catheterization here demonstrates a nearly totally occlusive lesion in the proximal portion of the LAD artery.

Transmural infarction results from total occlusion of the epicardial artery.

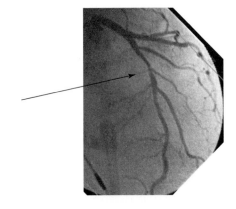

Transmural Infarction: Septum and Anterior Wall

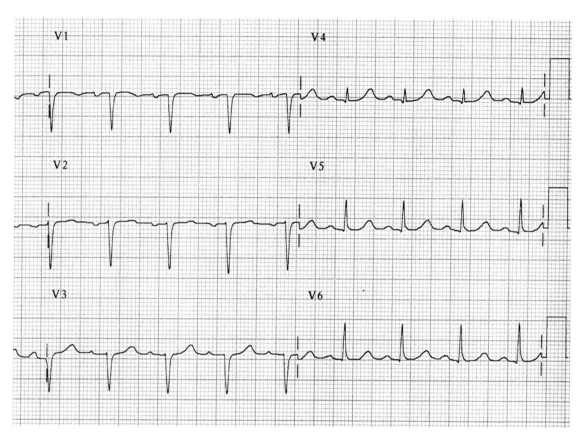

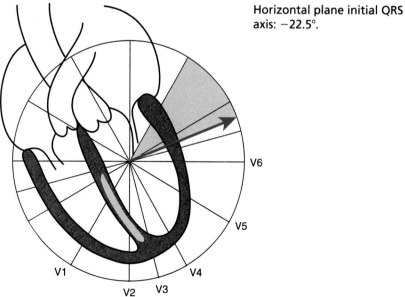

Horizontal plane initial QRS axis: −22.5°.

Concept: In transmural infarction of the septum and anterior wall, the initial part of the QRS points away from the damaged septum and anterior walls.

Axis: From −22.5° to −60° in the horizontal plane.

Pattern: The initial 0.04 seconds of the QRS in leads V1, V2, and V3 are negative.

Transmural Septal Infarction: Right Bundle Branch Block and LAHB

Septal infarctions are sometimes complicated by various conduction disturbances. The right and left bundle branches are located within the myocardial layer of the ventricular septum, and, when the septum is damaged, the bundle branches or parts of them may be damaged as well. Importantly, **RBBB does not affect the initial part of the QRS.** Examine the example below:

a) The **initial QRS** shows Q waves in leads V1 through V4 and indicates septal and anterior transmural infarction.

b) The **last part of the QRS** points anterior and rightward, indicating RBBB.

c) The **mean QRS** in the frontal plane is −90, indicating LAHB.

d) A single lesion in the LAD caused the infarction that resulted in all the above.

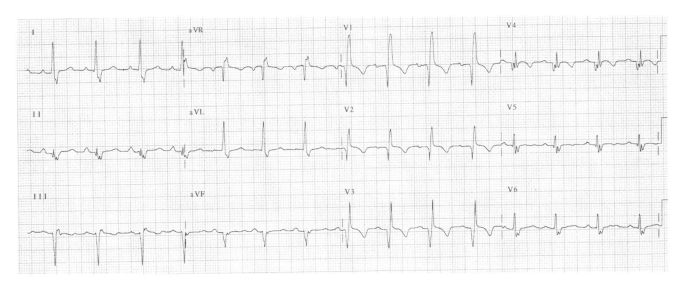

The most common conduction problems associated with septal infarctions are:

1) RBBB

2) LBBB

3) RBBB and left anterior hemiblock (LAHB)

4) RBBB and left posterior hemiblock (LPHB)

5) Complete heart block

Except for isolated RBBB, the above conduction diseases require a temporary ventricular pacemaker.

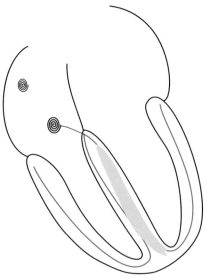

Septal infarction damaging the right bundle and the left anterior superior division of the left bundle.

Transmural Septal Infarction: Left Bundle Branch Block

There is no reliable way to diagnose infarction or ischemia in a patient with LBBB. The following patient *may* have had a septal infarction as the cause of the LBBB. There is just no useful way to decide that from the EKG. LBBB is LBBB. It indicates likely significant underlying pathology but creates a "fog of war" that prevents the use of the EKG to help diagnose its cause. The following EKG should *not* be read as septal infarction. It should *not* be read as transmural ischemia. It should be read as LBBB.

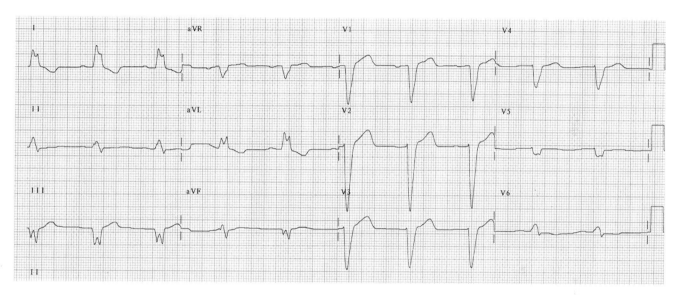

QRS interval: 0.16 seconds.

Last part of QRS: posterior and left.

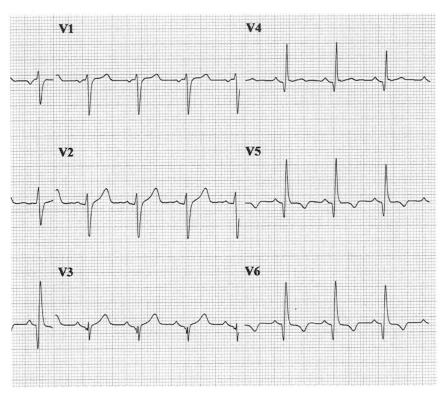

Horizontal plane initial QRS axis: +172.5°.

Concept: In transmural infarction of the anterior and lateral walls, the initial part of the QRS points away from the damaged anterior and lateral walls.

Initial QRS axis: From +165° to +180° in the horizontal plane.

Pattern: The initial 0.04 seconds of the QRS in leads V4, V5, and V6 are negative. V3 may be negative as well.

SUMMARY OF INITIAL QRS AXIS: HORIZONTAL PLANE

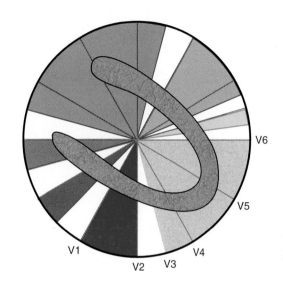

Location of Infarction	Concept to Understand	QRS$_{init.04}$ Axis to Translate the Concept (Don't Memorize)	Q Wave Pattern (Memorize)
Septal	QRS$_{init.04}$ axis points away from the septum	−75° to −15°	V1 and V2
Septal and anterior	QRS$_{init.04}$ axis points away from the septum and anterior walls	−22.5° to −60°	V1, V2, and V3 (+/− V4)
Septal anterior and lateral	QRS$_{init.04}$ axis points away from septum and anterior and lateral walls	−75° to −165°	V2 to V5 (+/− V1, +/− V6)
Anterior and lateral	QRS$_{init.04}$ axis points away from anterior and lateral wall	+165° to +180°	V4, V5 (+/− V3, +/− V6)
Lateral	QRS$_{init.04}$ axis points away from lateral wall	+135° to +150°	V5 and V6
Posterior	QRS$_{init.04}$ axis points away from the posterior wall	+90° to +120°	Wide R wave in V1 and V2
Normal	QRS$_{init.04}$ axis points toward the apex	0° to +75°	V1 or V6 only

SUMMARY OF INITIAL QRS: HORIZONTAL PLANE PATTERN

Patterns of Q Waves	Locations of Infarct
V1, V2	Septal
V3, V4	Anterior
V5, V6	Lateral
Tall wide R wave in V1 and V2	Posterior

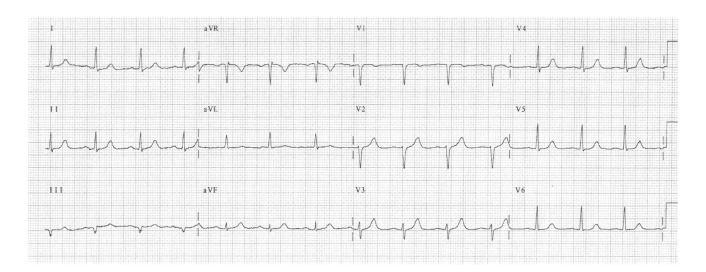

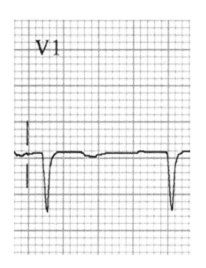

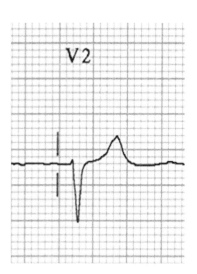

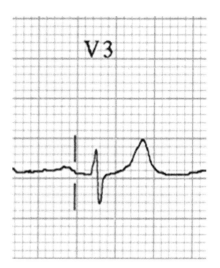

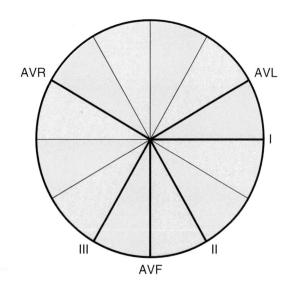

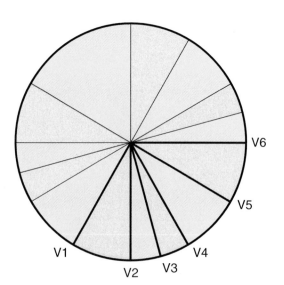

Heart Rate:

Rhythm:

Intervals (measured in the limb leads)

PR: short (< .12)
       normal (.12 to .20)
       long (>0.20 seconds); this is 1st degree AV
       block

QRS: normal (≤0.09 seconds)
       prolonged (.10 or .11); this is intraventricular
       conduction delay (IVCD)
       Bundle Branch Block (.12 seconds or greater)

QT:

P axis: normal
           rightward
           arm-lead reversal or dextrocardia
           junctional rhythm

QRS axis: normal
           left anterior hemiblock
           left posterior hemiblock
           indeterminate

T wave inversion (ischemia or infarction):

II,III,AVF	inferior
I, AVL	lateral
V1, without V2	nonspecific septal
V1 and V2	septal
V3 and V4	anterior
V5 and V6	lateral
V6, without V5	nonspecific lateral

ST Elevation (acute infarction):

II,III,AVF	inferior
I, AVL	lateral
V1, without V2	nonspecific septal
V1 and V2	septal
V3 and V4	anterior
V5 and V6	lateral
V6, without V5.	nonspecific lateral

ST Depression (ischemia or infarction):

I,II,III,AVL,AVF	diffuse subendocardial ischemia or infarction
V2,V3,V4,V5	diffuse subendocardial ischemia or infarction

Q waves (infarction):

II,III,AVF	inferior
I, AVL	lateral
V1, without V2	nonspecific septal
V1 and V2	septal
V3 and V4	anterior
V5 and V6	lateral
V6, without V5	nonspecific lateral

Hypertrophy:

Right atrial: Tall P wave 2.5 mm in II, III, or AVF

Left atrial: Deep negative part of P wave in V1

LVH: R wave in 1 + S wave in III ≥ 25mV
      S wave in V1 + R wave in V5 ≥ 35mV

RVH: Mean QRS either anterior, or rightward

The heart rate is 83 beats per minute. The PR interval is 0.18 seconds. The QT interval is 0.34 seconds. The P axis is normal (+60°). The mean QRS axis is +15° in the frontal plane and −15° in the horizontal plane. The initial QRS axis is normal in the frontal plane. **In the horizontal plane, the initial part of the QRS is negative in V1 and V2, indicating septal infarction.** The age is indeterminate, because the T waves and ST segments are essentially normal. Note that lead V2 doesn't really have a q wave. It has an embryonic r wave followed by an S wave. This is why pattern reading is tricky if you don't really understand axis. *Although there is no q present in V2, by axis, we would consider the initial 0.04 seconds, the initial part of the QRS, to be clearly negative, and therefore equivalent to a q wave.*

Parts of the answer sheets are "grayed out" because these sections have not yet been covered. Answer only the parts that are not highlighted.

Worksheet 15-2

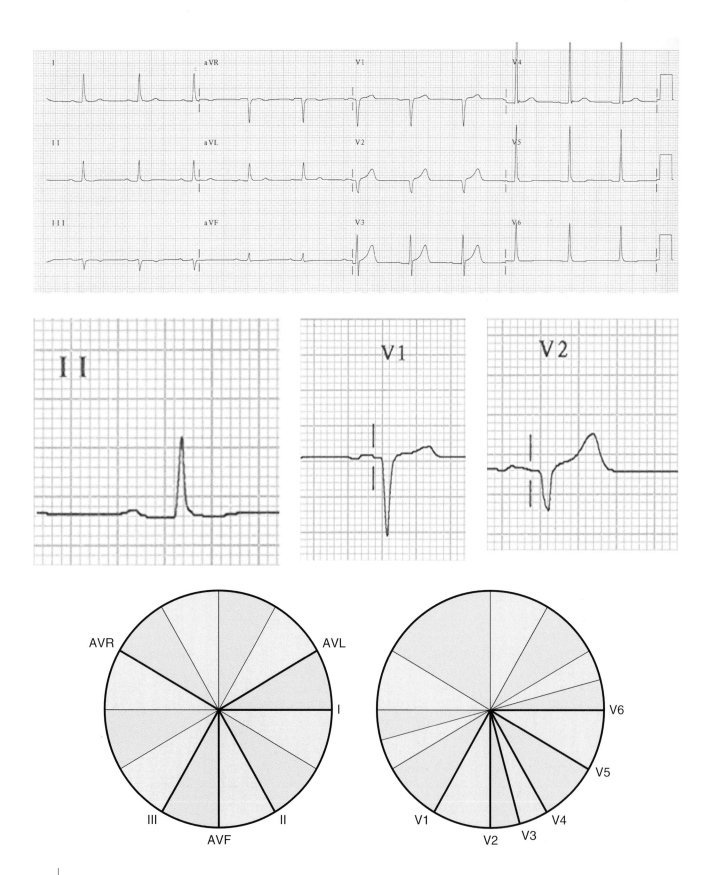

Heart Rate:

Rhythm:

Intervals (measured in the limb leads)

PR: short (< .12)
       normal (.12 to .20)
       long (>0.20 seconds); this is 1st degree AV
       block

QRS: normal (≤0.09 seconds)
       prolonged (.10 or .11); this is intraventricular
       conduction delay (IVCD)
       Bundle Branch Block (.12 seconds or greater)

QT:

P axis: normal
             rightward
             arm-lead reversal or dextrocardia
             junctional rhythm

QRS axis: normal
             left anterior hemiblock
             left posterior hemiblock
             indeterminate

T wave inversion (ischemia or infarction):

II,III,AVF	inferior
I, AVL	lateral
V1, without V2	nonspecific septal
V1 and V2	septal
V3 and V4	anterior
V5 and V6	lateral
V6, without V5	nonspecific lateral

ST Elevation (acute infarction):

II,III,AVF	inferior
I, AVL	lateral
V1, without V2	nonspecific septal
V1 and V2	septal
V3 and V4	anterior
V5 and V6	lateral
V6, without V5.	nonspecific lateral

ST Depression (ischemia or infarction):

I,II,III,AVL,AVF	diffuse subendocardial ischemia or infarction
V2,V3,V4,V5	diffuse subendocardial ischemia or infarction

Q waves (infarction):

II,III,AVF	inferior
I, AVL	lateral
V1, without V2	nonspecific septal
V1 and V2	septal
V3 and V4	anterior
V5 and V6	lateral
V6, without V5	nonspecific lateral

Hypertrophy:

Right atrial: Tall P wave 2.5 mm in II, III, or AVF

Left atrial: Deep negative part of P wave in V1

LVH: R wave in 1 + S wave in III ≥ 25mV
      S wave in V1 + R wave in V5 ≥ 35mV

RVH: Mean QRS either anterior, or rightward

The heart rate is 63 beats per minute. The PR interval measures .24 seconds, which is long and indicates 1° AV block. The QRS interval is 0.08 seconds. The QT interval measures 0.36 seconds, but it is difficult to measure due to low, amplitude T waves. The P axis (+30°) is normal. The mean QRS axis is +15° in the frontal plane and −7.5° in the horizontal plane. The initial QRS, the T axis, and the ST are all normal in the frontal plane. **In the horizontal plane, the initial part of the QRS points away from leads V1 and V2 (initial QRS axis is −7.5°) and indicates septal infarction.** The ST segment in the horizontal plane is slightly elevated and could be nonspecific. In the presence of the Q waves in V1 and V2, it suggests the possibility that the infarction may be recent or possibly acute.

Parts of the answer sheets are "grayed out" because these sections have not yet been covered. Answer only the parts that are not highlighted.

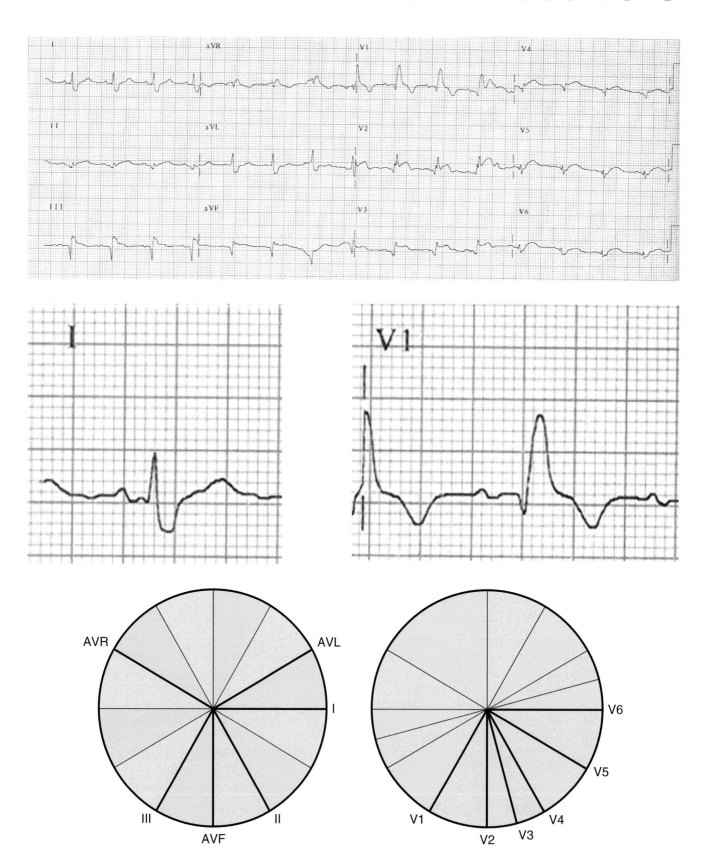

Heart Rate:

Rhythm:

Intervals (measured in the limb leads)

PR: short (< .12)
         normal (.12 to .20)
         long (>0.20 seconds); this is 1st degree AV
         block

QRS: normal (≤0.09 seconds)
         prolonged (.10 or .11); this is intraventricular
         conduction delay (IVCD)
         Bundle Branch Block (.12 seconds or greater)

QT:

P axis: normal
           rightward
           arm-lead reversal or dextrocardia
           junctional rhythm

QRS axis: normal
           left anterior hemiblock
           left posterior hemiblock
           indeterminate

T wave inversion (ischemia or infarction):

II,III,AVF	inferior
I, AVL	lateral
V1, without V2	nonspecific septal
V1 and V2	septal
V3 and V4	anterior
V5 and V6	lateral
V6, without V5	nonspecific lateral

ST Elevation (acute infarction):

II,III,AVF	inferior
I, AVL	lateral
V1, without V2	nonspecific septal
V1 and V2	septal
V3 and V4	anterior
V5 and V6	lateral
V6, without V5.	nonspecific lateral

ST Depression (ischemia or infarction):

I,II,III,AVL,AVF	diffuse subendocardial ischemia or infarction
V2,V3,V4,V5	diffuse subendocardial ischemia or infarction

Q waves (infarction):

II,III,AVF	inferior
I, AVL	lateral
V1, without V2	nonspecific septal
V1 and V2	septal
V3 and V4	anterior
V5 and V6	lateral
V6, without V5	nonspecific lateral

Hypertrophy:

Right atrial: Tall P wave 2.5 mm in II, III, or AVF

Left atrial: Deep negative part of P wave in V1

LVH: R wave in 1 + S wave in III ≥ 25mV
       S wave in V1 + R wave in V5 ≥ 35mV

RVH: Mean QRS either anterior, or rightward

The heart rate is 88 beats per minute. The PR interval is 0.14 seconds. The QRS interval measures 0.12 seconds, indicating BBB. The last part of the QRS points toward the right ventricle in both the frontal plane (in lead I, the last part of the QRS is rightward) and the horizontal plane (in lead V2, the last part of the QRS points anteriorly, and in V6 the last part of the QRS points rightward). **This indicates RBBB.** The QT interval is 0.36 seconds. The mean QRS axis is −30° and indicates left anterior hemiblock. The initial part of the QRS should be analyzed in RBBB. In the frontal plane, the initial part of the QRS is −60° (or Q waves are present in II, III, and AVF), indicating inferior infarction. The ST axis in the frontal plane points toward the inferior wall, indicating that the infarction is acute. In the horizontal plane, there are q waves in leads V1 through V4 (initial QRS axis of −60°), indicating transmural infarction of the anterior and lateral walls. The horizontal ST axis is positive in leads V1 through V6 (ST axis of +60°), indicating that the infarction is acute. *The infarction of the septum has likely caused the RBBB and LAHB, because both course through the septum.*

Parts of the answer sheets are "grayed out" because these sections have not yet been covered. Answer only the parts that are not highlighted.

Worksheet 15-4

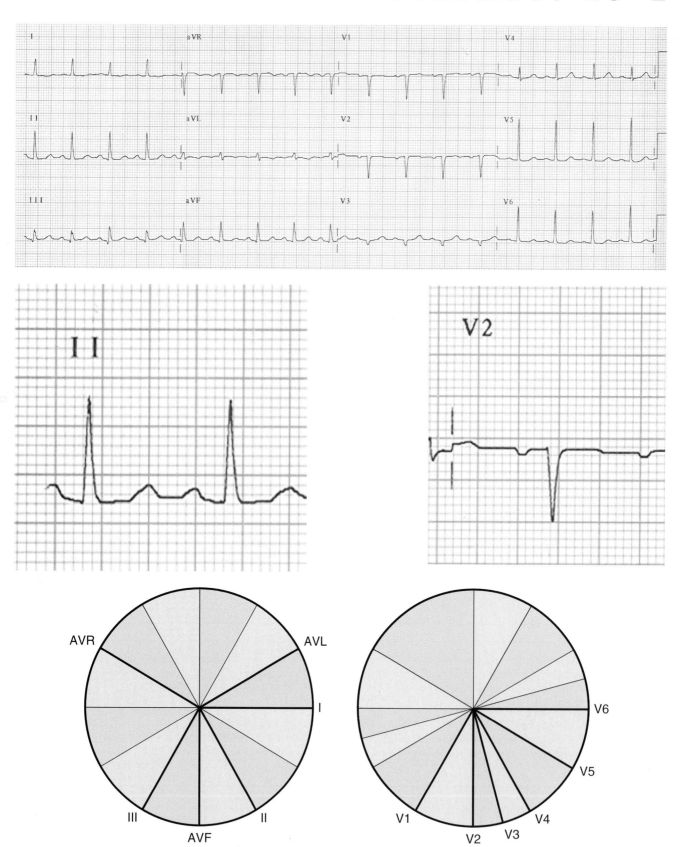

Heart Rate:

Rhythm:

Intervals (measured in the limb leads)

PR: short (< .12)
       normal (.12 to .20)
       long (>0.20 seconds); this is 1st degree AV
       block

QRS: normal (≤0.09 seconds)
       prolonged (.10 or .11); this is intraventricular
       conduction delay (IVCD)
       Bundle Branch Block (.12 seconds or greater)

QT:

P axis: normal
          rightward
          arm-lead reversal or dextrocardia
          junctional rhythm

QRS axis: normal
           left anterior hemiblock
           left posterior hemiblock
           indeterminate

T wave inversion (ischemia or infarction):

II,III,AVF	inferior
I, AVL	lateral
V1, without V2	nonspecific septal
V1 and V2	septal
V3 and V4	anterior
V5 and V6	lateral
V6, without V5	nonspecific lateral

ST Elevation (acute infarction):

II,III,AVF	inferior
I, AVL	lateral
V1, without V2	nonspecific septal
V1 and V2	septal
V3 and V4	anterior
V5 and V6	lateral
V6, without V5.	nonspecific lateral

ST Depression (ischemia or infarction):

I,II,III,AVL,AVF	diffuse subendocardial ischemia or infarction
V2,V3,V4,V5	diffuse subendocardial ischemia or infarction

Q waves (infarction):

II,III,AVF	inferior
I, AVL	lateral
V1, without V2	nonspecific septal
V1 and V2	septal
V3 and V4	anterior
V5 and V6	lateral
V6, without V5	nonspecific lateral

Hypertrophy:

Right atrial: Tall P wave 2.5 mm in II, III, or AVF

Left atrial: Deep negative part of P wave in V1

LVH: R wave in 1 + S wave in III ≥ 25mV
       S wave in V1 + R wave in V5 ≥ 35mV

RVH: Mean QRS either anterior, or rightward

The heart rate is 100 beats per minute. Although this is sinus rhythm, the rate of 100 suggests a problem. It indicates that the sympathetic/parasympathetic balance has tipped over towards a sympathetic tone. Is the patient in CHF? Shock? Septic? Bleeding? The PR interval measures 0.18 seconds. The QRS interval measures 0.08 seconds and is normal. The QT interval is 0.32 seconds. This is at the upper limits of normal. The P axis is normal at +75°. The mean QRS axis in the frontal plane is +45° and is normal. The initial QRS axis in the frontal plane points away from the inferior wall for only 0.02 seconds, and only in leads III and AVF, so these are "nonspecific inferior Q waves." In the horizontal plane, there is a septal and anterior wall infarction because the initial QRS points away from the septum and anterior wall leads (V1, V2, and V3 all have Q waves). The ST segments are abnormal but nonspecific. There are no ischemic changes shown by definite T wave or ST segment changes, thus the infarction is "old" or "age indeterminate."

Parts of the answer sheets are "grayed out" because these sections have not yet been covered. Answer only the parts that are not highlighted.

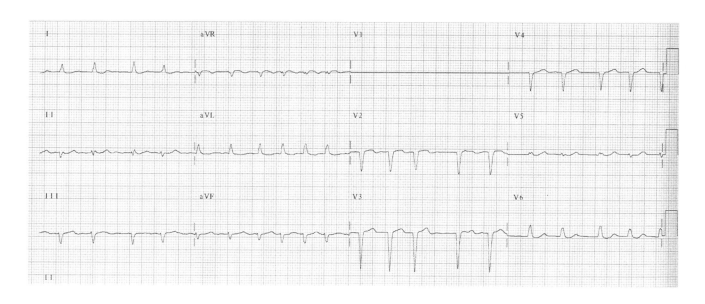

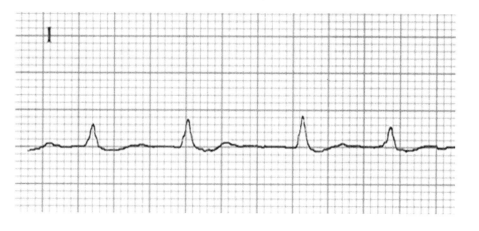

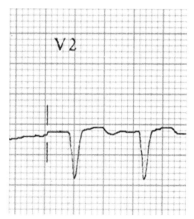

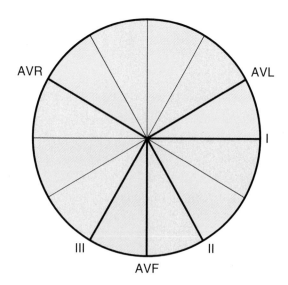

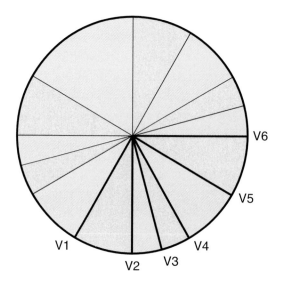

Heart Rate:

Rhythm:

ST Elevation (acute infarction):

II, III, AVF	inferior
I, AVL	lateral
V1, without V2	nonspecific septal
V1 and V2	septal
V3 and V4	anterior
V5 and V6	lateral
V6, without V5.	nonspecific lateral

Intervals (measured in the limb leads)

PR: short (< .12)
      normal (.12 to .20)
      long (>0.20 seconds); this is 1st degree AV
      block

QRS: normal (≤0.09 seconds)
       prolonged (.10 or .11); this is intraventricular
       conduction delay (IVCD)
       Bundle Branch Block (.12 seconds or greater)

QT:

ST Depression (ischemia or infarction):

I, II, III, AVL, AVF	diffuse subendocardial ischemia or infarction
V2, V3, V4, V5	diffuse subendocardial ischemia or infarction

P axis: normal
          rightward
          arm-lead reversal or dextrocardia
          junctional rhythm

QRS axis: normal
            left anterior hemiblock
            left posterior hemiblock
            indeterminate

Q waves (infarction):

II, III, AVF	inferior
I, AVL	lateral
V1, without V2	nonspecific septal
V1 and V2	septal
V3 and V4	anterior
V5 and V6	lateral
V6, without V5	nonspecific lateral

T wave inversion (ischemia or infarction):

II, III, AVF	inferior
I, AVL	lateral
V1, without V2	nonspecific septal
V1 and V2	septal
V3 and V4	anterior
V5 and V6	lateral
V6, without V5	nonspecific lateral

Hypertrophy:

Right atrial: Tall P wave 2.5 mm in II, III, or AVF

Left atrial: Deep negative part of P wave in V1

LVH: R wave in 1 + S wave in III ≥ 25mV
       S wave in V1 + R wave in V5 ≥ 35mV

RVH: Mean QRS either anterior, or rightward

The rhythm is **atrial fibrillation.** The ventricular rate is 110 beats per minute. The PR is undefined. The QRS interval is 0.08 seconds. The QT interval is 0.36 seconds. The T wave amplitude is low. The P axis is undefined. The mean QRS axis is −30° in the frontal plane and −60° in the horizontal plane. The initial QRS axis in the frontal plane is abnormal but nonspecific (initial QRS axis is −30°, there are q waves in II and III, but not AVF). In the horizontal plane, the initial QRS axis is abnormal and points away from the septum (V2) and anterior walls (V3 and V4), consistent with septal and anterior wall infarction. The ST segment points toward the septum (V2) and anterior wall (V3 and V4) and indicates that the infarction may be acute.

Parts of the answer sheets are "grayed out" because these sections have not yet been covered. Answer only the parts that are not highlighted.

Atrial Abnormalities

P wave analysis identifies atrial abnormalities. Both right atrial abnormality (RAA) and left atrial abnormality (LAA) can be distinguished by analyzing the P wave.

The right atrium is to the right and in front of the left atrium. In fact, the right atrium is the most rightward chamber of the heart. As the right atrium is subjected to the stress of pressure or volume, it enlarges as a compensatory mechanism to handle the increased work. Increased pressure in the right ventricle can be present from pulmonary hypertension secondary to chronic obstructive lung disease or pulmonary embolism. To handle the stiff muscular right ventricle, the right atrium has to "bulk up" in response. Increased volume in the right atrium can result from tricuspid regurgitation, commonly seen after pacemaker implantation, or from long-standing pulmonary hypertension. To handle the volume overload, the right atrium has to "make space" and dilates.

KEY CONCEPT

RAA can be diagnosed by change in the P wave axis to a rightward direction.

RAA can also be diagnosed by an increase in the P wave amplitude to 2.5 little boxes in leads II, III, and AVF.

Right atrial abnormality on the EKG identifies enlargement in cavity size or muscle mass of the right atrium.

Enlargement (bigger chamber) or hypertrophy (thicker walls) of the right atrium can change the P axis to a rightward direction. It can also increase the amplitude of the P wave.

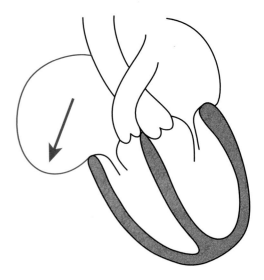

Right Atrial Abnormality

A normal range for the P wave axis in the frontal plane is anywhere from −30° to +75°. The normal P axis electrical depolarization should point in this range. Right atrial abnormality on the electrocardiogram (EKG) identifies enlargement in cavity size or muscle mass of the right atrium. Enlargement (bigger chamber) or hypertrophy (thicker walls) of the right atrium can change the P axis to a rightward direction

A P axis of +90° to +105° indicates RAA.

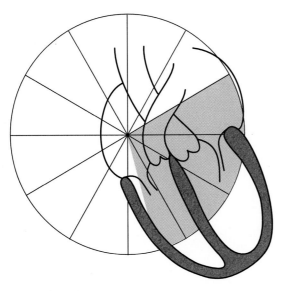

Normal P axis.

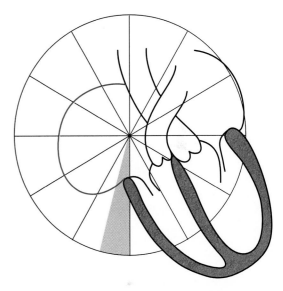

Enlargement of the right atrium produces a bigger electrical force in the right atrium and moves the P axis to the right in the range of +90° to +105°.

Right Atrial Abnormality

The right atrium is depolarized by an electrical impulse that begins in the sinus node and travels inferiorly toward the AV node. If the right atrium is enlarged, the P wave may demonstrate increased voltage due to the increased right atrium electrical force. **An increase in the P wave amplitude of 2.5 little boxes high in any one of leads II, III, or AVF indicates RAA.**

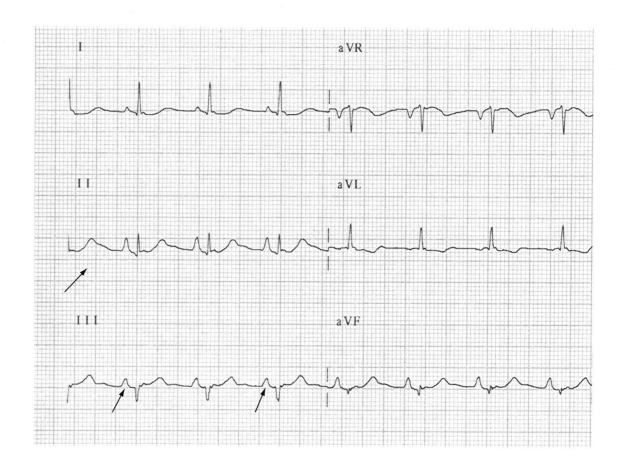

Left Atrial Abnormality

The left atrium is located behind the right atrium. In fact, **the left atrium is the most posterior chamber of the heart.** As the left atrium is subjected to the stress of pressure or volume it enlarges as a compensatory mechanism to handle the increased work. Increased pressure in the left ventricle can be present from hypertension, aortic stenosis, or hypertrophic obstructive cardiomyopathy. To handle the stiff muscular left ventricle, the left atrium has to "bulk up" in response. Increased pressure in the left atrium can directly result from **mitral stenosis.** Increased volume in the left atrium can result from **mitral regurgitation.** To handle the volume overload, the left atrium has to "make space" and dilates. The small pouchlike sack attached to the left atrium is called the **left atrial appendage.** It is a critical structure clinically, because it can harbor thrombus formation in low-flow states such as atrial fibrillation. Part of the thrombus can fragment and embolize to the systemic circulation where it can cause stroke, bowel infarction, or limb embolus. **Left atrial abnormality is a tiny part of the EKG that provides important clinical clues about disease on the left side of the heart.**

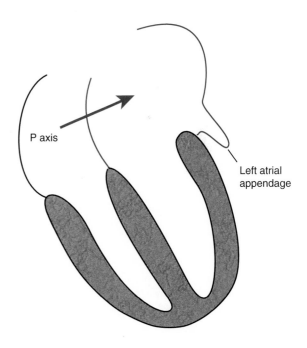

P axis

Left atrial
appendage

The direction of normal left atrial depolarization is posterior. The atrial depolarization force is represented on the EKG by the P wave. An increase in left atrial mass will increase the left atrium component of the P wave. **Lead V1 is usually the best lead for determining whether the left atrium is enlarged.** LAA creates a visible negative part to the P wave in V1. Because the left atrium is further away from the sinus node than the right atrium, the second half of the P wave usually represents the left atrial component. **In LAA, the P wave in V1 is negative by at least 1 little box. The negative part of the P wave in V1 must also be 1 little box wide (0.04 seconds).**

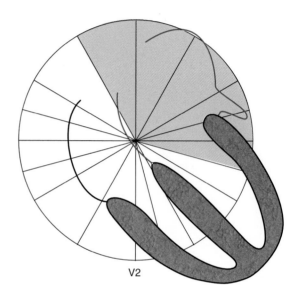

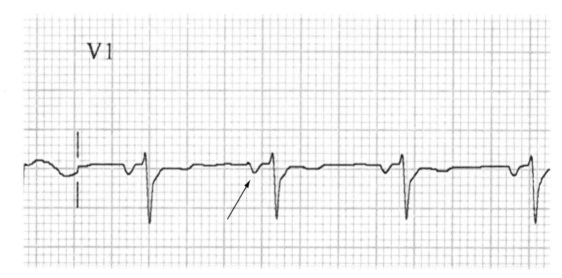

Valvular Heart Disease

Diseased or malfunctioning heart valves cause increased burdens on the atria and ventricles (either volume or pressure) that can produce suggestive EKG changes. When valves leak (regurgitate) or become narrowed (stenose), they put a strain on at least one of the four chambers of the heart. This strain leads to increased mass of the involved chamber as it tries to adapt to the new added workload. **The increased mass of any cardiac chamber creates a larger electrical force on the EKG, and this is how we detect hypertrophy of any of the heart chambers.**

Regurgitation typically causes an added burden in the form of extra volume, which requires more space. The involved chambers of the heart respond by dilatation. This adaptation works well to the volume overload of regurgitation, as long as it develops slowly.

Stenosis is quite a different matter. It creates an added burden in the form of increased resistance to flow, which requires pressure-generating ability. The involved chambers behind the stenosis typically develop thicker walls.

In the adult, the four most common valvular heart diseases that cause abnormalities on the EKG are mitral stenosis, mitral regurgitation, aortic regurgitation, and aortic stenosis.

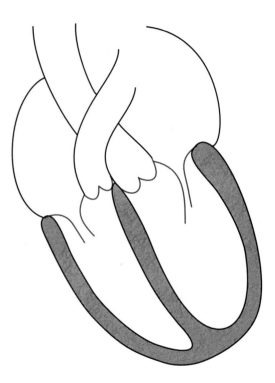

Mitral Stenosis

The mitral valve separates the left atrium from the left ventricle. When the valve is stenosed, it becomes constricted and narrowed, interfering with the flow of blood from the left atrium into the left ventricle. This increases the workload of the heart and eventually causes the left atrium to become enlarged. As the pressure backs up to the lungs, the right ventricle and right atrium also enlarge. Mitral stenosis is almost always a result of acute rheumatic fever. LAA, right ventricular hypertrophy (RVH), and RAA, can be seen in mitral stenosis. The left ventricle is not involved. Treatment is surgical and is aimed at reducing the resistance to flow through the mitral valve.

Mitral stenosis causes blood to back up into the left atrium. The blood backs up from the left atrium into the lungs, causing shortness of breath (dyspnea). Eventually the blood backs up into the right ventricle and right atrium. The results are dilated left atrium, right ventricular hypertrophy, and right atrial hypertrophy.

Meanwhile, the left ventricle doesn't see any problem. There is no extra work for the left ventricle. Mitral stenosis does not affect the left ventricle!

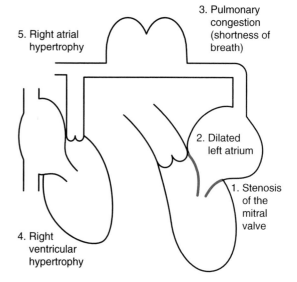

5. Right atrial hypertrophy

3. Pulmonary congestion (shortness of breath)

2. Dilated left atrium

1. Stenosis of the mitral valve

4. Right ventricular hypertrophy

Mitral Regurgitation

Mitral regurgitation is most commonly caused by mitral valve prolapse or rheumatic heart disease. Mitral regurgitation occurs when the mitral valve allows the backflow of blood from the left ventricle into the left atrium. The left atrium and left ventricle become dilated and hypertrophied trying to accommodate the extra blood volume. The EKG can demonstrate LAA and left ventricular hypertrophy (LVH).

Mitral regurgitation allows for a backward movement of blood between the left ventricle and left atrium during ventricular systole.

The left atrium dilates to accommodate the extra blood volume. The left atrium fills from blood pumped from the right ventricle but has no extra room to accommodate the regurgitant volume from the left ventricle and dilates to compensate.

The left ventricle dilates to accommodate the extra blood volume. The left ventricle fills with blood pumped from the right ventricle but has no extra room to accommodate the regurgitant volume and dilates to compensate.

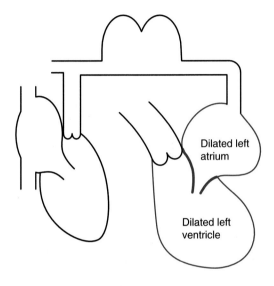

Dilated left atrium

Dilated left ventricle

Worksheet 16-1

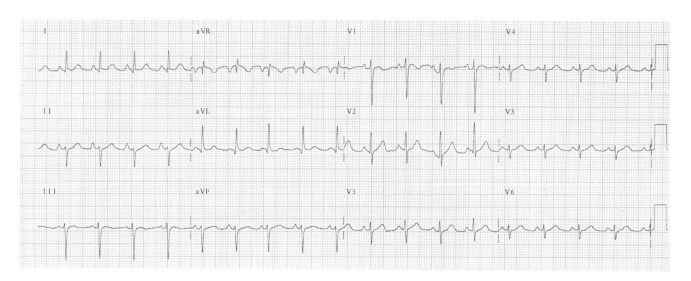

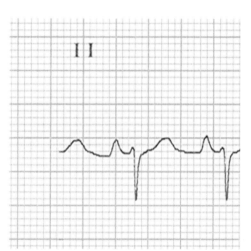

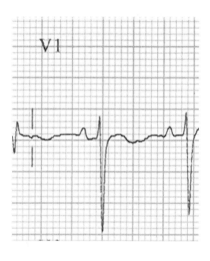

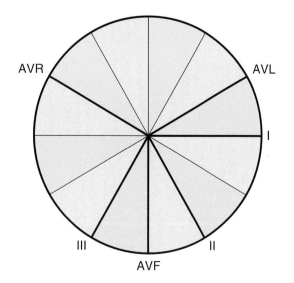

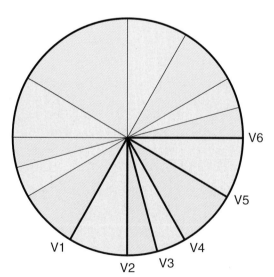

Heart Rate:

Rhythm:

Intervals (measured in the limb leads)

PR: short (< .12)
       normal (.12 to .20)
       long (>0.20 seconds); this is 1st degree AV
       block

QRS: normal (≤0.09 seconds)
       prolonged (.10 or .11); this is intraventricular
       conduction delay (IVCD)
       Bundle Branch Block (.12 seconds or greater)

QT:

P axis:	normal
	rightward
	arm-lead reversal or dextrocardia
	junctional rhythm
QRS axis:	normal
	left anterior hemiblock
	left posterior hemiblock
	indeterminate

T wave inversion (ischemia or infarction):

II,III,AVF	inferior
I, AVL	lateral
V1, without V2	nonspecific septal
V1 and V2	septal
V3 and V4	anterior
V5 and V6	lateral
V6, without V5	nonspecific lateral

ST Elevation (acute infarction):

II,III,AVF	inferior
I, AVL	lateral
V1, without V2	nonspecific septal
V1 and V2	septal
V3 and V4	anterior
V5 and V6	lateral
V6, without V5.	nonspecific lateral

ST Depression (ischemia or infarction):

| I,II,III,AVL,AVF | diffuse subendocardial ischemia or infarction |
| V2,V3,V4,V5 | diffuse subendocardial ischemia or infarction |

Q waves (infarction):

II,III,AVF	inferior
I, AVL	lateral
V1, without V2	nonspecific septal
V1 and V2	septal
V3 and V4	anterior
V5 and V6	lateral
V6, without V5	nonspecific lateral

Hypertrophy:

Right atrial: Tall P wave 2.5 mm in II, III, or AVF

Left atrial: Deep negative part of P wave in V1

LVH: R wave in 1 + S wave in III ≥ 25mV
      S wave in V1 + R wave in V5 ≥ 35mV

RVH: Mean QRS either anterior, or rightward

The heart rate is 107 beats per minute. The PR interval measures 0.12 seconds, which is normal. The QRS interval measures 0.08 seconds, which is normal. The QT interval measures 0.32 seconds. The P axis is normal (+45°). The mean QRS axis is −60° in the frontal plane and indicates left anterior hemiblock. The mean QRS axis in the horizontal plane is −22.5°. The T axis is +30° in the frontal plane and +30° in the horizontal plane and is in the normal range. There is no significant ST elevation more than 1 mm above or below baseline. **There are peaked P waves in lead II, which measure 2.5 little boxes. This indicates right atrial abnormality (RAA).**

Parts of the answer sheets are "grayed out" because these sections have not yet been covered. Answer only the parts that are not highlighted.

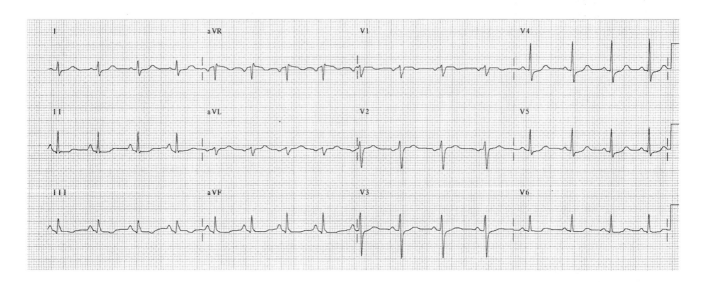

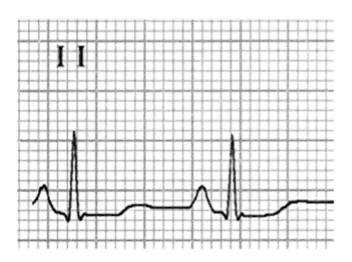

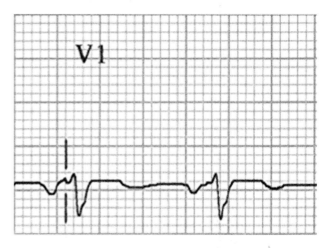

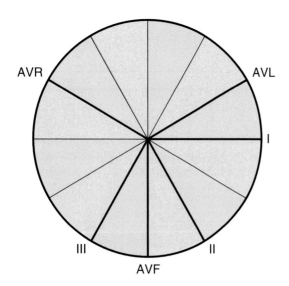

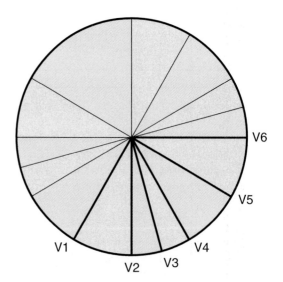

Heart Rate:

Rhythm:

Intervals (measured in the limb leads)

PR: short (< .12)
       normal (.12 to .20)
       long (>0.20 seconds); this is 1st degree AV
       block

QRS: normal (≤0.09 seconds)
       prolonged (.10 or .11); this is intraventricular
       conduction delay (IVCD)
       Bundle Branch Block (.12 seconds or greater)

QT:

P axis: normal
            rightward
            arm-lead reversal or dextrocardia
            junctional rhythm

QRS axis: normal
            left anterior hemiblock
            left posterior hemiblock
            indeterminate

T wave inversion (ischemia or infarction):

II,III,AVF	inferior
I, AVL	lateral
V1, without V2	nonspecific septal
V1 and V2	septal
V3 and V4	anterior
V5 and V6	lateral
V6, without V5	nonspecific lateral

ST Elevation (acute infarction):

II,III,AVF	inferior
I, AVL	lateral
V1, without V2	nonspecific septal
V1 and V2	septal
V3 and V4	anterior
V5 and V6	lateral
V6, without V5.	nonspecific lateral

ST Depression (ischemia or infarction):

I,II,III,AVL,AVF	diffuse subendocardial ischemia or infarction
V2,V3,V4,V5	diffuse subendocardial ischemia or infarction

Q waves (infarction):

II,III,AVF	inferior
I, AVL	lateral
V1, without V2	nonspecific septal
V1 and V2	septal
V3 and V4	anterior
V5 and V6	lateral
V6, without V5	nonspecific lateral

Hypertrophy:

Right atrial: Tall P wave 2.5 mm in II, III, or AVF

Left atrial: Deep negative part of P wave in V1

LVH: R wave in 1 + S wave in III ≥ 25mV
      S wave in V1 + R wave in V5 ≥ 35mV

RVH: Mean QRS either anterior, or rightward

The heart rate is 94 beats per minute. The PR interval measures 0.14 seconds and is normal. The QRS interval measures 0.08 seconds and is normal. The QT interval measures 0.36 seconds and is normal. The P axis is normal at +60°. The mean QRS axis is +75° in the frontal plane and −22.5° in the horizontal plane and is normal. The T axis is 0° in the frontal plane and 0° in the horizontal plane. In the frontal plane, the ST segment is depressed in leads I, II, III, AVL, and AVF but isoelectric in lead AVR. This combination points to −120° and indicates subendocardial ischemia or infarction. In the horizontal plane, the ST segment is isoelectric in lead V2 but slightly depressed in leads V3 through V6. This combination points to 180°, also consistent with subendocaridal ischemia or infarction. The P wave amplitude in lead II measures 2.5 little boxes and indicates right atrial abnormality. The negative component of the P wave in lead V1 measures 1 little box wide by 1 little box deep, indicating left atrial abnormality (LAA).

Parts of the answer sheets are "grayed out" because these sections have not yet been covered. Answer only the parts that are not highlighted.

Worksheet 16-3

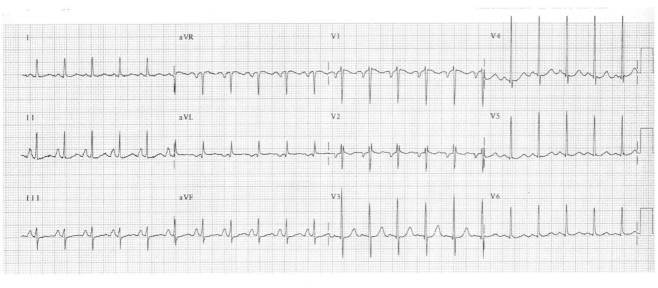

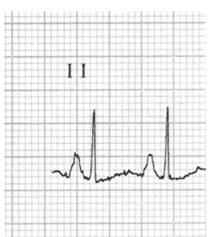

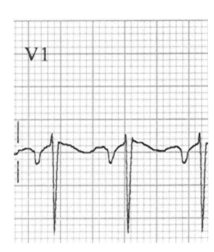

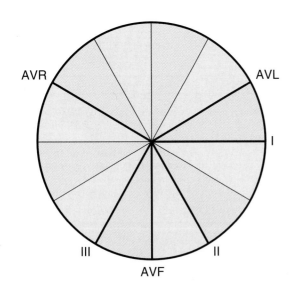

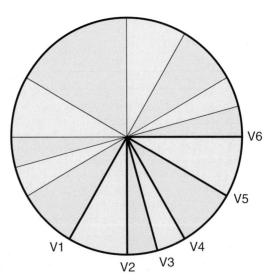

Heart Rate:

Rhythm:

Intervals (measured in the limb leads)

PR: short (< .12)
     normal (.12 to .20)
     long (>0.20 seconds); this is 1st degree AV block

QRS: normal (≤0.09 seconds)
      prolonged (.10 or .11); this is intraventricular conduction delay (IVCD)
      Bundle Branch Block (.12 seconds or greater)

QT:

P axis: normal
         rightward
         arm-lead reversal or dextrocardia
         junctional rhythm

QRS axis: normal
           left anterior hemiblock
           left posterior hemiblock
           indeterminate

T wave inversion (ischemia or infarction):

II,III,AVF	inferior
I, AVL	lateral
V1, without V2	nonspecific septal
V1 and V2	septal
V3 and V4	anterior
V5 and V6	lateral
V6, without V5	nonspecific lateral

ST Elevation (acute infarction):

II,III,AVF	inferior
I, AVL	lateral
V1, without V2	nonspecific septal
V1 and V2	septal
V3 and V4	anterior
V5 and V6	lateral
V6, without V5.	nonspecific lateral

ST Depression (ischemia or infarction):

I,II,III,AVL,AVF	diffuse subendocardial ischemia or infarction
V2,V3,V4,V5	diffuse subendocardial ischemia or infarction

Q waves (infarction):

II,III,AVF	inferior
I, AVL	lateral
V1, without V2	nonspecific septal
V1 and V2	septal
V3 and V4	anterior
V5 and V6	lateral
V6, without V5	nonspecific lateral

Hypertrophy:

Right atrial: Tall P wave 2.5 mm in II, III, or AVF

Left atrial: Deep negative part of P wave in V1

LVH: R wave in 1 + S wave in III ≥ 25mV
      S wave in V1 + R wave in V5 ≥ 35mV

RVH: Mean QRS either anterior, or rightward

The heart rate is 136 beats per minute. The PR interval measures 0.14 seconds. The QRS interval measures 0.08 seconds. The QT interval measures 0.32 seconds, which is long. The T amplitude is low in the frontal plane. Both suggest hypokalemia. Hypocalcemia is another possibility. (Both are discussed in Chapter 19.) Clinically, sinus tachycardia plus hypokalemia suggests the possibility of hypovolemia due to overdiuresis or excessive GI fluid loss (vomiting or diarrhea). The combination of sinus tachycardia plus hypocalcemia suggests the possibility of hypovolemia due to blood loss, with secondary hypocalcemia associated with multiple transfusions.

Continuing, the P axis is normal at +75°. The mean QRS axis is +15° in the frontal plane and −7.5° in the horizontal plane. The T axis is +30° in the frontal plane and 0° in the horizontal plane. There are tall P waves in leads II, III, and AVF, and the P wave reaches 3 little boxes in lead II, indicating RAA. The negative component of the P wave in lead V1 is negative (1 box wide by 1 box deep), also indicating left atrial abnormality (LAA).

Parts of the answer sheets are "grayed out" because these sections have not yet been covered. Answer only the parts that are not highlighted.

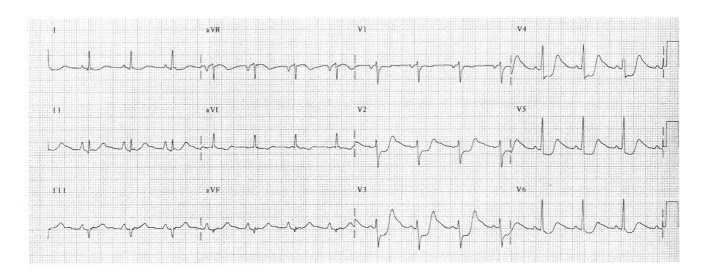

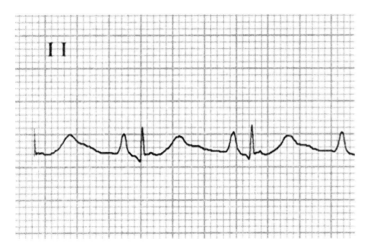

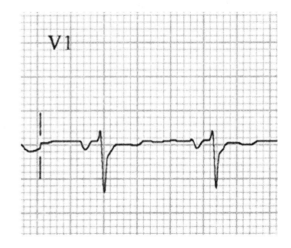

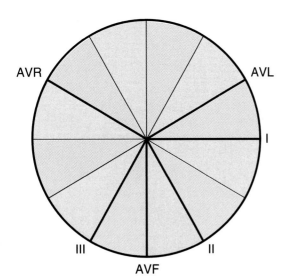

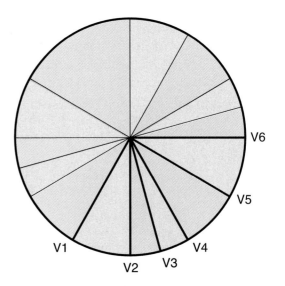

Heart Rate:

Rhythm:

Intervals (measured in the limb leads)

PR: short (< .12)
normal (.12 to .20)
long (>0.20 seconds); this is 1st degree AV block

QRS: normal (≤0.09 seconds)
prolonged (.10 or .11); this is intraventricular conduction delay (IVCD)
Bundle Branch Block (.12 seconds or greater)

QT:

P axis: normal
rightward
arm-lead reversal or dextrocardia
junctional rhythm

QRS axis: normal
left anterior hemiblock
left posterior hemiblock
indeterminate

T wave inversion (ischemia or infarction):

II,III,AVF	inferior
I, AVL	lateral
V1, without V2	nonspecific septal
V1 and V2	septal
V3 and V4	anterior
V5 and V6	lateral
V6, without V5	nonspecific lateral

ST Elevation (acute infarction):

II,III,AVF	inferior
I, AVL	lateral
V1, without V2	nonspecific septal
V1 and V2	septal
V3 and V4	anterior
V5 and V6	lateral
V6, without V5.	nonspecific lateral

ST Depression (ischemia or infarction):

I,II,III,AVL,AVF	diffuse subendocardial ischemia or infarction
V2,V3,V4,V5	diffuse subendocardial ischemia or infarction

Q waves (infarction):

II,III,AVF	inferior
I, AVL	lateral
V1, without V2	nonspecific septal
V1 and V2	septal
V3 and V4	anterior
V5 and V6	lateral
V6, without V5	nonspecific lateral

Hypertrophy:

Right atrial: Tall P wave 2.5 mm in II, III, or AVF

Left atrial: Deep negative part of P wave in V1

LVH: R wave in 1 + S wave in III ≥ 25mV
S wave in V1 + R wave in V5 ≥ 35mV

RVH: Mean QRS either anterior, or rightward

The heart rate is 88 beats per minute. The PR interval measures 0.14 seconds. The QRS interval measures 0.08 seconds. The QT interval measures 0.36 seconds. The P axis is normal (+75°). The mean QRS axis is 0° in the frontal plane and −22.5° in the horizontal plane. The T axis is +45° in the frontal plane. The ST segment in the frontal plane is abnormal. It is depressed slightly in leads I and AVL, pointing away (+150°) from the apical wall, indicating subendocardial ischemia. In the horizontal plane, the T axis is +30° but the ST segment is abnormal. The ST segment points away from the septum and anterior and lateral walls (−105°) and indicates subendocardial ischemia or infarction. The initial QRS axis in the frontal plane is negative in III and borderline in AVF. This is nonspecific inferior Q wave. (This nomenclature is designed to call attention to the possibility of an abnormality, while acknowledging that the error rate or false positivity for this is high). There is a tall P wave in lead II, and this indicates RAA. There is a negative component to the P wave in lead V1 that is 1 box wide by 1 box deep, indicating LAA as well. This patient likely has obstructive CAD, and if not chronic, now has an acute coronary syndrome, caused by a ruptured plaque in the LAD artery. The heart rate of 88 is too fast for either of these conditions. If no contraindications are present, therapy to lower heart rate should be given, typically in the form of a beta blocker.

Parts of the answer sheets are "grayed out" because these sections have not yet been covered. Answer only the parts that are not highlighted.

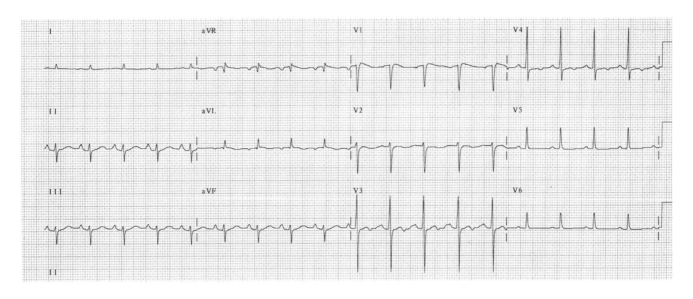

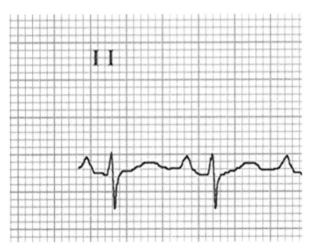

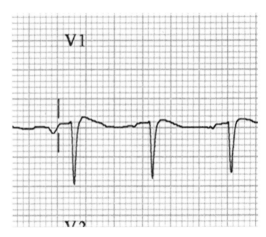

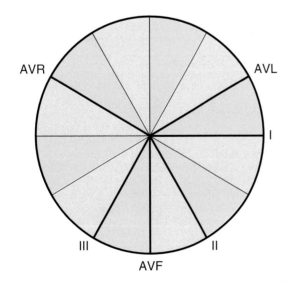

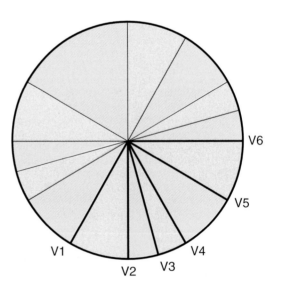

Heart Rate:

Rhythm:

Intervals (measured in the limb leads)

PR: short (< .12)
       normal (.12 to .20)
       long (>0.20 seconds); this is 1st degree AV block

QRS: normal (≤0.09 seconds)
       prolonged (.10 or .11); this is intraventricular conduction delay (IVCD)
       Bundle Branch Block (.12 seconds or greater)

QT:

P axis: normal
           rightward
           arm-lead reversal or dextrocardia
           junctional rhythm

QRS axis: normal
           left anterior hemiblock
           left posterior hemiblock
           indeterminate

T wave inversion (ischemia or infarction):

II,III,AVF	inferior
I, AVL	lateral
V1, without V2	nonspecific septal
V1 and V2	septal
V3 and V4	anterior
V5 and V6	lateral
V6, without V5	nonspecific lateral

ST Elevation (acute infarction):

II,III,AVF	inferior
I, AVL	lateral
V1, without V2	nonspecific septal
V1 and V2	septal
V3 and V4	anterior
V5 and V6	lateral
V6, without V5.	nonspecific lateral

ST Depression (ischemia or infarction):

I,II,III,AVL,AVF	diffuse subendocardial ischemia or infarction
V2,V3,V4,V5	diffuse subendocardial ischemia or infarction

Q waves (infarction):

II,III,AVF	inferior
I, AVL	lateral
V1, without V2	nonspecific septal
V1 and V2	septal
V3 and V4	anterior
V5 and V6	lateral
V6, without V5	nonspecific lateral

Hypertrophy:

Right atrial: Tall P wave 2.5 mm in II, III, or AVF

Left atrial: Deep negative part of P wave in V1

LVH: R wave in 1 + S wave in III ≥ 25mV
       S wave in V1 + R wave in V5 ≥ 35mV

RVH: Mean QRS either anterior, or rightward

The heart rate is 107 beats per minute. This is sinus tachycardia. The PR interval measures 0.16 seconds. The QRS interval measures 0.08 seconds. The QT interval measures 0.34 seconds. The QT interval is long. The P axis is normal (+75°). The mean QRS axis is −60° in the frontal plane, indicating left anterior hemiblock. The mean QRS is −22.5° in the horizontal plane. The T waves are flattened laterally (I, AVL, V5, and V6) but they are not negative by 1 little box. These are nonspecific T wave abnormalities. Good terminology for these is "nonspecific T wave changes" or "nonspecific lateral T wave changes." The notion here is that ischemia *could* be present, but other causes could be present as well. The ST segments are slightly elevated in V1 and V2, biphasic in V2 and V3, and flat in V5 and V6. These do not meet our criteria for ischemia, so they are termed nonspecific ST changes. Good terminology for this is "nonspecific ST changes" or "nonspecific septal, anterior, and lateral ST changes." If you are concerned about the possibility of ischemia, repeat the EKG in 20 minutes; it may show more definitive changes. When the ST and T waves are diffusely but nospecifically abnormal, the ultimate hedge of diffuse nonspecific ST and T changes is appropriate. In Chapter 19, the effect of electrolytes and drugs on the ST and T segments is addressed. Continuing, RAA is present but not LAA.

Parts of the answer sheets are "grayed out" because these sections have not yet been covered. Answer only the parts that are not highlighted.

Left Ventricular Hypertrophy

Left ventricular hypertrophy (LVH) is often the result of an increase in pressure or volume within the left ventricle. When the pressure in the left ventricle increases, it adapts by developing a concentrically thicker wall. However, as the ventricular wall thickness increases, the cavity size becomes smaller. Increased pressure in the left ventricle is seen in **systemic hypertension, aortic stenosis, or hypertrophic cardiomyopathy.** When the left ventricle is strained from volume overload, it compensates by making extra space or dilating. Volume overload is often seen in **mitral or aortic regurgitation.**

Increased pressure in the left ventricle can be present from systemic hypertension, aortic stenosis, or hypertrophic cardiomyopathy. The left ventricle adaptation to increased pressure load is a concentrically increased wall thickness with a small left ventricular cavity size.

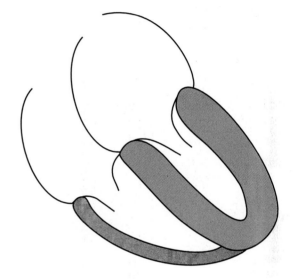

Increased volume in the left ventricle can result from mitral or aortic regurgitation. To handle the volume overload, the left ventricle has to "make space" and dilates.

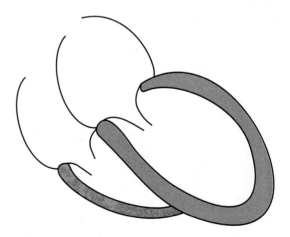

Aortic Stenosis

Aortic stenosis develops when the opening of the aortic valve becomes narrowed, restricting the flow of blood out of the left ventricle. The left ventricle hypertrophies to provide the extra force to push the blood through the aortic valve. The most common causes of aortic stenosis are rheumatic heart disease, congenital malformation, or calcification of the bicuspid valve.

Aortic stenosis restricts the flow of blood out of the left ventricle. The left ventricle hypertrophies to provide extra force to push the blood across the aortic valve. The left atrium hypertrophies as well, because it needs to force blood into a thick muscular ventricle. This causes left ventricular hypertrophy (LVH) on the EKG.

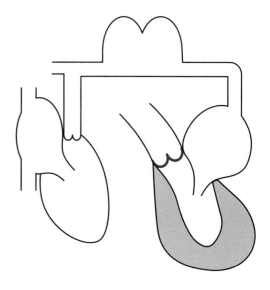

EKG Criteria for LVH

LVH increases the amplitude of the left ventricular forces. However, the *mean QRS axis is not really affected because the left ventricular forces already predominate over the force generated by the right ventricle.* In the following example of LVH, the mean QRS axis in the frontal and horizontal planes lies within the normal range. The increased mass of the left ventricle (whether concentric with a small cavity or eccentric with a dilated cavity) increases the amplitude of the QRS force. Both the frontal plane and the horizontal plane may show the increased amplitude of LVH. There are separate criteria for each.

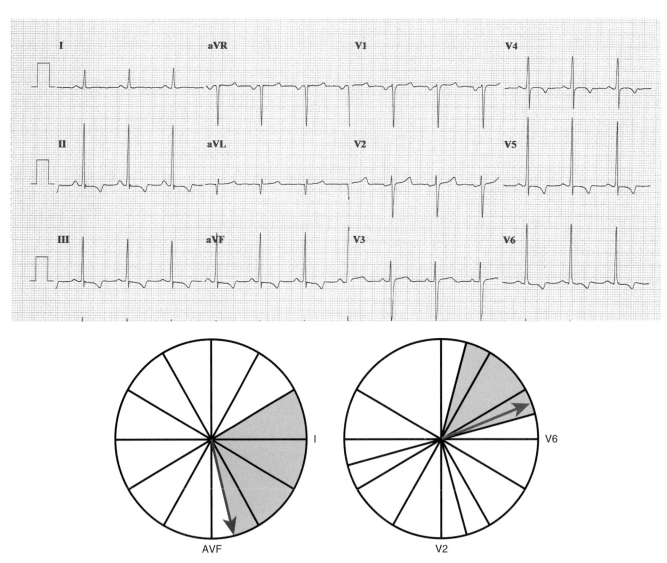

Concept: The QRS axis points leftward and posterior as usual.

Axis: The mean QRS axis points to the left ventricle, but it does that anyway. Axis doesn't really help diagnose LVH.

Pattern: The QRS voltage is increased.

EKG Criteria for LVH in the Frontal Plane

Concept: LVH increases the amplitude of the left ventricular forces toward the left ventricle, leftward (I positive and III negative).

Criteria: The depth of the S wave in lead III added to the height of the R wave in lead I equals 25 little boxes or more. Here the sum is 31 little boxes.

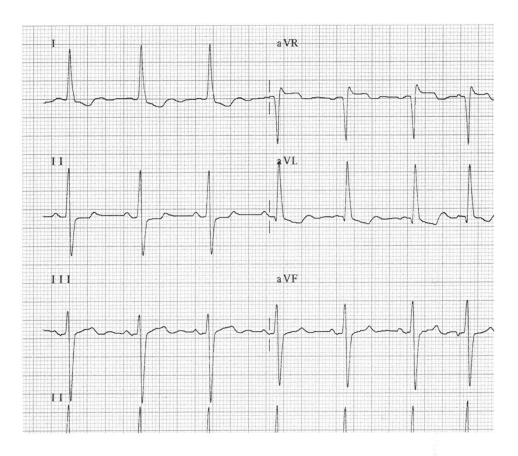

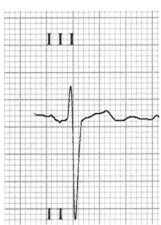

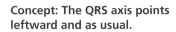

Concept: The QRS axis points leftward and as usual.

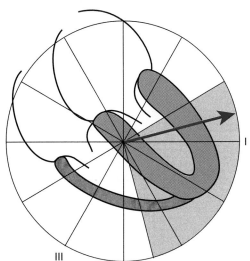

Axis: The mean QRS axis points to the left ventricle, but it does that anyway. Axis doesn't really help diagnose LVH.

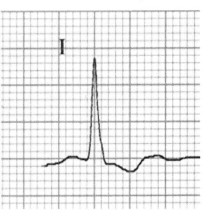

Pattern: The QRS voltage is increased.

EKG Criteria for LVH in the Horizontal Plane

Concept: LVH increases the amplitude of the left ventricular forces toward the left ventricle, posterior (V1 negative) and leftward (V5 positive).

Criteria: The depth of the S wave in lead VI added to the height of the R wave in lead V5 equals 35 little boxes or more. Here the sum is 44 little boxes.

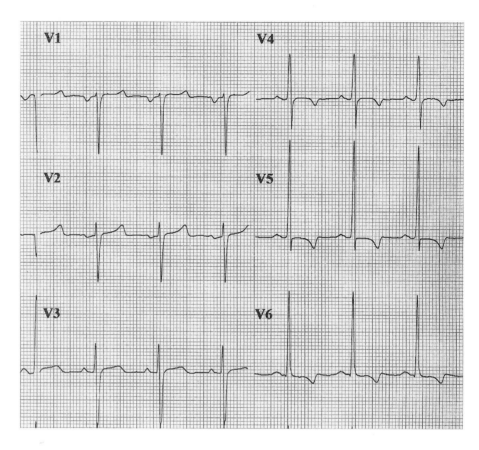

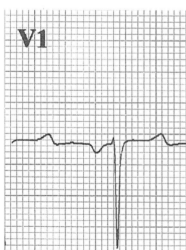

Concept: The QRS axis points leftward and posterior as usual.

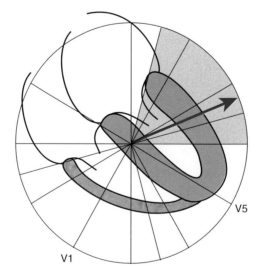

Axis: The mean QRS axis points to the left ventricle, but it does that anyway. Axis doesn't really help diagnose LVH.

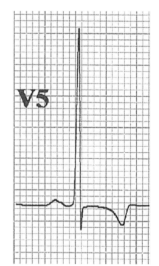

Pattern: The QRS voltage is increased.

ST Segment Changes in LVH

In LVH, the ST segment may point opposite the mean QRS axis. This is sometimes referred to as "strain pattern." These ST segment changes can be seen in the frontal plane, the horizontal plane, or both. In either plane, the ST segment points away from the left ventricle, as it would in left bundle branch block or subendocardial ischemia of the lateral wall. ST elevation in leads III, V1, and V2 may be reciprocal changes due to the ST depression in the lateral leads and not an indication of transmural ischemia or infarction.

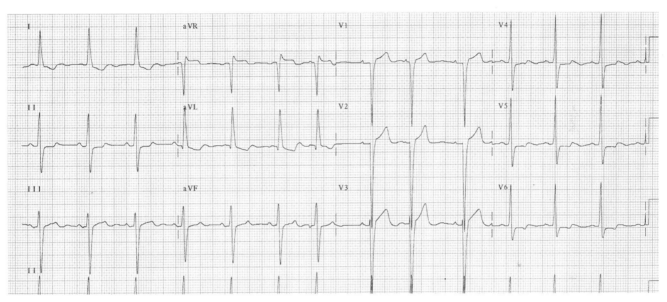

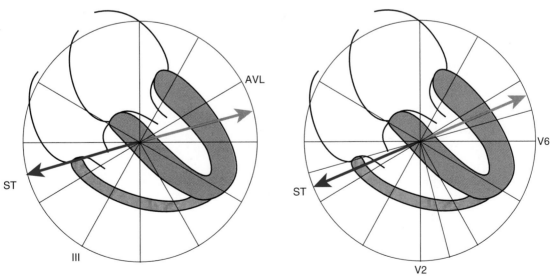

Concept: LVH can cause the ST axis to point opposite the mean QRS axis.

Axis: The ST axis points opposite the mean QRS axis.

Pattern: ST depression in leads I, AVL, V5, and V6. There may be ST elevation in leads III, V1, and V2.

LVH Simulating Anterior Wall Infarction

As the left ventricle mass increases, it creates larger negative voltages in leads V1 and V2. A point can be reached at which the negative voltage washes out the R waves in these leads and gives the appearance of septal infarction. **The Q waves in V1 and V2 may be due solely to LVH.** The ST segment changes in LVH, which point away from the lateral walls, can cause the appearance of ST elevation, **simulating transmural ischemia of the inferior wall and septum.** On the other hand, hypertension frequently is the underlying cause of LVH, and hypertension is a major risk factor for coronary artery disease. LVH, by creating its own ST segment depression and elevation, as well as Q waves in the septal leads, complicates the interpretation of ischemia in these patients. Further testing and information are almost always necessary.

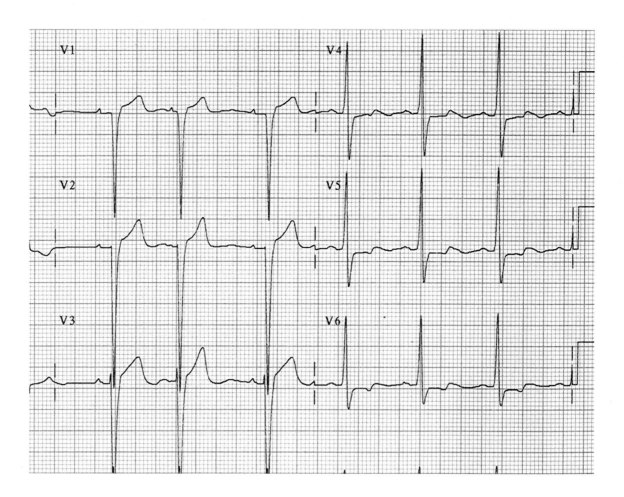

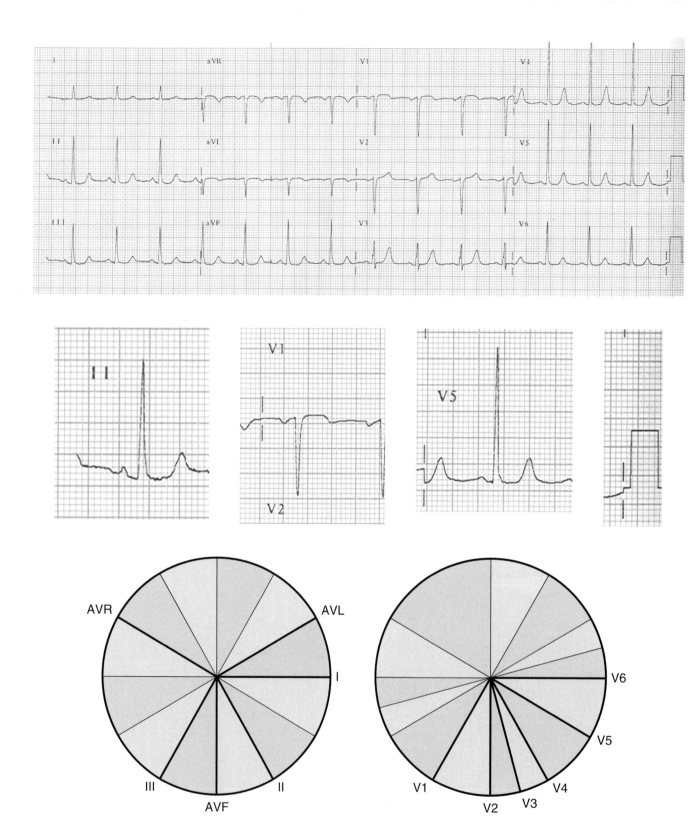

Heart Rate:

Rhythm:

ST Elevation (acute infarction):

II,III,AVF	inferior
I, AVL	lateral
V1, without V2	nonspecific septal
V1 and V2	septal
V3 and V4	anterior
V5 and V6	lateral
V6, without V5.	nonspecific lateral

Intervals (measured in the limb leads)

PR: short (< .12)
        normal (.12 to .20)
        long (>0.20 seconds); this is 1st degree AV
        block

QRS: normal (≤0.09 seconds)
        prolonged (.10 or .11); this is intraventricular
        conduction delay (IVCD)
        Bundle Branch Block (.12 seconds or greater)

QT:

ST Depression (ischemia or infarction):

I,II,III,AVL,AVF	diffuse subendocardial ischemia or infarction
V2,V3,V4,V5	diffuse subendocardial ischemia or infarction

P axis: normal
            rightward
            arm-lead reversal or dextrocardia
            junctional rhythm

QRS axis: normal
            left anterior hemiblock
            left posterior hemiblock
            indeterminate

Q waves (infarction):

II,III,AVF	inferior
I, AVL	lateral
V1, without V2	nonspecific septal
V1 and V2	septal
V3 and V4	anterior
V5 and V6	lateral
V6, without V5	nonspecific lateral

T wave inversion (ischemia or infarction):

II,III,AVF	inferior
I, AVL	lateral
V1, without V2	nonspecific septal
V1 and V2	septal
V3 and V4	anterior
V5 and V6	lateral
V6, without V5	nonspecific lateral

Hypertrophy:

Right atrial: Tall P wave 2.5 mm in II, III, or AVF

Left atrial: Deep negative part of P wave in V1

LVH: R wave in 1 + S wave in III ≥ 25mV
      S wave in V1 + R wave in V5 ≥ 35mV

RVH: Mean QRS either anterior, or rightward

The heart rate is 83 beats per minute. The PR interval measures 0.16 seconds. The QRS interval measures 0.08 seconds. The QT interval measures 0.38 seconds. The P axis is normal at +75°. The mean QRS axis is +75° in the frontal plane and −7.5° in the horizontal plane. The T axis is +60° in the frontal plane and +30° in the horizontal plane. In the frontal plane, the ST segments are slightly depressed in II, III, and AVF. This may represent inferior subendocardial ischemia or infarction. The depth of the S wave in lead V1 (15 mm) plus the height of the R wave in lead V5 (25 mm) adds up to 40 mm, above the **criteria for left ventricular hypertrophy (LVH)**. *LVH is most commonly caused by hypertension.* If the patient has hypertension, then the diagnosis of hypertensive heart disease can be supported by this EKG. If the patient does not have hypertension, then pressure or overload conditions must be ruled out. These include *aortic stenosis, aortic regurgitation, mitral regurgitation, and hypertrophic cardiomyopathy.* An echocardiogram in the setting of LVH is always appropriate to separate each of these causes. *The murmur or aortic stenosis may not be clinically appreciated, but the presence of LVH on the EKG unattended by clinical hypertension always suggests the possibility of aortic stenosis. Always figure out why the patient has LVH.* The nonspecific EKG changes on this EKG may be caused by ischemia or hypertension or drugs used to treat hypertension (see Chapter 19).

Parts of the answer sheets are "grayed out" because these sections have not yet been covered. Answer only the parts that are not highlighted.

Worksheet 17-2

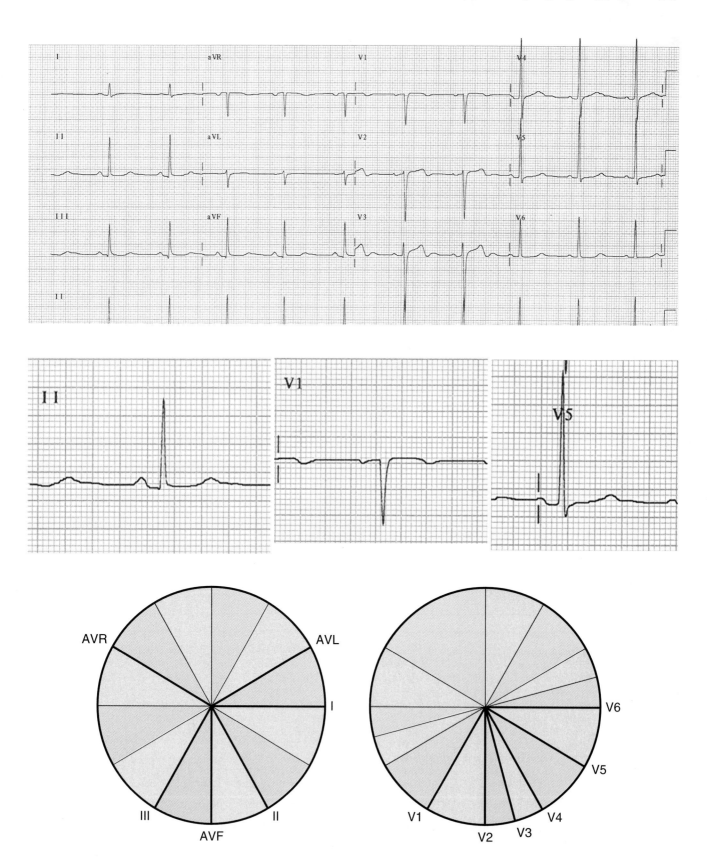

Heart Rate:

Rhythm:

Intervals (measured in the limb leads)

PR: short (< .12)
       normal (.12 to .20)
       long (>0.20 seconds); this is 1st degree AV block

QRS: normal (≤0.09 seconds)
       prolonged (.10 or .11); this is intraventricular conduction delay (IVCD)
       Bundle Branch Block (.12 seconds or greater)

QT:

P axis: normal
          rightward
          arm-lead reversal or dextrocardia
          junctional rhythm

QRS axis: normal
           left anterior hemiblock
           left posterior hemiblock
           indeterminate

T wave inversion (ischemia or infarction):

II,III,AVF	inferior
I, AVL	lateral
V1, without V2	nonspecific septal
V1 and V2	septal
V3 and V4	anterior
V5 and V6	lateral
V6, without V5	nonspecific lateral

ST Elevation (acute infarction):

II,III,AVF	inferior
I, AVL	lateral
V1, without V2	nonspecific septal
V1 and V2	septal
V3 and V4	anterior
V5 and V6	lateral
V6, without V5.	nonspecific lateral

ST Depression (ischemia or infarction):

I,II,III,AVL,AVF	diffuse subendocardial ischemia or infarction
V2,V3,V4,V5	diffuse subendocardial ischemia or infarction

Q waves (infarction):

II,III,AVF	inferior
I, AVL	lateral
V1, without V2	nonspecific septal
V1 and V2	septal
V3 and V4	anterior
V5 and V6	lateral
V6, without V5	nonspecific lateral

Hypertrophy:

Right atrial: Tall P wave 2.5 mm in II, III, or AVF

Left atrial: Deep negative part of P wave in V1

LVH: R wave in 1 + S wave in III ≥ 25mV
      S wave in V1 + R wave in V5 ≥ 35mV

RVH: Mean QRS either anterior, or rightward

The heart rate is 60 beats per minute. The PR interval measures 0.18 seconds. The QRS interval measures 0.08 seconds. The QT interval measures 0.44 seconds. The prominent U wave is noted in lead V3 after the T wave, and this suggests hypokalemia. The P axis is normal (+60°). The mean QRS axis is +75° in the frontal plane and −22.5° in the horizontal plane. The initial QRS is normal in the frontal and horizontal planes. The T axis +90° in the frontal plane and +30° in the horizontal plane. The ST segments are not significantly abnormal in the frontal plane. In the horizontal plane, the ST segments are abnormal and point toward the septum and anterior walls. This can be due to transmural ischemia or infarction of the septum and anterior walls. The S wave in lead V1 (13 mm) added to the R wave in lead V5 (24 mm) total 37 mm, indicating LVH. LVH by changing the depolarization of the ventricles (it changes the QRS) can change the repolarization as well. This is called secondary ST changes. In LVH (as in LBBB), the ST segment can point away from the lateral wall and toward the septum solely as a consequence of the LVH. *In this EKG then, the ST segment abnormality may be due to either transmural ischemia of the septum or LVH.*

Importantly, LVH frequently is due to hypertension. Its presence on the EKG suggests it has not been well controlled. Hypertension is a major risk factor for coronary artery disease. Most of the EKG readings from now on should contain a differential of clinical possibilities. The U waves and long QT suggest that this patient is on a diuretic (possibly for hypertension) and has hypokalemia, a common side effect of diuretic therapy. If this patient doesn't have hypertension, he or she may have an important degree of aortic stenosis, aortic regurgitation, or mitral regurgitation. He or she does have heart disease. LVH is not a disease of the EKG.

Parts of the answer sheets are "grayed out" because these sections have not yet been covered. Answer only the parts that are not highlighted.

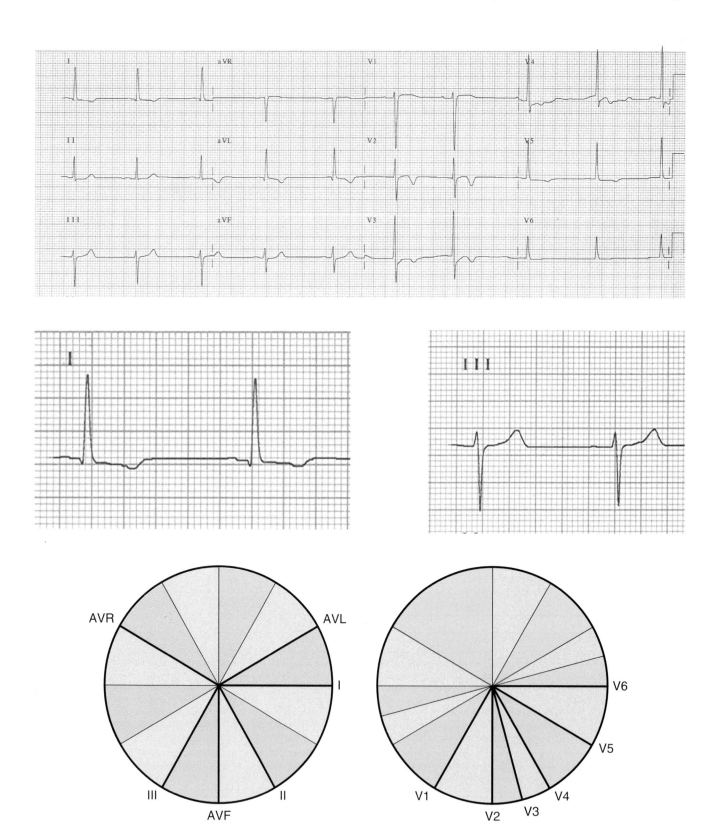

Heart Rate:

Rhythm:

Intervals (measured in the limb leads)

PR: short (< .12)
normal (.12 to .20)
long (>0.20 seconds); this is 1st degree AV block

QRS: normal (≤0.09 seconds)
prolonged (.10 or .11); this is intraventricular conduction delay (IVCD)
Bundle Branch Block (.12 seconds or greater)

QT:

P axis: normal
rightward
arm-lead reversal or dextrocardia
junctional rhythm

QRS axis: normal
left anterior hemiblock
left posterior hemiblock
indeterminate

T wave inversion (ischemia or infarction):

II,III,AVF	inferior
I, AVL	lateral
V1, without V2	nonspecific septal
V1 and V2	septal
V3 and V4	anterior
V5 and V6	lateral
V6, without V5	nonspecific lateral

ST Elevation (acute infarction):

II,III,AVF	inferior
I, AVL	lateral
V1, without V2	nonspecific septal
V1 and V2	septal
V3 and V4	anterior
V5 and V6	lateral
V6, without V5.	nonspecific lateral

ST Depression (ischemia or infarction):

I,II,III,AVL,AVF	diffuse subendocardial ischemia or infarction
V2,V3,V4,V5	diffuse subendocardial ischemia or infarction

Q waves (infarction):

II,III,AVF	inferior
I, AVL	lateral
V1, without V2	nonspecific septal
V1 and V2	septal
V3 and V4	anterior
V5 and V6	lateral
V6, without V5	nonspecific lateral

Hypertrophy:

Right atrial: Tall P wave 2.5 mm in II, III, or AVF

Left atrial: Deep negative part of P wave in V1

LVH: R wave in 1 + S wave in III ≥ 25mV
S wave in V1 + R wave in V5 ≥ 35mV

RVH: Mean QRS either anterior, or rightward

The heart rate varies from 53 to 60 beats per minute. This is sinus arrhythmia. The PR interval measures 0.16 seconds. The QRS interval measures 0.10 seconds (LIVCD). The QT interval measures 0.40 seconds. The P axis is normal (+60°, although it is difficult to determine it is positive in I and AVF). The mean QRS axis in the frontal plane is −15° and in the horizontal plane is 0°. The initial QRS axis is normal in the frontal and horizontal planes. The ST segment in the frontal plane is abnormal (−165°) and points away from the lateral wall. The ST segment in the horizontal plane is abnormal and points toward the septum (+165°). The R wave in lead I (12 mm) plus the S wave in lead III (12 mm) totals 25 mm and indicates LVH. The S wave in lead V1 (21 mm) plus the R wave in V5 (15 mm) totals 36 mm and indicates LVH as well. In LVH, the ST segment can be abnormal and points opposite the mean QRS axis in the frontal and horizontal planes. As a shortcut, if the mean QRS is positive in a given lead, the expected ST segment would be negative. Therefore, the ST segments in LVH appear similar to lateral subendocardial ischemia or transmural septal ischemia.

A useful differential would be "the ST segments are abnormal and are consistent with LVH, with transmural septal ischemia, or with lateral subendocardial ischemia."

Parts of the answer sheets are "grayed out" because these sections have not yet been covered. Answer only the parts that are not highlighted.

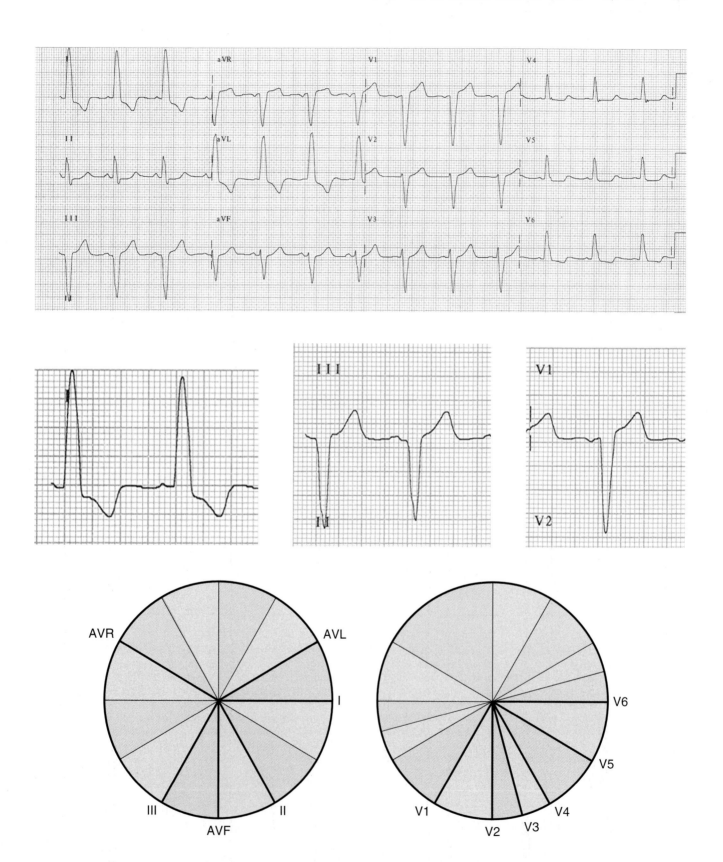

Heart Rate:

Rhythm:

Intervals (measured in the limb leads)

PR: short (< .12)
      normal (.12 to .20)
      long (>0.20 seconds); this is 1st degree AV block

QRS: normal (≤0.09 seconds)
      prolonged (.10 or .11); this is intraventricular conduction delay (IVCD)
      Bundle Branch Block (.12 seconds or greater)

QT:

P axis: normal
           rightward
           arm-lead reversal or dextrocardia
           junctional rhythm

QRS axis: normal
           left anterior hemiblock
           left posterior hemiblock
           indeterminate

T wave inversion (ischemia or infarction):

II,III,AVF	inferior
I, AVL	lateral
V1, without V2	nonspecific septal
V1 and V2	septal
V3 and V4	anterior
V5 and V6	lateral
V6, without V5	nonspecific lateral

ST Elevation (acute infarction):

II,III,AVF	inferior
I, AVL	lateral
V1, without V2	nonspecific septal
V1 and V2	septal
V3 and V4	anterior
V5 and V6	lateral
V6, without V5.	nonspecific lateral

ST Depression (ischemia or infarction):

I,II,III,AVL,AVF	diffuse subendocardial ischemia or infarction
V2,V3,V4,V5	diffuse subendocardial ischemia or infarction

Q waves (infarction):

II,III,AVF	inferior
I, AVL	lateral
V1, without V2	nonspecific septal
V1 and V2	septal
V3 and V4	anterior
V5 and V6	lateral
V6, without V5	nonspecific lateral

Hypertrophy:

Right atrial: Tall P wave 2.5 mm in II, III, or AVF

Left atrial: Deep negative part of P wave in V1

LVH: R wave in 1 + S wave in III ≥ 25mV
      S wave in V1 + R wave in V5 ≥ 35mV

RVH: Mean QRS either anterior, or rightward

The heart rate is 75 beats per minute. The PR interval measures 0.12 seconds. The QRS interval measures 0.12 seconds. There is BBB. The last part of the QRS is (positive in lead I) leftward in the frontal plane (−45°). It is leftward (positive in lead V6) and posterior (negative in lead V2) in the horizontal plane (−22.5°). This indicates LBBB. The ST segment points away from the last part of the QRS as expected.

Do not evaluate the QRS for hypertrophy or infarction in the presence of LBBB.

The ST segments are abnormal (they point leftward and anterior, away from the last part of the QRS, as expected in LBBB). *However, don't diagnose transmural septal ischemia, lateral subendocardial ischemia, or LVH in the presence of LBBB.*

Atrial hypertrophy could be diagnosed but is not present on this EKG.

Parts of the answer sheets are "grayed out" because these sections have not yet been covered. Answer only the parts that are not highlighted.

Worksheet 17-5

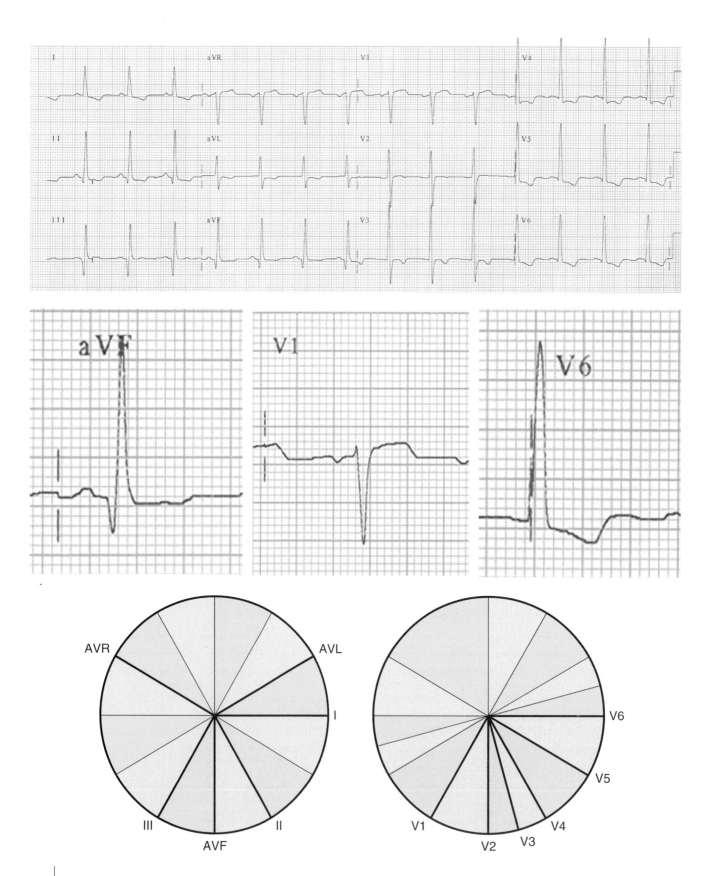

Heart Rate:

Rhythm:

Intervals (measured in the limb leads)

PR: short (< .12)
        normal (.12 to .20)
        long (>0.20 seconds); this is 1st degree AV block

QRS: normal (≤0.09 seconds)
        prolonged (.10 or .11); this is intraventricular conduction delay (IVCD)
        Bundle Branch Block (.12 seconds or greater)

QT:

P axis: normal
           rightward
           arm-lead reversal or dextrocardia
           junctional rhythm

QRS axis: normal
           left anterior hemiblock
           left posterior hemiblock
           indeterminate

T wave inversion (ischemia or infarction):

II,III,AVF	inferior
I, AVL	lateral
V1, without V2	nonspecific septal
V1 and V2	septal
V3 and V4	anterior
V5 and V6	lateral
V6, without V5	nonspecific lateral

ST Elevation (acute infarction):

II,III,AVF	inferior
I, AVL	lateral
V1, without V2	nonspecific septal
V1 and V2	septal
V3 and V4	anterior
V5 and V6	lateral
V6, without V5.	nonspecific lateral

ST Depression (ischemia or infarction):

I,II,III,AVL,AVF	diffuse subendocardial ischemia or infarction
V2,V3,V4,V5	diffuse subendocardial ischemia or infarction

Q waves (infarction):

II,III,AVF	inferior
I, AVL	lateral
V1, without V2	nonspecific septal
V1 and V2	septal
V3 and V4	anterior
V5 and V6	lateral
V6, without V5	nonspecific lateral

Hypertrophy:

Right atrial: Tall P wave 2.5 mm in II, III, or AVF

Left atrial: Deep negative part of P wave in V1

LVH: R wave in 1 + S wave in III ≥ 25mV
       S wave in V1 + R wave in V5 ≥ 35mV

RVH: Mean QRS either anterior, or rightward

The heart rate is 83 beats per minute. The PR interval measures 0.14 seconds. The QRS interval measures 0.11 seconds. This is IVCD, which is commonly seen in LVH. (The slurred downstroke in II, III, and AVF makes the true QRS difficult to measure in these leads. If you call this 0.12 seconds, you will have to call it LBBB, and then be unable to read further into the EKG.) Because the last part of the QRS is posterior and leftward, it represents LIVCD. This reduces the specificity of EKG readings but not as much as LBBB does. The QT interval measures 0.34 seconds. The P axis is normal (+60°). The mean QRS axis is +45° in the frontal plane and 0° in the horizontal plane. The initial QRS axis in the frontal plane points away from the inferior wall (−45°), with q waves in II, III, and AVF, representing transmural infarction of the inferior wall. Whenever abnormal Q waves are present, any abnormality of the ST segment or T wave in any plane or lead should always suggest the possibility that the infarction may be acute. The S wave in lead VI (11 mm) and the S wave in lead V5 (22 mm) total 33 mm and do not meet the criteria given for LVH. To indicate that the QRS voltage is high but doesn't quite meet LVH criteria, the terminology "high QRS voltage" can be used. The ST segments are abnormal, and point away from the lateral wall and toward the septum. This may represent LVH or be due to ischemia.

Parts of the answer sheets are "grayed out" because these sections have not yet been covered. Answer only the parts that are not highlighted.

Right Ventricular Hypertrophy

KEY CONCEPT

Because the left ventricle is normally more massive than the right ventricle, any shift of the mean QRS axis—either rightward *or* anterior— indicates right ventricular hypertrophy.

The QRS complex represents depolarization of the right and left ventricles. Because the left ventricle is more massive than the right ventricle, the mean QRS axis normally points toward the left ventricle. Therefore, in the frontal plane, the normal mean QRS points posterior and leftward. In the horizontal plane, the normal mean QRS also points to the left ventricle, which is posterior and leftward. **The diagnosis of right ventricular hypertrophy (RVH) is made by identifying a mean QRS axis that points either rightward or anterior or both.**

In the frontal plane, the normal mean QRS points posterior and leftward, toward the more massive left ventricle.

In the horizontal plane, the normal mean QRS also points to the more massive left ventricle, which is posterior and leftward.

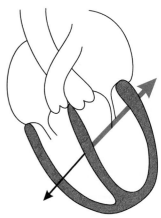

The diagnosis of right ventricular hypertrophy is made by identifying a mean QRS axis that points either rightward or anterior or both.

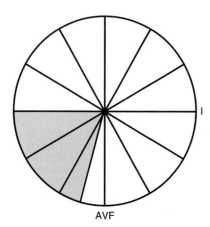

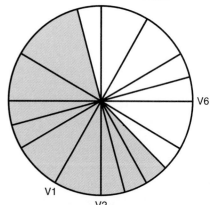

Right Ventricular Hypertrophy

As the right ventricle is subjected to the stress of pressure or volume, its mass increases as a compensatory mechanism to handle the increased work. Increased pressure in the right ventricle can be present from pulmonary hypertension. **In adults this is commonly due to obstructive lung disease or pulmonary emboli.** The right ventricular adaptation is to increase its mass. Increased volume in the right ventricle can result from tricuspid regurgitation or an intracardiac shunt such as an **atrial septal defect (ASD).** To handle the volume overload, the right ventricle has to "make space" and dilates.

Increased pressure in the right ventricle can be present from chronic obstructive pulmonary disease or pulmonary embolism. The right ventricle adaptation to increased pressure load is increased wall thickness and cavity size.

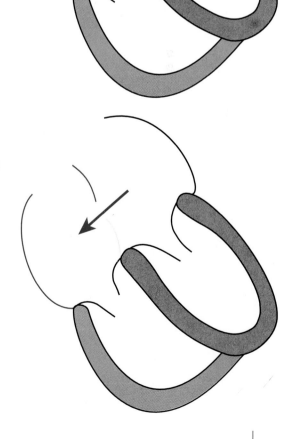

Increased volume in the right ventricle can result from an atrial septal defect (ASD) shown or tricuspid regurgitation. To handle the volume overload, the right ventricle has to "make space" and dilates.

EKG Criteria for RVH in the Frontal Plane

The left ventricle is leftward and posterior, and as it depolarizes simultaneously with the right ventricle, its more massive forces predominate, so the mean QRS axis points toward the left ventricle. **If the right ventricle can achieve enough mass to pull the mean QRS rightward in the frontal plane, then this indicates right ventricular hypertrophy. If lead I demonstrates the mean QRS axis in the frontal plane as rightward, this by itself indicates RVH.** Chapter 8 demonstrates left posterior hemiblock (LPHB) as an otherwise unexplained right axis. **Now there is a differential diagnosis when an EKG has a mean QRS that points rightward: LPHB, RVH, or a large lateral wall infarction.** Other clues must be examined to help narrow the diagnosis.

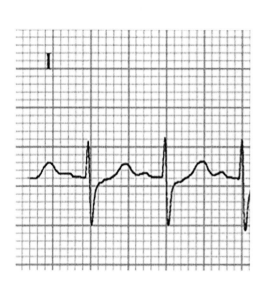

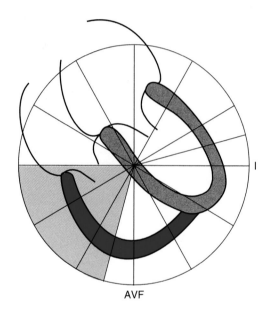

Concept: If the right ventricle can achieve enough mass to pull the mean QRS axis rightward, then this indicates right ventricular hypertrophy.

Axis: The mean QRS axis in the frontal plane points rightward, greater than +90°.

Pattern: The QRS is negative in lead I.

EKG Criteria for RVH in the Horizontal Plane

The left ventricle is leftward and posterior, and as it depolarizes simultaneously with the right ventricle, its more massive forces predominate, so the mean QRS axis points toward the left ventricle. If the right ventricle can achieve enough mass to **pull the mean QRS *either* rightward *or* anterior,** in either the frontal plane or the horizontal plane, then this indicates RVH. If lead I demonstrates the mean QRS axis in the frontal plane as rightward, this indicates RVH. Notice that the mean QRS in the horizontal plane is also rightward and also anterior. Cut the right ventricle some slack. It's up against the left ventricle. If the right ventricle can pull the QRS **either anterior or rightward,** then this indicates RVH.

The colored pie shape indicates regions where either V1 is positive or V6 is negative.

Only one of these conditions needs to be met.

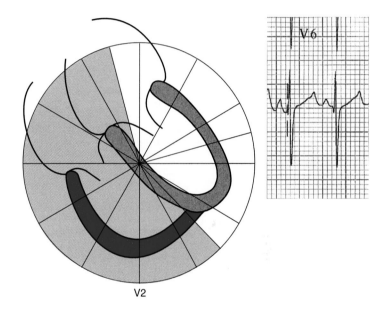

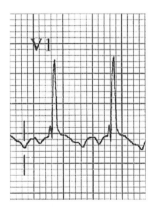

Concept: If the right ventricle can achieve enough mass to pull the mean QRS rightward or anterior, in the horizontal plane then this indicates right ventricular hypertrophy.

Axis: The mean QRS axis in the horizontal plane points rightward or anterior, less than −90° or greater than +30°.

Pattern: The QRS is positive in lead V1 or negative in lead V6.

ST Segment Changes in RVH

In RVH, the ST segment or T wave axis may point away from the right ventricle. These ST or T wave changes can happen in the frontal plane, the horizontal plane, or both. In either plane, the ST or T points away from the right ventricle, as it would in right bundle branch block or subendocardial ischemia of the septum.

The mean QRS axis in the horizontal plane points rightward. Notice the T axis in the horizontal plane. It points away from the septum and the right ventricle.

To determine whether there is ischemia of the septum or a pulmonary embolus, clinical information is necessary.

A casual examination of this EKG would suggest septal ischemia but might miss the QRS axis pointing at the right ventricle. Be complete!

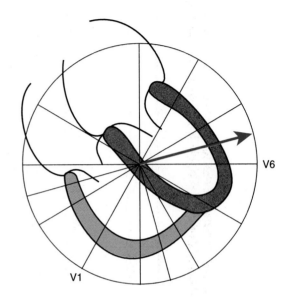

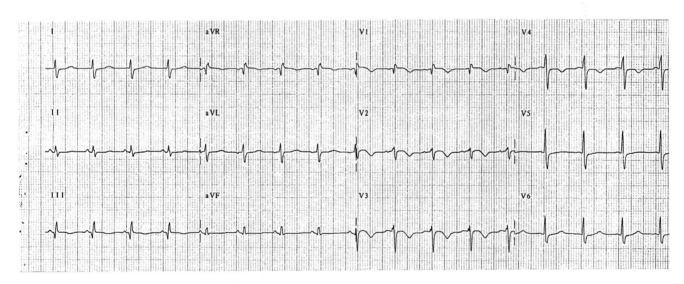

Obstructive Lung Disease

Obstructive lung disease (COPD), commonly caused by smoking, increases the pulmonary resistance to blood flow from the pulmonary artery. When the resistance to blood flow rises, the pressure builds up in the right ventricle. The increased pressure must be generated by the right ventricle, which hypertrophies to meet the new increased workload. The right atrium eventually becomes involved, as the right ventricle struggles to meet its new burdens. The EKG shows RVH and RAA. COPD traps a large volume of air inside the lungs. This air is a terrible conductor of electricity and interferes with the recording of the EKG. This can cause *low voltage* to appear on the EKG, as shown.

COPD reduces the cross-sectional area of blood flow through the lungs. This increases the pressure in the pulmonary artery, which the right ventricle must match and exceed or the pulmonary valve will never open. The right atrium hypertrophies as well to assist the right ventricle meet its new workload.

When the level of trapped air becomes severe, the EKG shows low voltage as shown. If the sum of the QRS amplitude in leads I, II, and III is less than 15 little boxes, low voltage is present. If none of the QRS complexes in leads V1, V2, or V3 is 15 little boxes by itself, then low voltage is present.

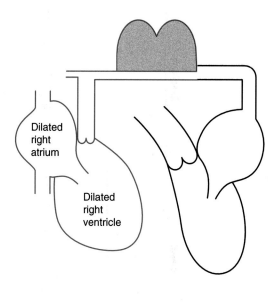

Dilated right atrium

Dilated right ventricle

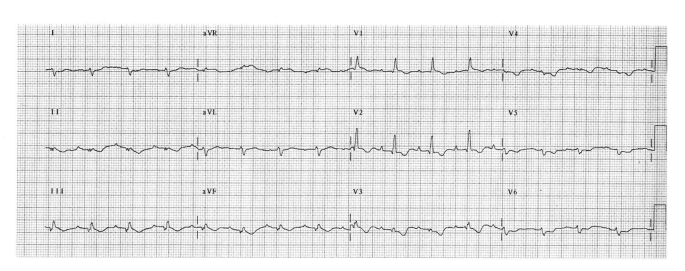

Pulmonary Embolism

Pulmonary embolism is usually part of the disease process termed venous thromboembolism, or VTE. Because of a hypercoagulable state, trauma to a blood vessel, or low flow states, thrombus can form in the venous system and then embolize to the pulmonary artery. Pulmonary embolism can develop as a single event but can also become recurrent. The embolus in the pulmonary artery obstructs blood flow to part of the lungs and increases the pressure behind the clot. The right ventricle typically dilates rapidly in response to this. In the acute setting, the EKG can (but may not) demonstrate sinus tachycardia, RVH, and RAA. If the pressure overload is severe, there can be a supply and demand mismatch for the right ventricle, and abnormal T waves can result. **The EKG can show a T axis that points posterior, not away from the septum but away from the free wall of the right ventricle, as in the following example.**

Pulmonary embolism obstructs blood flow through the lungs. This raises the pressure in the pulmonary artery, which the right ventricle must immediately handle.

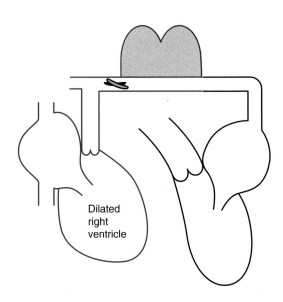

Dilated right ventricle

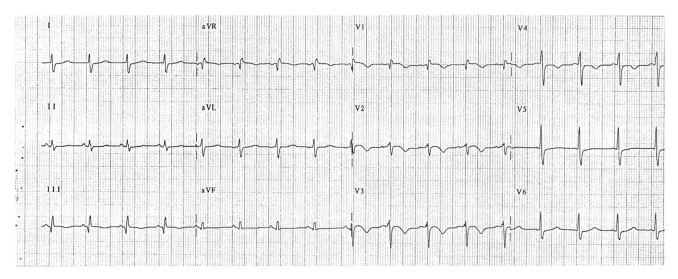

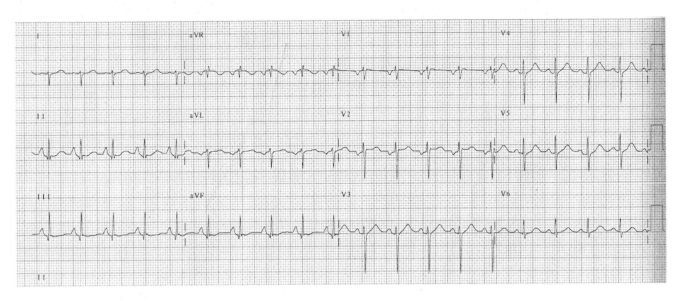

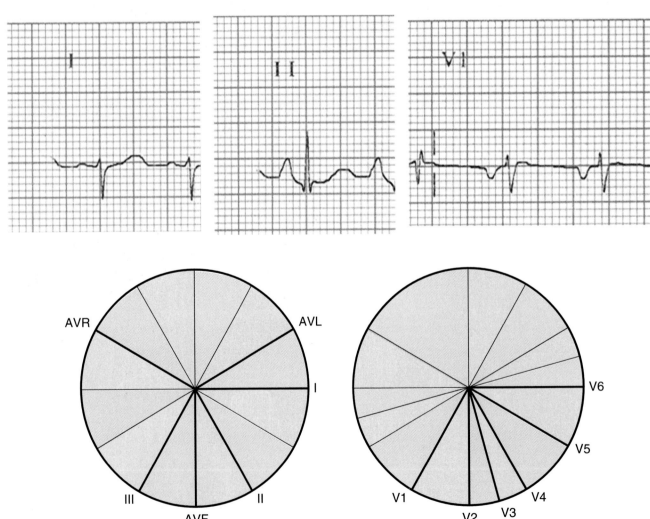

Heart Rate:

Rhythm:

Intervals (measured in the limb leads)

PR: short (< .12)
        normal (.12 to .20)
        long (>0.20 seconds); this is 1st degree AV block

QRS: normal (≤0.09 seconds)
        prolonged (.10 or .11); this is intraventricular conduction delay (IVCD)
        Bundle Branch Block (.12 seconds or greater)

QT:

P axis: normal
             rightward
             arm-lead reversal or dextrocardia
             junctional rhythm

QRS axis: normal
             left anterior hemiblock
             left posterior hemiblock
             indeterminate

T wave inversion (ischemia or infarction):

II,III,AVF   inferior
I, AVL   lateral
V1, without V2   nonspecific septal
V1 and V2   septal
V3 and V4   anterior
V5 and V6   lateral
V6, without V5   nonspecific lateral

ST Elevation (acute infarction):

II,III,AVF   inferior
I, AVL   lateral
V1, without V2   nonspecific septal
V1 and V2   septal
V3 and V4   anterior
V5 and V6   lateral
V6, without V5.   nonspecific lateral

ST Depression (ischemia or infarction):

I,II,III,AVL,AVF   diffuse subendocardial ischemia or infarction

V2,V3,V4,V5   diffuse subendocardial ischemia or infarction

Q waves (infarction):

II,III,AVF   inferior
I, AVL   lateral
V1, without V2   nonspecific septal
V1 and V2   septal
V3 and V4   anterior
V5 and V6   lateral
V6, without V5   nonspecific lateral

Hypertrophy:

Right atrial: Tall P wave 2.5 mm in II, III, or AVF

Left atrial: Deep negative part of P wave in V1

LVH: R wave in 1 + S wave in III ≥ 25mV
      S wave in V1 + R wave in V5 ≥ 35mV

RVH: Mean QRS either anterior, or rightward

The heart rate is 115 beats per minute. The PR interval measures 0.14 seconds. The QRS interval measures 0.08 seconds. The QT interval measures 0.30 seconds. The P axis is normal (+75°). In the frontal plane, the mean QRS axis points toward the right ventricle at +105°. In the horizontal plane, the mean QRS is posterior (V2 is negative) (note: V6 should always look like lead I. When it doesn't, it usually means that V6 was incorrectly placed and should have been further toward the patient's left). *This rightward mean QRS axis indicates right ventricular hypertrophy or left posterior hemiblock. Either is possible.* The T axis is normal in the frontal (+30°) and horizontal (+30°) planes. The ST segments are nonspecifically abnormal at most. There is a tall P wave in lead II, indicating right atrial abnormality (RAA). There is a negative component to the P wave in V1 that is 1 little box wide and 1 little box deep. This indicates left atrial abnormality.

Mitral stenosis could cause LAA, RVH, and RAA. A pulmonary embolus could acutely cause sinus tachycardia, RAA, and RVH. In view of the RAA and LAA, it is less likely that the rightward QRS represents left posterior hemiblock.

Parts of the answer sheets are "grayed out" because these sections have not yet been covered. Answer only the parts that are not highlighted.

Worksheet 18-2

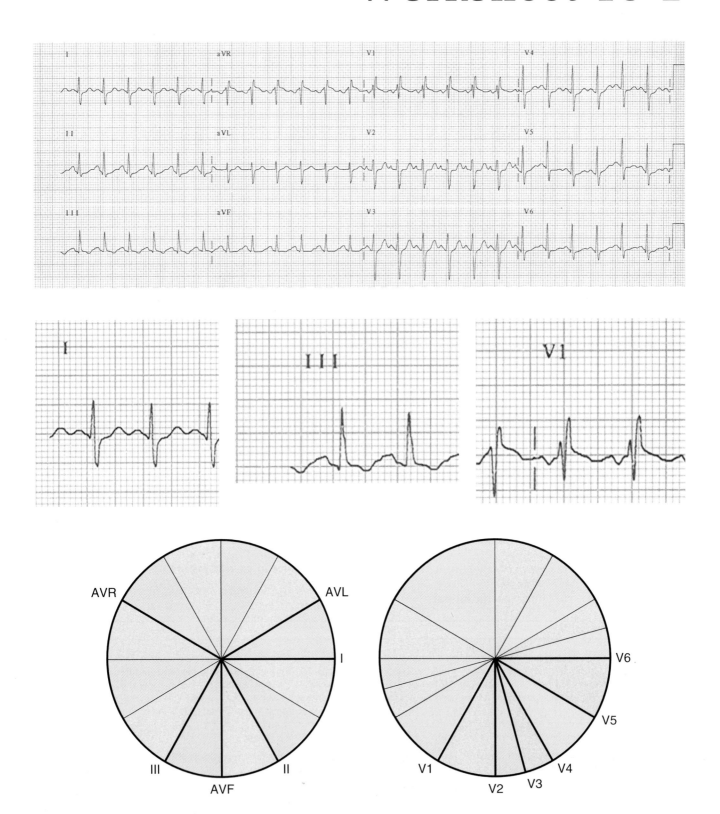

Heart Rate:

Rhythm:

Intervals (measured in the limb leads)

PR: short (< .12)
normal (.12 to .20)
long (>0.20 seconds); this is 1st degree AV block

QRS: normal (≤0.09 seconds)
prolonged (.10 or .11); this is intraventricular conduction delay (IVCD)
Bundle Branch Block (.12 seconds or greater)

QT:

P axis: normal
rightward
arm-lead reversal or dextrocardia
junctional rhythm

QRS axis: normal
left anterior hemiblock
left posterior hemiblock
indeterminate

T wave inversion (ischemia or infarction):

II,III,AVF	inferior
I, AVL	lateral
V1, without V2	nonspecific septal
V1 and V2	septal
V3 and V4	anterior
V5 and V6	lateral
V6, without V5	nonspecific lateral

ST Elevation (acute infarction):

II,III,AVF	inferior
I, AVL	lateral
V1, without V2	nonspecific septal
V1 and V2	septal
V3 and V4	anterior
V5 and V6	lateral
V6, without V5.	nonspecific lateral

ST Depression (ischemia or infarction):

I,II,III,AVL,AVF	diffuse subendocardial ischemia or infarction
V2,V3,V4,V5	diffuse subendocardial ischemia or infarction

Q waves (infarction):

II,III,AVF	inferior
I, AVL	lateral
V1, without V2	nonspecific septal
V1 and V2	septal
V3 and V4	anterior
V5 and V6	lateral
V6, without V5	nonspecific lateral

Hypertrophy:

Right atrial: Tall P wave 2.5 mm in II, III, or AVF

Left atrial: Deep negative part of P wave in V1

LVH: R wave in 1 + S wave in III ≥ 25mV
S wave in V1 + R wave in V5 ≥ 35mV

RVH: Mean QRS either anterior, or rightward

The heart rate is 150 beats per minute. This is sinus tachycardia. The PR interval measures 0.14 seconds. The QRS interval measures 0.08 seconds (*note: in lead V1 there is an RSR pattern. Because the QRS duration is normal, there is no BBB or IVCD. This RSR in V1 has three common associations: normal variation, secundum ASD, and pulmonary embolus*). The QT interval measures 0.26 seconds. The P axis is normal (+60°). The mean QRS axis in the frontal plane is rightward (+105°) and points to the right ventricle. In the horizontal plane the mean QRS points toward the right ventricle as well (−165°). This indicates RVH. The ST segments are abnormal and point opposite the QRS and could be due to RVH. Clinically, the combination of RVH, RSR′, and sinus tachycardia all suggest the diagnosis of acute pulmonary embolism.

A specific pattern of changes is present on this EKG. An S wave in lead I, a tiny q wave in lead III, and an inverted T wave in lead III are given the name McGinn-White and suggest acute pulmonary embolism.

Parts of the answer sheets are "grayed out" because these sections have not yet been covered. Answer only the parts that are not highlighted.

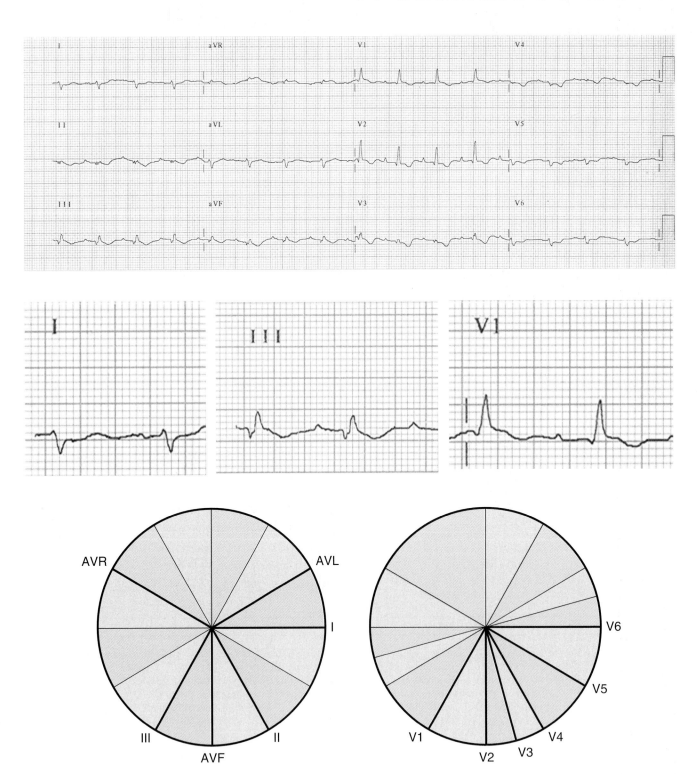

Heart Rate:

Rhythm:

ST Elevation (acute infarction):

II,III,AVF	inferior
I, AVL	lateral
V1, without V2	nonspecific septal
V1 and V2	septal
V3 and V4	anterior
V5 and V6	lateral
V6, without V5.	nonspecific lateral

Intervals (measured in the limb leads)

PR: short (< .12)
        normal (.12 to .20)
        long (>0.20 seconds); this is 1st degree AV block

QRS: normal ($\leq$0.09 seconds)
        prolonged (.10 or .11); this is intraventricular conduction delay (IVCD)
        Bundle Branch Block (.12 seconds or greater)

QT:

ST Depression (ischemia or infarction):

I,II,III,AVL,AVF	diffuse subendocardial ischemia or infarction
V2,V3,V4,V5	diffuse subendocardial ischemia or infarction

P axis: normal
             rightward
             arm-lead reversal or dextrocardia
             junctional rhythm

QRS axis: normal
                left anterior hemiblock
                left posterior hemiblock
                indeterminate

Q waves (infarction):

II,III,AVF	inferior
I, AVL	lateral
V1, without V2	nonspecific septal
V1 and V2	septal
V3 and V4	anterior
V5 and V6	lateral
V6, without V5	nonspecific lateral

T wave inversion (ischemia or infarction):

II,III,AVF	inferior
I, AVL	lateral
V1, without V2	nonspecific septal
V1 and V2	septal
V3 and V4	anterior
V5 and V6	lateral
V6, without V5	nonspecific lateral

Hypertrophy:

Right atrial: Tall P wave 2.5 mm in II, III, or AVF

Left atrial: Deep negative part of P wave in V1

LVH: R wave in 1 + S wave in III $\geq$ 25mV
       S wave in V1 + R wave in V5 $\geq$ 35mV

RVH: Mean QRS either anterior, or rightward

The heart rate is 94 beats per minute. There is low voltage of the QRS present, suggesting chronic obstructive pulmonary disease (COPD), pericardial effusion, or pneumothorax. The PR interval measures 0.18 seconds but is difficult to measure. The QRS interval measures 0.11 seconds and indicates IVCD. The last part of the QRS points rightward and anteriorly and indicates RIVCD. (If the QRS were 0.12 seconds, it would represent RBBB. RVH should not be diagnosed in the presence of RBBB; however, hypertrophy and ischemia should be evaluated.) The P axis is normal at +60°. The mean QRS axis is indeterminate in the frontal plane because most of the complexes are isoelectric. In the horizontal plane it points rightward and anteriorly at +165°. This indicates RVH. The ST segment is abnormal in the frontal plane (−120°), representing diffuse subendocardial ischemia or infarction or changes due to RVH. In the horizontal plane, the ST axis is abnormal (−150°) and does not point way from the QRS (+165°). Therefore, the ST segments indicate subendocardial ischemia or infarction, as well. Note that there is an S wave in lead I and a q wave with an inverted T wave in lead III: the McGinn-White pattern indicates pulmonary embolism. Acute pulmonary embolism could precipitate diffuse myocardial ischemia. This may also represent a patient with chronic COPD (low voltage), possibly a smoker, who now has coronary disease as well.

Parts of the answer sheets are "grayed out" because these sections have not yet been covered. Answer only the parts that are not highlighted.

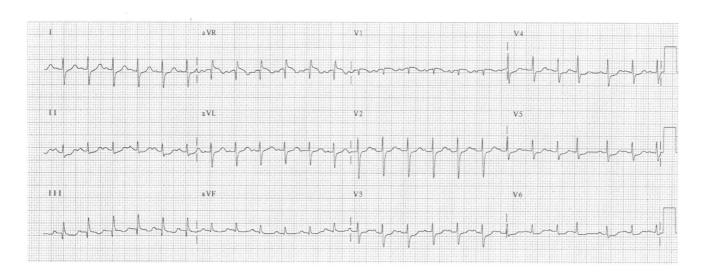

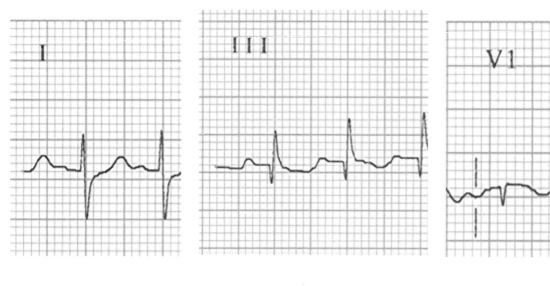

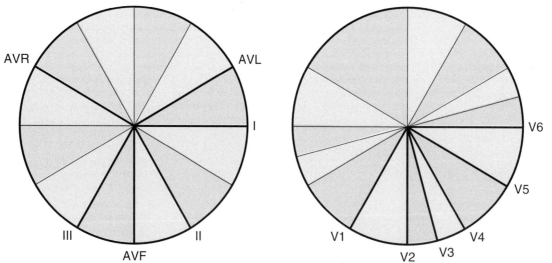

Heart Rate:

Rhythm:

ST Elevation (acute infarction):

II,III,AVF	inferior
I, AVL	lateral
V1, without V2	nonspecific septal
V1 and V2	septal
V3 and V4	anterior
V5 and V6	lateral
V6, without V5.	nonspecific lateral

Intervals (measured in the limb leads)

PR: short (< .12)
        normal (.12 to .20)
        long (>0.20 seconds); this is 1st degree AV
        block

QRS: normal (≤0.09 seconds)
        prolonged (.10 or .11); this is intraventricular
        conduction delay (IVCD)
        Bundle Branch Block (.12 seconds or greater)

QT:

ST Depression (ischemia or infarction):

| I,II,III,AVL,AVF | diffuse subendocardial ischemia or infarction |
| V2,V3,V4,V5 | diffuse subendocardial ischemia or infarction |

P axis: normal
            rightward
            arm-lead reversal or dextrocardia
            junctional rhythm

QRS axis: normal
            left anterior hemiblock
            left posterior hemiblock
            indeterminate

Q waves (infarction):

II,III,AVF	inferior
I, AVL	lateral
V1, without V2	nonspecific septal
V1 and V2	septal
V3 and V4	anterior
V5 and V6	lateral
V6, without V5	nonspecific lateral

T wave inversion (ischemia or infarction):

II,III,AVF	inferior
I, AVL	lateral
V1, without V2	nonspecific septal
V1 and V2	septal
V3 and V4	anterior
V5 and V6	lateral
V6, without V5	nonspecific lateral

Hypertrophy:

Right atrial: Tall P wave 2.5 mm in II, III, or AVF

Left atrial: Deep negative part of P wave in V1

LVH: R wave in 1 + S wave in III ≥ 25mV
     S wave in V1 + R wave in V5 ≥ 35mV

RVH: Mean QRS either anterior, or rightward

The heart rate is 150 beats per minute. The PR interval measures 0.14 seconds. The QRS interval measures 0.08 seconds. The QT interval measures 0.26 seconds. The P axis in the frontal plane is normal (+45°). The mean QRS axis in the frontal plane is +120° and indicates RVH or LPHB. The mean QRS axis in the horizontal plane is −22.5° which is leftward and posterior (meaning V6 was incorrectly placed). The ST axis is diffusely abnormal in the frontal and horizontal planes, indicating subendocardial ischemia or infarction. Again, there is an S wave in lead I, with a q wave and an inverted T wave in lead III (McGinn-White pattern), indicating pulmonary embolism. The fast heart rate suggests hemodynamic compromise and may be precipitating the subendocardial ischemia as well.

Parts of the answer sheets are "grayed out" because these sections have not yet been covered. Answer only the parts that are not highlighted.

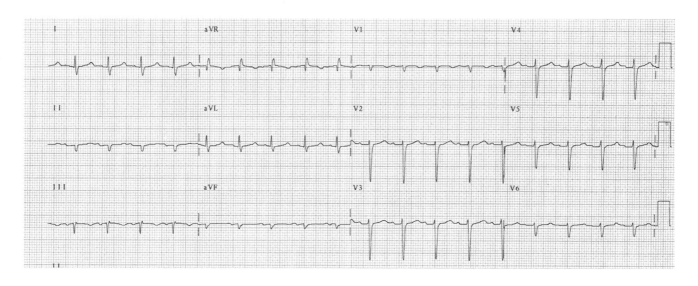

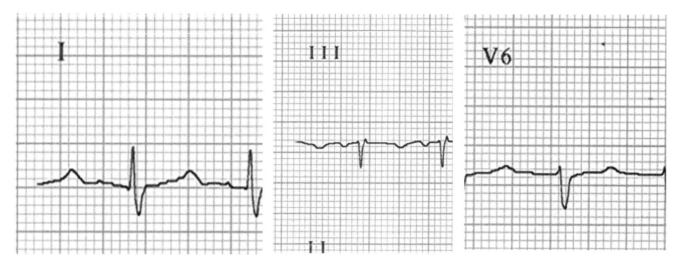

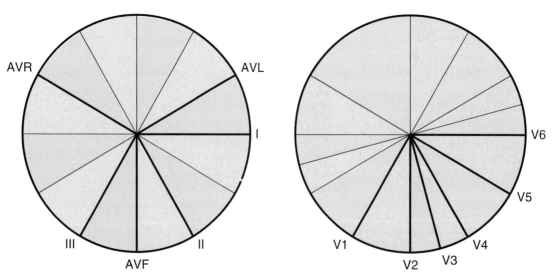

Heart Rate:

Rhythm:

Intervals (measured in the limb leads)

PR: short (< .12)
     normal (.12 to .20)
     long (>0.20 seconds); this is 1st degree AV
     block

QRS: normal (≤0.09 seconds)
      prolonged (.10 or .11); this is intraventricular
      conduction delay (IVCD)
      Bundle Branch Block (.12 seconds or greater)

QT:

P axis: normal
           rightward
           arm-lead reversal or dextrocardia
           junctional rhythm

QRS axis: normal
           left anterior hemiblock
           left posterior hemiblock
           indeterminate

T wave inversion (ischemia or infarction):

II,III,AVF	inferior
I, AVL	lateral
V1, without V2	nonspecific septal
V1 and V2	septal
V3 and V4	anterior
V5 and V6	lateral
V6, without V5	nonspecific lateral

ST Elevation (acute infarction):

II,III,AVF	inferior
I, AVL	lateral
V1, without V2	nonspecific septal
V1 and V2	septal
V3 and V4	anterior
V5 and V6	lateral
V6, without V5.	nonspecific lateral

ST Depression (ischemia or infarction):

I,II,III,AVL,AVF	diffuse subendocardial ischemia or infarction
V2,V3,V4,V5	diffuse subendocardial ischemia or infarction

Q waves (infarction):

II,III,AVF	inferior
I, AVL	lateral
V1, without V2	nonspecific septal
V1 and V2	septal
V3 and V4	anterior
V5 and V6	lateral
V6, without V5	nonspecific lateral

Hypertrophy:

Right atrial: Tall P wave 2.5 mm in II, III, or AVF

Left atrial: Deep negative part of P wave in V1

LVH: R wave in 1 + S wave in III ≥ 25mV
      S wave in V1 + R wave in V5 ≥ 35mV

RVH: Mean QRS either anterior, or rightward

The heart rate is 107 beats per minute. The PR interval measures 0.16 seconds. The QRS interval measures 0.08 seconds. The QT interval measures 0.36 seconds. There is borderline low voltage in the frontal plane (COPD, pericardial effusion, pneumothorax, pleural effusion). The P axis is 0°. The mean QRS axis in the frontal plane is −105°, indicating LAHB. In the horizontal plane, the QRS is rightward (−120°), indicating RVH. The initial QRS axis is abnormal and points away from the inferior wall, indicating transmural infarction of the inferior wall. The T waves and ST segments are not all normal, so the infarction may be acute. Again, note the pattern of an S wave in lead I, with q wave and an inverted T wave in lead III. This indicates acute pulmonary embolism.

Parts of the answer sheets are "grayed out" because these sections have not yet been covered. Answer only the parts that are not highlighted.

Clinical Conditions Affecting the EKG

The EKG not only provides valuable information on the electrical events of the heart but also can be useful in the diagnosis of medical and surgical conditions that affect the heart. Drugs, electrolyte imbalances, trauma, pericardial diseases, cancer, and systemic diseases are conditions that can cause specific changes on the EKG.

The heart lies in the chest in the mediastinum, slightly to the left of the midline. There are certain diseases and conditions that alter the normal anatomy of the chest cavity and can cause changes in the EKG. Some examples of this are a pneumothorax, pleural effusion, and dextrocardia.

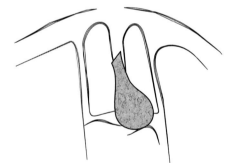

Limb leads: The sum of QRS amplitude in leads I, II, and III should be at least 15 little boxes.

Precordial (V leads): The QRS amplitude should be at least 15 little boxes in at least one of leads V1, V2, or V3.

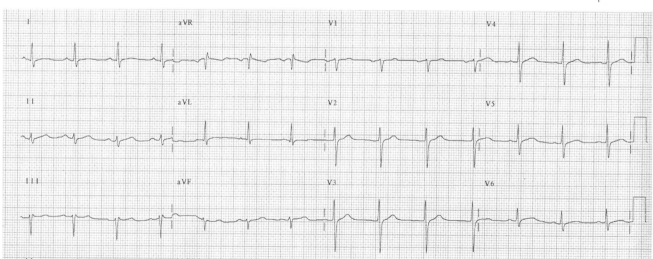

Pneumothorax

A pneumothorax occurs when air seeps into the pleural space. The air interferes with the negative pressure in the pleural space and causes the lung to collapse. A pneumothorax can occur spontaneously (without any specific cause). It can also occur secondary to some form of chest trauma. The air in pleural space pushes the heart away from the chest wall and because air is a poor conductor of electricity, it makes all the waveforms on the EKG smaller. Sinus tachycardia may be present and may indicate hemodynamic compromise, chest pain, or anxiety.

Free air inside the lung cavity (called the pleural space) squeezes the left lung.

It also reduces the size of the voltage on the EKG.

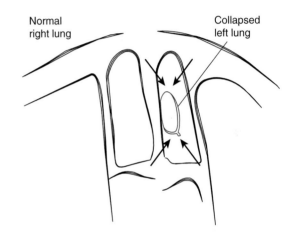

None of the QRS complexes in leads I, II, **or** III is greater than 5 little boxes.

None of the QRS complexes in leads V1, V2, or V3 is greater than 15 little boxes.

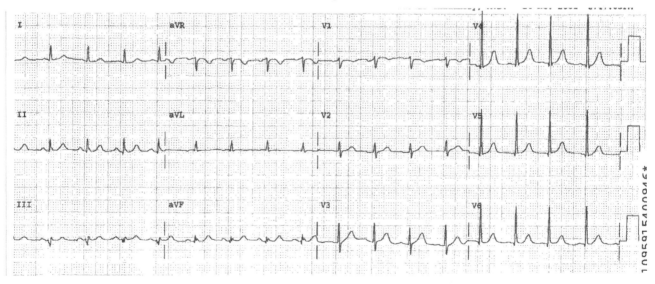

Pleural Effusion

A **pleural effusion** is another condition that causes smaller waveforms on the EKG. A pleural effusion is the term used for the buildup of fluid in the pleural space. The buildup of fluid in the pleural space is often associated with certain carcinomas, infection, congestive heart failure, or hemorrhage. In this instance, the fluid pushes the heart away from the chest wall and EKG leads. This is especially seen in a left-sided pleural effusion.

The EKG below does not technically meet criteria for low voltage. Compared to an EKG taken 6 weeks earlier, it now has less voltage.

If you wait for criteria before checking the patient, you're missing the point. **Don't wait for criteria!**

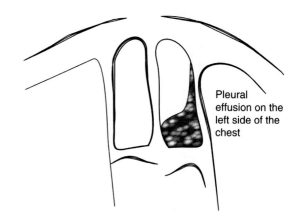

Pleural effusion on the left side of the chest

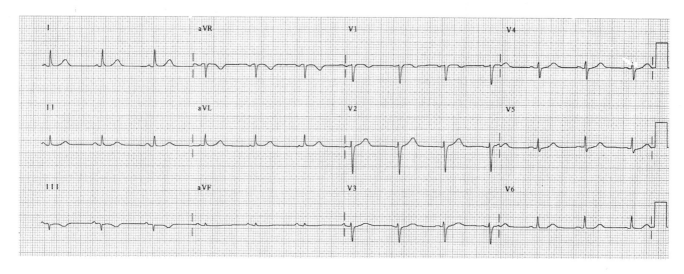

Dextrocardia

Dextrocardia is another condition that may produce low-voltage waves on the EKG. Dextrocardia is a congenital defect that places the heart on the right side of the chest instead of the left side. This opposite position puts a greater distance between the heart and the precordial (chest) leads.

Dextrocardia is a congenital condition in which the heart is reversed in the frontal view in a mirror image of normal.

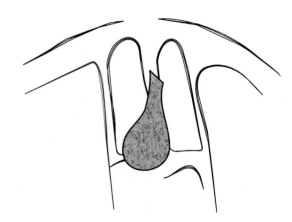

This EKG shows decreased waveform voltages as the leads progress from lead V1 to V6. Because the leads were placed on the left side of the patient's chest, lead V2 is further from the heart than V1. V2 is further than V3, and so on. V6 is the furthest from the heart, and therefore has the lowest voltage of all. The P axis, which is rightward at +135°, suggests the diagnosis.

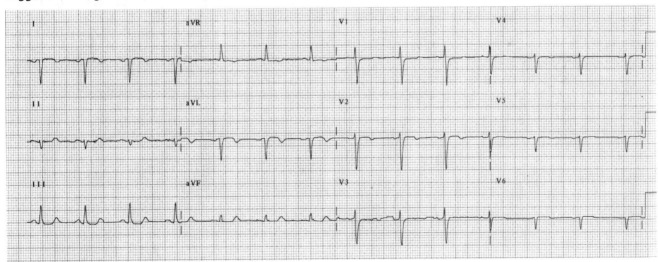

Pericardial Disease

KEY CONCEPT

Inflammation of the pericardium can cause changes on the EKG that can mimic ischemia or infarction.

Disorders of the pericardium can also produce specific changes in the EKG. **Pericarditis** occurs when the pericardium becomes inflamed. Although the cause of pericarditis is not fully understood, it is associated with other disease processes such as connective tissue disorders and infection. The inflammation of the pericardium can directly injure the underlying myocardium and mimic ischemia on the EKG. Sinus tachycardia may be present.

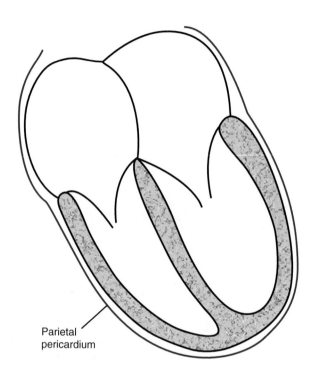

Parietal pericardium

EKG in Pericarditis

Inflammation of the pericardium can cause changes on the EKG that can mimic ischemia or infarction. A rapid look at this EKG could give the impression that the ST segment is elevated above baseline in the limb leads. An overly rapid interpretation of the EKG would describe the ST as elevated and pointing toward the inferior wall, consistent with transmural ischemia or infarction. However, after closer inspection, there is no ST segment elevation in the frontal plane. Rather it is an optical illusion caused by the presence of PT segment depression.

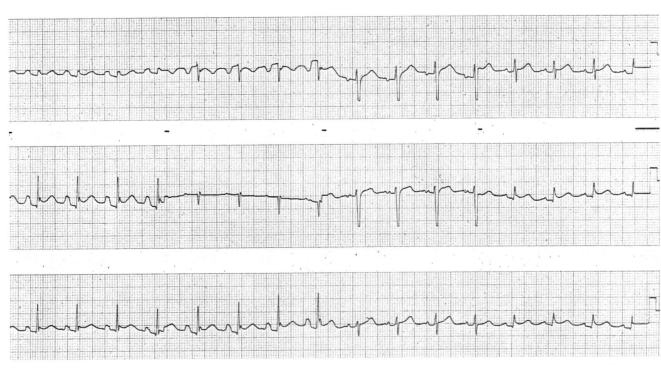

Now, look more carefully at the close-up of lead II, as shown. *The true baseline (arbitrarily, by definition) runs through the end of the T wave to the beginning of the P wave. There is no elevation of the ST segment in this lead.* There is depression of the segment between the end of the P wave and the beginning of the QRS complex. This is PT segment depression, which is seen in pericarditis.

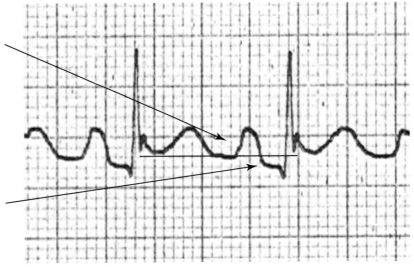

Pericardial Effusion

A pericardial effusion is a condition in which the pericardial space fills with fluid, exudates, or blood. It is often the result of infection, trauma, carcinoma, hypothyroidism, or rheumatoid disease. The fluid in the pericardial space decreases the voltage that reaches the EKG leads, producing smaller waveforms. Large or rapidly accumulating effusions can affect the hemodynamic status of the patient. Sinus tachycardia suggests hemodynamic compromise.

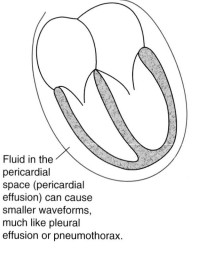

Fluid in the pericardial space (pericardial effusion) can cause smaller waveforms, much like pleural effusion or pneumothorax.

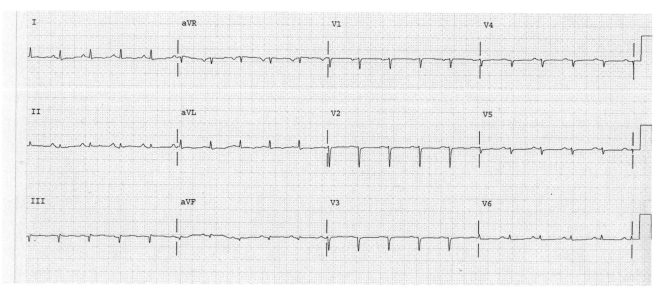

Dilated Cardiomyopathy

The EKG frequently demonstrates abnormalities in many of the cardiomyopathies. Dilated cardiomyopathy is the diagnostic term used to describe a dilated, diffusely weakened heart muscle. Although in most cases the cause of cardiomyopathy is unknown, there are certain diseases such as hypertension, viral infections, and alcoholism, that may contribute to it. The EKG may demonstrate left bundle branch block. Left atrial abnormality is another helpful clue.

Dilated hypokinetic right and left ventricles.

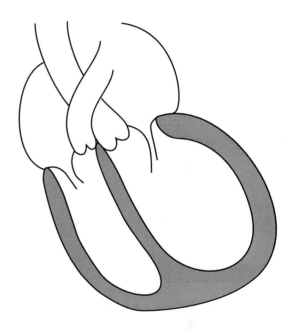

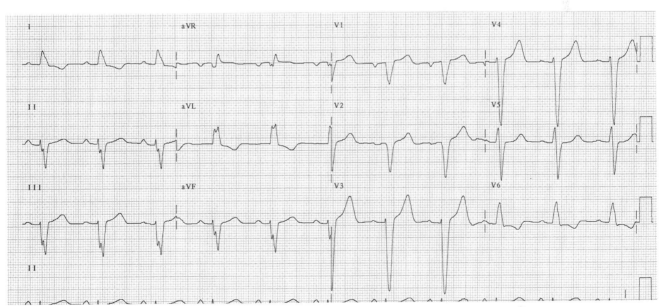

LAA and LBBB

Hypothyroidism

Hypothyroidism occurs when the thyroid gland does not produce enough of thyroid hormones T3 and T4. Hypothyroidism affects the heart as well as most other body systems. Low levels of T3 and T4 result in a decreased energy metabolism and a slow metabolic rate. Hypothyroidism is manifested on the EKG by sinus bradycardia, conduction disturbances, low voltage, and prolonged QT intervals.

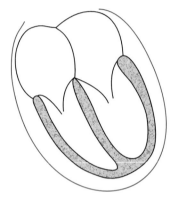

Thyroid disease.

Hypothyroidism can cause pericardial effusion, which produces low voltage on the EKG. Bradycardia, conduction disturbances, and prolonged QT intervals are frequently associated with hypothyrodism.

Electrolytes: Hyperkalemia

The normal electrical activity of the heart is dependent on the proper balance of specific serum electrolytes. Abnormal potassium (K^+) and calcium (CA^{++}) levels have a direct effect on the normal electrical activity of the heart and myocardium.

High serum potassium levels, or hyperkalemia, depresses conduction and impulse formation throughout the entire myocardium. **This produces flattened P waves, wide QRS complexes, and peaked T waves on the EKG.**

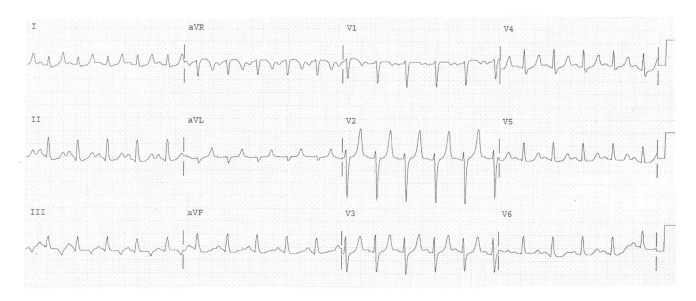

If the potassium level is higher, or increases more acutely, a wide, bizarre-looking sine wave–like pattern appears as shown.

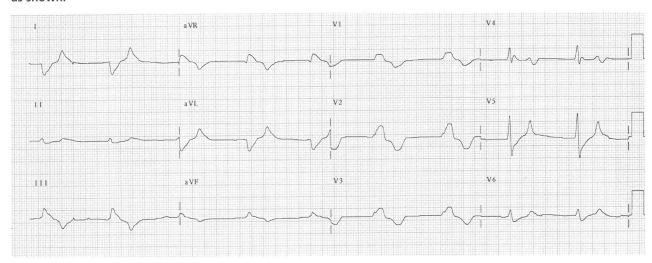

Electrolytes: Hypokalemia

A low serum potassium level, or hypokalemia, increases irritability of the conduction system and myocardium, increasing the likelihood and frequency of ventricular ectopy. Hypokalemia produces flattened T waves. **The QT interval becomes prolonged.** *A low-amplitude T wave due to hypokalemia is a common reason that the QT interval may be difficult to measure with confidence.* There can be diffuse ST segment depression, which looks like diffuse subendocardial ischemia. **U waves** (positive waves seen after the ST segment returns to baseline in the V leads) as well can sometimes be seen on the EKG. It's always clinically correct to worry about ischemia when ST depression or T wave inversion is present. It's essential to check the possibility of hypokalemia as well. The potassium level below was 1.7.

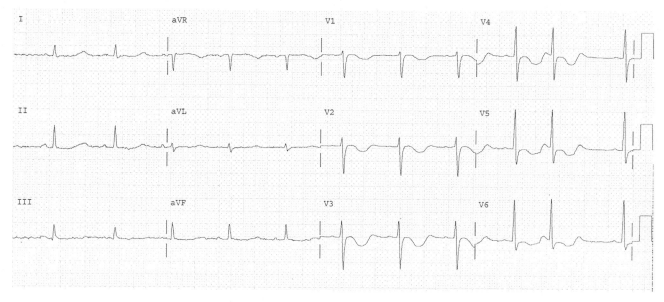

K^+ level 1.7 mEq/L, with dramatically long QT and QTc (more than 500 msec).

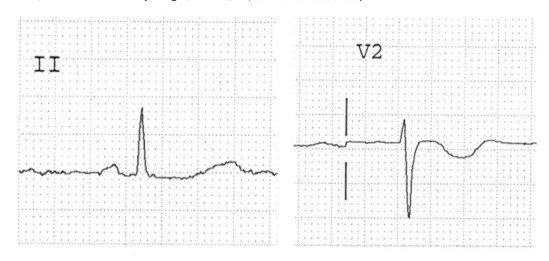

Electrolytes: Hypercalcemia

Hypercalcemia, or high serum calcium levels, significantly increases myocardial irritability and produces **shortened QT intervals** on the EKG. The serum calcium level was 12.8 in this patient. The QT interval here is 0.30 seconds.

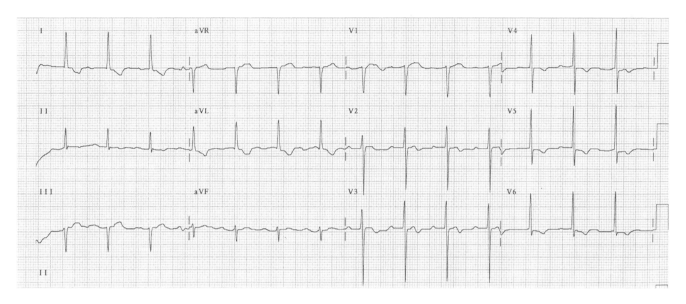

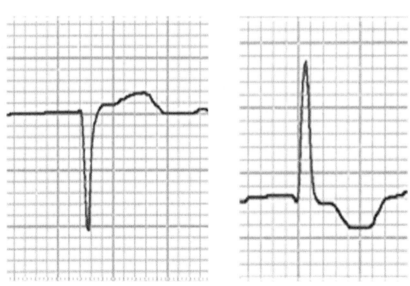

Electrolytes: Hypocalcemia

Low serum calcium levels, or hypocalcemia has the opposite effect on the myocardium. Hypocalcemia produces a prolonged QT interval. In the following example, the serum calcium level was 6.1. The QT measures 0.30 seconds, which is long for this rate.

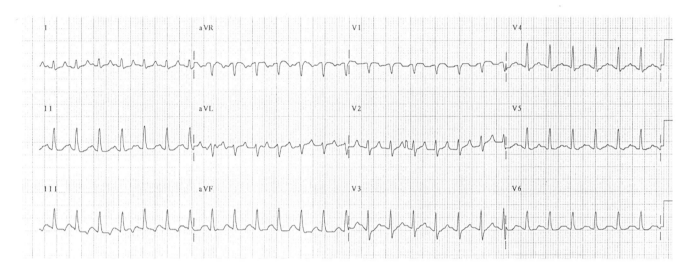

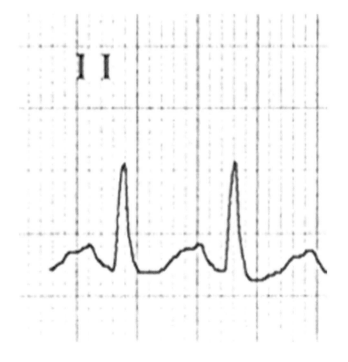

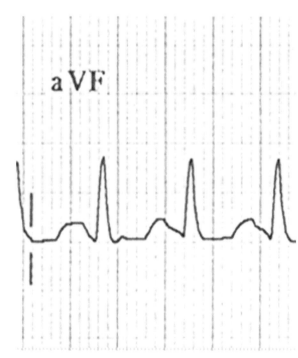

Medications: Digitalis

Digitalis is one of the oldest and most commonly used cardiac medications. In therapeutic doses, digitalis effectively inhibits the SA node from firing as often and slows conduction through the AV node. When the blood levels of digitalis exceed the therapeutic range, lethal dysrhythmia and EKG changes can occur. Digitalis toxicity produces various heart blocks, as well as ventricular dysrhythmias such as ventricular bigeminy and ventricular tachycardia. Digitalis toxicity produces a characteristic down sloping of the ST segment on the EKG. The following EKG demonstrates junctional rhythm, a short QT interval, and diffuse "cheshire cat smile" ST depression in the lateral leads. The appearance of U waves in V2 represents coexisting hypokalemia, which exacerbates the digitalis effect.

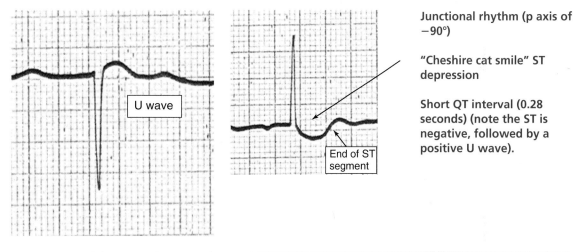

Junctional rhythm (p axis of −90°)

"Cheshire cat smile" ST depression

Short QT interval (0.28 seconds) (note the ST is negative, followed by a positive U wave).

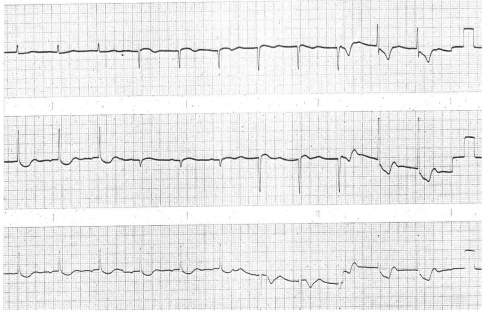

Chronic Lung Disease: Low Voltage

Chronic obstructive pulmonary disease (COPD) is a common disease. Diseased airways trap excessive air in the lungs. Air is a poor conductor of electrical forces and lowers the voltage of some or all leads on the EKG.

Low voltage on the EKG should always be explained.

Causes include
  COPD
  Pericardial effusion
  Left pneumothorax

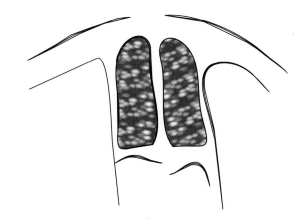

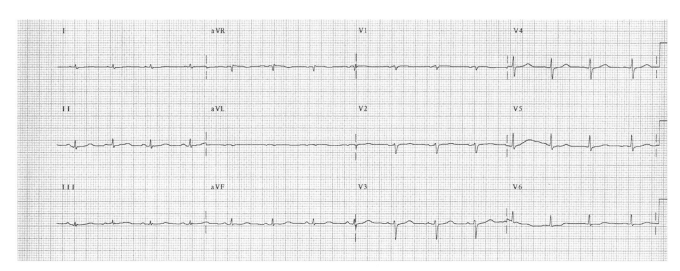

Chronic Lung Disease: Hypoxia

Hypoxia, or low oxygen level in the blood, is a common cause of bradycardia. All patients on ventilator support or those with chronic lung disease who develop sudden bradycardia should be evaluated immediately for hypoxia.

Pneumonia, COPD, pulmonary embolus, and congestive heart failure cause respiratory distress and sinus tachycardia.

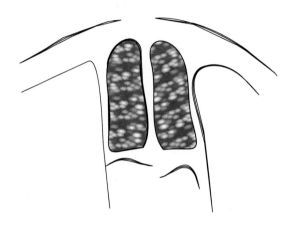

Postoperative Patients: Sinus Tachycardia

When evaluating a patient with sinus tachycardia, the nurse or physician should assess the patient's level of pain. Pain stimulates the sympathetic nervous system, which causes the heart rate to rise. For example, postoperative patients who are experiencing pain or those patients maintained on mechanical ventilators and not properly sedated often develop sinus tachycardia. Once the patient is properly medicated and made comfortable, the heart rate often returns to normal.

Pneumothorax.

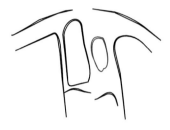

Hypovolemia, possibly secondary to bleeding.

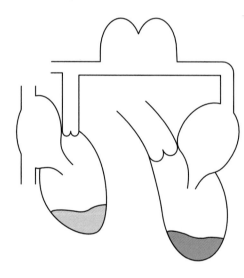

Pulmonary embolus.

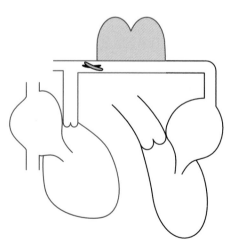

Cancer Effects on the EKG

Malignant carcinomas and some cancer treatment modalities directly affect the heart and cause specific changes on the EKG. Pericardial effusions, tamponade, increased heart size, heart failure, and new heart murmurs are manifestations of malignant invasion of the heart. Radiation therapy can cause pericarditis. Chemotherapy can cause myocardial depression. Metastatic disease may also cause renal failure and electrolyte disturbances, which can adversely affect the cardiac electrical system and cause observable EKG changes. Some common EKG changes are low voltage from pericardial effusion, hyperkalemia, hypercalcemia, and sinus tachycardia.

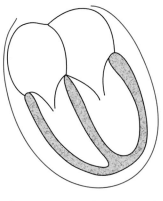

Metastatic cancer, especially from the breast (in women) and the lung (in men), can cause large pericardial effusions, which produce smaller waveforms on the EKG. Sinus tachycardia may be present as well.

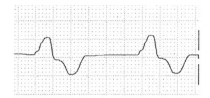

Cancer can cause renal failure from obstruction or chemotherapy. Renal failure increases the risk of hyperkalemia, which, if left untreated, can be fatal.

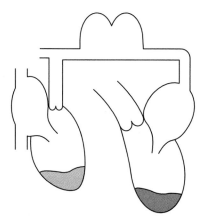

Cancer causes hypovolemia from bleeding and infection, enteropathies, and vomiting. This produces tachycardia.

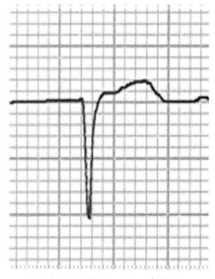

Metastatic disease (typically from lung, prostate, kidney, thyroid, or breast) that spreads to bone can cause hypercalcemia. This is manifested on the EKG by shortened QT intervals.

Love

Love can cause a broken heart.
Love can also heal a broken heart.

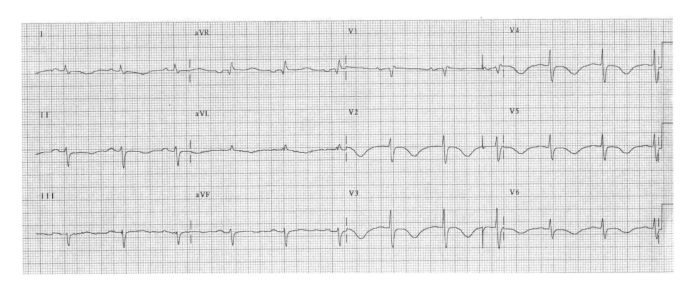

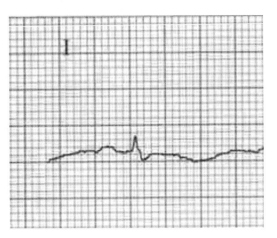

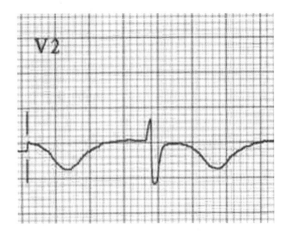

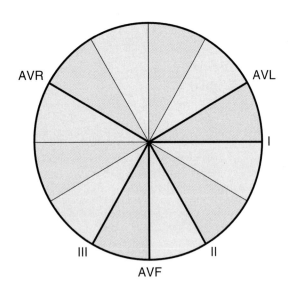

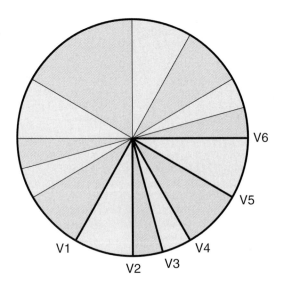

Heart Rate:

Rhythm:

Intervals (measured in the limb leads)

PR: short (< .12)
normal (.12 to .20)
long (>0.20 seconds); this is 1st degree AV block

QRS: normal (≤0.09 seconds)
prolonged (.10 or .11); this is intraventricular conduction delay (IVCD)
Bundle Branch Block (.12 seconds or greater)

QT:

P axis: normal
rightward
arm-lead reversal or dextrocardia
junctional rhythm

QRS axis: normal
left anterior hemiblock
left posterior hemiblock
indeterminate

T wave inversion (ischemia or infarction):

II,III,AVF	inferior
I, AVL	lateral
V1, without V2	nonspecific septal
V1 and V2	septal
V3 and V4	anterior
V5 and V6	lateral
V6, without V5	nonspecific lateral

ST Elevation (acute infarction):

II,III,AVF	inferior
I, AVL	lateral
V1, without V2	nonspecific septal
V1 and V2	septal
V3 and V4	anterior
V5 and V6	lateral
V6, without V5.	nonspecific lateral

ST Depression (ischemia or infarction):

I,II,III,AVL,AVF	diffuse subendocardial ischemia or infarction
V2,V3,V4,V5	diffuse subendocardial ischemia or infarction

Q waves (infarction):

II,III,AVF	inferior
I, AVL	lateral
V1, without V2	nonspecific septal
V1 and V2	septal
V3 and V4	anterior
V5 and V6	lateral
V6, without V5	nonspecific lateral

Hypertrophy:

Right atrial: Tall P wave 2.5 mm in II, III, or AVF

Left atrial: Deep negative part of P wave in V1

LVH: R wave in 1 + S wave in III ≥ 25mV
S wave in V1 + R wave in V5 ≥ 35mV

RVH: Mean QRS either anterior, or rightward

The heart rate is 65 beats per minute. The PR interval measures 0.20 seconds. The QRS interval measures 0.11 seconds, indicating IVCD. The last part of the QRS points toward the right ventricle, making this RIVCD. The mean QRS axis in the frontal plane is −75°, indicating LAHB. The QT interval measures 0.56 seconds. *Because the QT interval crosses the midpoint between the R-R intervals, it is long just by inspection.* Long QT interval is caused by many drugs (sotalol, quinidine, diisopyramide, and procainamide are but a few) and electrolyte disturbances (hypokalemia and hypocalcemia). Diffuse ST or T wave segment changes associated with a long QT interval may be secondary to the drug or electrolyte effect. However, the possibility of ischemia should be included in the reading. Here, the T axis is +180° in the frontal plane. In the horizontal plane, the T axis is abnormal (−150°) and points away from the septum and anterior and lateral walls. This indicates the possibility of subendocardial ischemia or infarction. A good clinical approach is to check the patient's medications and electrolytes immediately. The long QT interval predisposes the patient to polymorphous ventricular tachycardia (torsade de pointes).

The above patient was on sotalol, a drug known to prolong the QT interval.

Parts of the answer sheets are "grayed out" because these sections have not yet been covered. Answer only the parts that are not highlighted.

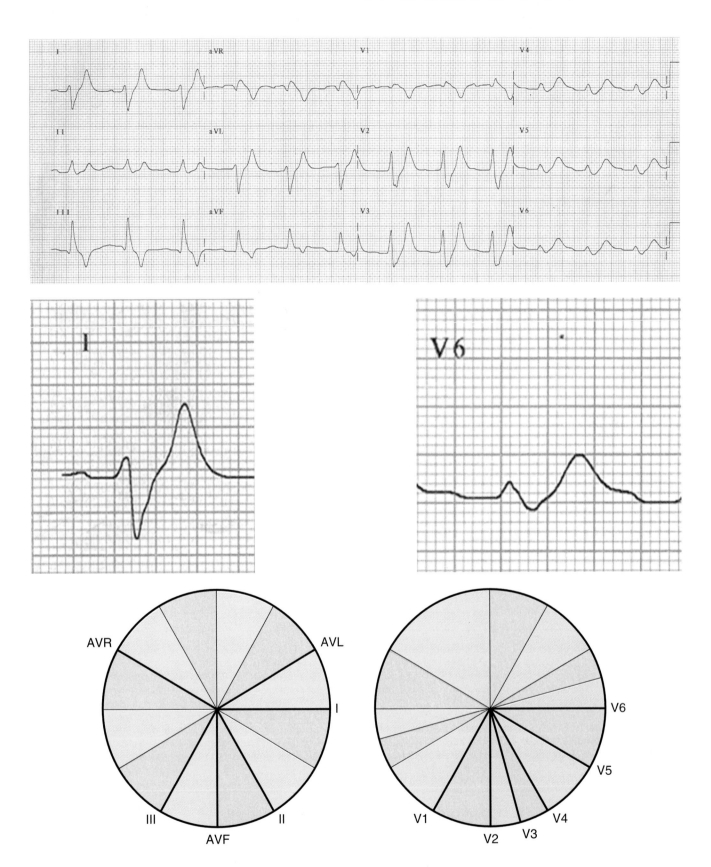

Heart Rate:

Rhythm:

Intervals (measured in the limb leads)

PR: short (< .12)
normal (.12 to .20)
long (>0.20 seconds); this is 1st degree AV block

QRS: normal (≤0.09 seconds)
prolonged (.10 or .11); this is intraventricular conduction delay (IVCD)
Bundle Branch Block (.12 seconds or greater)

QT:

P axis: normal
rightward
arm-lead reversal or dextrocardia
junctional rhythm

QRS axis: normal
left anterior hemiblock
left posterior hemiblock
indeterminate

T wave inversion (ischemia or infarction):

II,III,AVF	inferior
I, AVL	lateral
V1, without V2	nonspecific septal
V1 and V2	septal
V3 and V4	anterior
V5 and V6	lateral
V6, without V5	nonspecific lateral

ST Elevation (acute infarction):

II,III,AVF	inferior
I, AVL	lateral
V1, without V2	nonspecific septal
V1 and V2	septal
V3 and V4	anterior
V5 and V6	lateral
V6, without V5.	nonspecific lateral

ST Depression (ischemia or infarction):

I,II,III,AVL,AVF	diffuse subendocardial ischemia or infarction
V2,V3,V4,V5	diffuse subendocardial ischemia or infarction

Q waves (infarction):

II,III,AVF	inferior
I, AVL	lateral
V1, without V2	nonspecific septal
V1 and V2	septal
V3 and V4	anterior
V5 and V6	lateral
V6, without V5	nonspecific lateral

Hypertrophy:

Right atrial: Tall P wave 2.5 mm in II, III, or AVF

Left atrial: Deep negative part of P wave in V1

LVH: R wave in 1 + S wave in III ≥ 25mV
S wave in V1 + R wave in V5 ≥ 35mV

RVH: Mean QRS either anterior, or rightward

The heart rate is 65 beats per minute. The rhythm is sinus. The PR interval measures 0.24 seconds and indicates 1° AV block (pronounced "first degree AV block"). The QRS interval measures 0.20 seconds. The QRS is bizarrely wide and has the appearance of a sine wave in several of the leads. This could be severe hyperkalemia, which should be ruled out immediately. Further analyzing the EKG is pointless until the serum potassium level has been determined.

The serum potassium level for this patient was 8.8 mEq/L.

Normalizing the serum potassium returns all the changes to normal.

Parts of the answer sheets are "grayed out" because these sections have not yet been covered. Answer only the parts that are not highlighted.

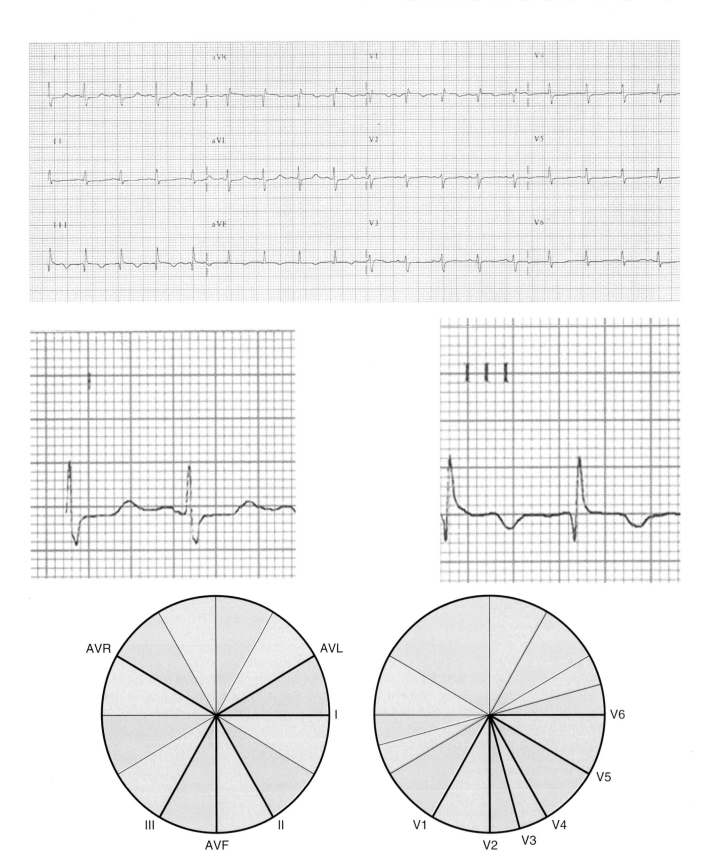

Heart Rate:

Rhythm:

ST Elevation (acute infarction):

II, III, AVF	inferior
I, AVL	lateral
V1, without V2	nonspecific septal
V1 and V2	septal
V3 and V4	anterior
V5 and V6	lateral
V6, without V5.	nonspecific lateral

Intervals (measured in the limb leads)

PR: short (< .12)
normal (.12 to .20)
long (>0.20 seconds); this is 1st degree AV block

QRS: normal (≤0.09 seconds)
prolonged (.10 or .11); this is intraventricular conduction delay (IVCD)
Bundle Branch Block (.12 seconds or greater)

QT:

ST Depression (ischemia or infarction):

I, II, III, AVL, AVF	diffuse subendocardial ischemia or infarction
V2, V3, V4, V5	diffuse subendocardial ischemia or infarction

P axis: normal
rightward
arm-lead reversal or dextrocardia
junctional rhythm

QRS axis: normal
left anterior hemiblock
left posterior hemiblock
indeterminate

Q waves (infarction):

II, III, AVF	inferior
I, AVL	lateral
V1, without V2	nonspecific septal
V1 and V2	septal
V3 and V4	anterior
V5 and V6	lateral
V6, without V5	nonspecific lateral

T wave inversion (ischemia or infarction):

II, III, AVF	inferior
I, AVL	lateral
V1, without V2	nonspecific septal
V1 and V2	septal
V3 and V4	anterior
V5 and V6	lateral
V6, without V5	nonspecific lateral

Hypertrophy:

Right atrial: Tall P wave 2.5 mm in II, III, or AVF

Left atrial: Deep negative part of P wave in V1

LVH: R wave in 1 + S wave in III ≥ 25mV
S wave in V1 + R wave in V5 ≥ 35mV

RVH: Mean QRS either anterior, or rightward

The heart rate is 107 beats per minute. The PR interval is 0.14 seconds. The QRS interval measures 0.10 seconds, indicating IVCD. The last part of the QRS points rightward in I and V6 and toward the right ventricle in lead V1, indicating RIVCD. The QT interval is 0.36 seconds. The P axis is +90°. The mean QRS axis in the frontal plane is +105° indicating RVH or LPHB. The mean QRS axis in the horizontal plane is −30°. The T axis in the frontal plane is −30° pointing away from the inferior wall. The T axis in the horizontal plane is of low amplitude and is nonspecific. The ST axis in the frontal plane is 180° but of low amplitude, making it nonspecific.

There is an S wave in lead I and a q wave with an inverted T wave in lead III (McGinn-White). This indicates pulmonary embolism. Inferior wall ischemia may be present as well, or this may reflect secondary changes because of RVH.

Parts of the answer sheets are "grayed out" because these sections have not yet been covered. Answer only the parts that are not highlighted.

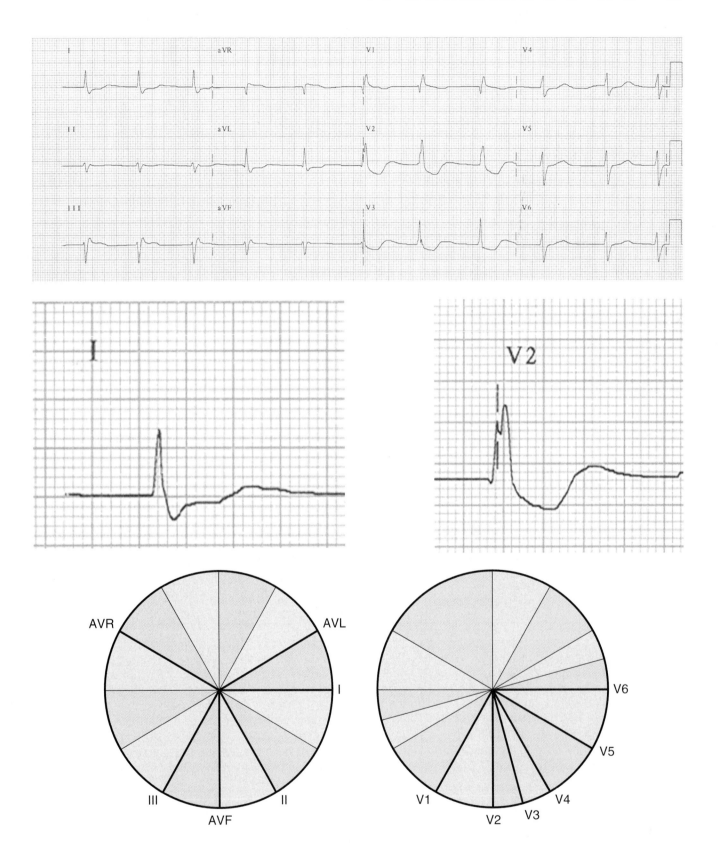

Heart Rate:

Rhythm:

Intervals (measured in the limb leads)

PR: short (< .12)
        normal (.12 to .20)
        long (>0.20 seconds); this is 1st degree AV
        block

QRS: normal (≤0.09 seconds)
        prolonged (.10 or .11); this is intraventricular
        conduction delay (IVCD)
        Bundle Branch Block (.12 seconds or greater)

QT:

P axis: normal
                rightward
                arm-lead reversal or dextrocardia
                junctional rhythm

QRS axis: normal
                left anterior hemiblock
                left posterior hemiblock
                indeterminate

T wave inversion (ischemia or infarction):

II,III,AVF	inferior
I, AVL	lateral
V1, without V2	nonspecific septal
V1 and V2	septal
V3 and V4	anterior
V5 and V6	lateral
V6, without V5	nonspecific lateral

ST Elevation (acute infarction):

II,III,AVF	inferior
I, AVL	lateral
V1, without V2	nonspecific septal
V1 and V2	septal
V3 and V4	anterior
V5 and V6	lateral
V6, without V5.	nonspecific lateral

ST Depression (ischemia or infarction):

I,II,III,AVL,AVF	diffuse subendocardial ischemia or infarction
V2,V3,V4,V5	diffuse subendocardial ischemia or infarction

Q waves (infarction):

II,III,AVF	inferior
I, AVL	lateral
V1, without V2	nonspecific septal
V1 and V2	septal
V3 and V4	anterior
V5 and V6	lateral
V6, without V5	nonspecific lateral

Hypertrophy:

Right atrial: Tall P wave 2.5 mm in II, III, or AVF

Left atrial: Deep negative part of P wave in V1

LVH: R wave in 1 + S wave in III ≥ 25mV
      S wave in V1 + R wave in V5 ≥ 35mV

RVH: Mean QRS either anterior, or rightward

The heart rate is 68 beats per minute. There is no P wave. The rhythm is junctional. Digitalis toxicity should be considered in patients with junctional rhythm. The PR interval is undefined. The QRS interval measures 0.12 seconds, indicating BBB. The last part of the QRS complex points toward the right ventricle, indicating RBBB. The T waves are of low amplitude, suggesting possible hypokalemia. The QT interval is 0.40 seconds. The mean QRS axis in the frontal plane is −60°, indicating LAHB is also present. RVH is not diagnosed in the presence of RBBB. The ST axis in the frontal plane is abnormal (+150°) and points toward the inferior wall. This may reflect transmural inferior wall ischemia or infarction. This is not the expected range in RBBB, where the ST segments should point away from the last part of the QRS complex. The ST segments diffusely appear scooped out in a "cheshire cat smile" suggestive of digitalis toxicity.

Parts of the answer sheets are "grayed out" because these sections have not yet been covered. Answer only the parts that are not highlighted.

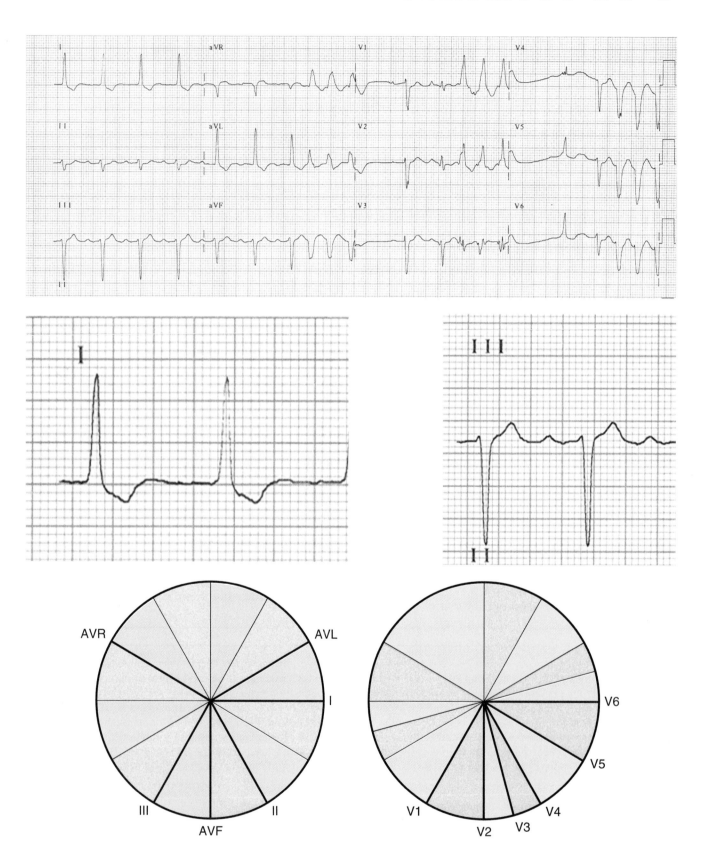

Heart Rate:

Rhythm:

Intervals (measured in the limb leads)

PR: short (< .12)
       normal (.12 to .20)
       long (>0.20 seconds); this is 1st degree AV
       block

QRS: normal (≤0.09 seconds)
       prolonged (.10 or .11); this is intraventricular
       conduction delay (IVCD)
       Bundle Branch Block (.12 seconds or greater)

QT:

P axis:	normal
	rightward
	arm-lead reversal or dextrocardia
	junctional rhythm
QRS axis:	normal
	left anterior hemiblock
	left posterior hemiblock
	indeterminate

T wave inversion (ischemia or infarction):

II,III,AVF	inferior
I, AVL	lateral
V1, without V2	nonspecific septal
V1 and V2	septal
V3 and V4	anterior
V5 and V6	lateral
V6, without V5	nonspecific lateral

ST Elevation (acute infarction):

II,III,AVF	inferior
I, AVL	lateral
V1, without V2	nonspecific septal
V1 and V2	septal
V3 and V4	anterior
V5 and V6	lateral
V6, without V5.	nonspecific lateral

ST Depression (ischemia or infarction):

| I,II,III,AVL,AVF | diffuse subendocardial ischemia or infarction |
| V2,V3,V4,V5 | diffuse subendocardial ischemia or infarction |

Q waves (infarction):

II,III,AVF	inferior
I, AVL	lateral
V1, without V2	nonspecific septal
V1 and V2	septal
V3 and V4	anterior
V5 and V6	lateral
V6, without V5	nonspecific lateral

Hypertrophy:

Right atrial: Tall P wave 2.5 mm in II, III, or AVF

Left atrial: Deep negative part of P wave in V1

LVH: R wave in 1 + S wave in III ≥ 25mV
      S wave in V1 + R wave in V5 ≥ 35mV

RVH: Mean QRS either anterior, or rightward

The heart rate is 93 beats per minute. The rhythm is sinus, with three episodes of wide QRS tachycardia. The PR interval measures 0.24 seconds, indicating 1° AV block. The QRS interval measures 0.08 seconds. The QT interval measures 0.26 seconds, which is short. Short or long QT interval indicates drug or electrolyte toxicity. *The combination of 1° AV block and short QT are hallmarks of digitalis toxicity. Diffuse ST segment changes, typically ST depression in the lateral leads, are a third association. Atrial or ventricular tachycardia is also a common manifestation.* The P axis is +90°. The mean QRS axis in the frontal plane is −45°, indicating LAHB. The mean QRS axis in the horizontal plane is −22.5°. The ST axis in the frontal plane is 180° consistent with lateral subendocardial ischemia or infarction, digitalis toxicity, or LVH. The sum of the R wave in lead I (13 mm) and the S wave in lead III (16 mm) totals 29, which indicates LVH.

Parts of the answer sheets are "grayed out" because these sections have not yet been covered. Answer only the parts that are not highlighted.

Putting It All Together: Practice EKGs

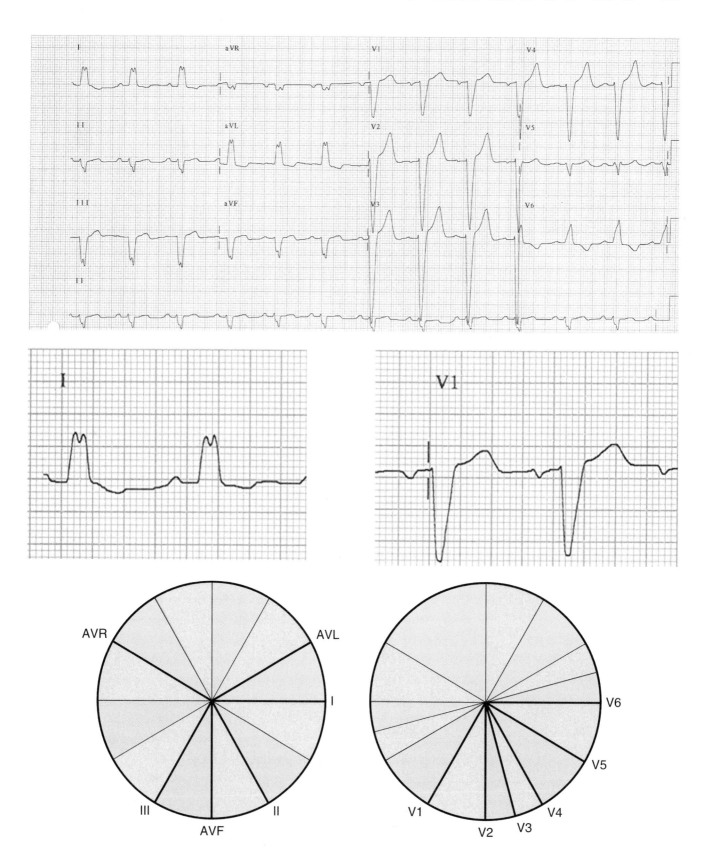

Heart Rate:

Rhythm:

Intervals (measured in the limb leads)

PR: short (< .12)
normal (.12 to .20)
long (>0.20 seconds); this is 1st degree AV block

QRS: normal (≤0.09 seconds)
prolonged (.10 or .11); this is intraventricular conduction delay (IVCD)
Bundle Branch Block (.12 seconds or greater)

QT:

P axis: normal
rightward
arm-lead reversal or dextrocardia
junctional rhythm

QRS axis: normal
left anterior hemiblock
left posterior hemiblock
indeterminate

T wave inversion (ischemia or infarction):

II,III,AVF	inferior
I, AVL	lateral
V1, without V2	nonspecific septal
V1 and V2	septal
V3 and V4	anterior
V5 and V6	lateral
V6, without V5	nonspecific lateral

ST Elevation (acute infarction):

II,III,AVF	inferior
I, AVL	lateral
V1, without V2	nonspecific septal
V1 and V2	septal
V3 and V4	anterior
V5 and V6	lateral
V6, without V5.	nonspecific lateral

ST Depression (ischemia or infarction):

I,II,III,AVL,AVF	diffuse subendocardial ischemia or infarction
V2,V3,V4,V5	diffuse subendocardial ischemia or infarction

Q waves (infarction):

II,III,AVF	inferior
I, AVL	lateral
V1, without V2	nonspecific septal
V1 and V2	septal
V3 and V4	anterior
V5 and V6	lateral
V6, without V5	nonspecific lateral

Hypertrophy:

Right atrial: Tall P wave 2.5 mm in II, III, or AVF

Left atrial: Deep negative part of P wave in V1

LVH: R wave in 1 + S wave in III ≥ 25mV
S wave in V1 + R wave in V5 ≥ 35mV

RVH: Mean QRS either anterior, or rightward

The heart rate is 71 beats per minute. The PR interval measures 0.20 seconds. The QRS interval measures 0.16 seconds and indicates BBB. The last part of the QRS points leftward in the frontal plane (−45°). It points leftward and posterior (−75°) in the horizontal plane. This indicates LBBB. The QT interval measures 0.40 seconds. The P axis is normal (at +30°). The mean QRS axis (−45°) is not analyzed in LBBB. The ST segments point opposite the last part of the QRS (+120°) in the frontal plane and in the horizontal plane (+105°). The ST segment deviation is as expected for a LBBB, but would not be analyzed further even it wasn't. A left atrial abnormality is present in lead V1.

Ischemia, infarction, RVH, LVH, and hemiblock cannot be read with confidence when LBBB is present. So don't!

The most common diseases associated with LBBB are ischemic heart disease, valvular heart disease and hypertension, cardiomyopathy, and primary conduction disease.

Worksheet 20-2

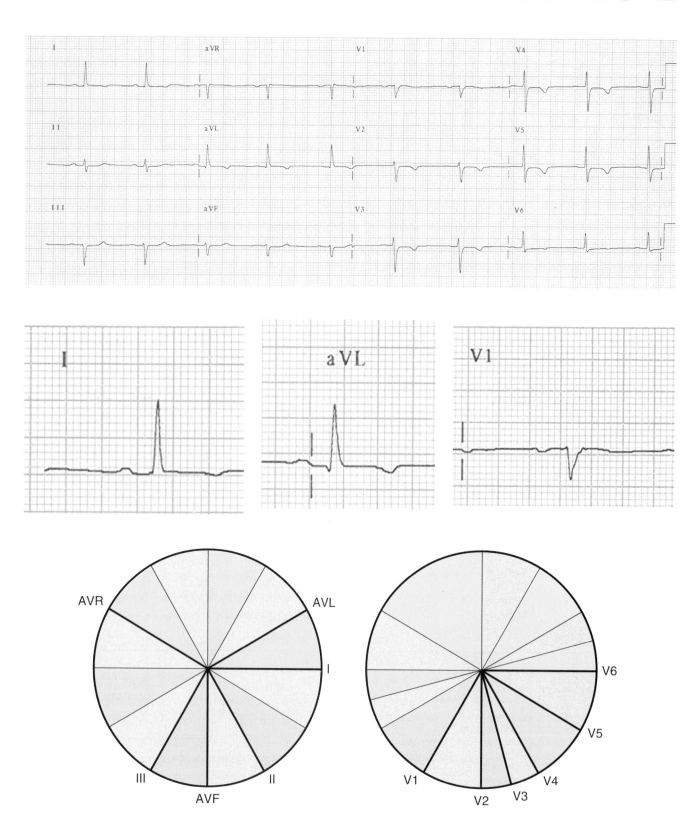

Heart Rate:

Rhythm:

Intervals (measured in the limb leads)

PR: short (< .12)
        normal (.12 to .20)
        long (>0.20 seconds); this is 1st degree AV
        block

QRS: normal (≤0.09 seconds)
        prolonged (.10 or .11); this is intraventricular
        conduction delay (IVCD)
        Bundle Branch Block (.12 seconds or greater)

QT:

P axis: normal
            rightward
            arm-lead reversal or dextrocardia
            junctional rhythm

QRS axis: normal
            left anterior hemiblock
            left posterior hemiblock
            indeterminate

T wave inversion (ischemia or infarction):

II,III,AVF	inferior
I, AVL	lateral
V1, without V2	nonspecific septal
V1 and V2	septal
V3 and V4	anterior
V5 and V6	lateral
V6, without V5	nonspecific lateral

ST Elevation (acute infarction):

II,III,AVF	inferior
I, AVL	lateral
V1, without V2	nonspecific septal
V1 and V2	septal
V3 and V4	anterior
V5 and V6	lateral
V6, without V5.	nonspecific lateral

ST Depression (ischemia or infarction):

I,II,III,AVL,AVF	diffuse subendocardial ischemia or infarction
V2,V3,V4,V5	diffuse subendocardial ischemia or infarction

Q waves (infarction):

II,III,AVF	inferior
I, AVL	lateral
V1, without V2	nonspecific septal
V1 and V2	septal
V3 and V4	anterior
V5 and V6	lateral
V6, without V5	nonspecific lateral

Hypertrophy:

Right atrial: Tall P wave 2.5 mm in II, III, or AVF

Left atrial: Deep negative part of P wave in V1

LVH: R wave in 1 + S wave in III ≥ 25mV
        S wave in V1 + R wave in V5 ≥ 35mV

RVH: Mean QRS either anterior, or rightward

The heart rate is 60 beats per minute. The rhythm is sinus. The PR interval measures 0.24 seconds and indicates 1° AV block. The QRS interval measures 0.08 seconds. The QT interval measures 0.40 seconds. The P axis is normal (+60°). The mean QRS axis is −30° in the frontal plane and −22.5° in the horizontal plane. The T axis is abnormal (although of low amplitude so less specific) and points away from the lateral wall (+120°), indicating nonspecific lateral T wave changes (or lateral subendocardial ischemia or infarction). In the horizontal plane, the T axis is abnormal and points away from the septum (inverted T wave in V1 and V2), anterior wall (inverted T wave in V3 and V4), and lateral walls (inverted T wave in V5), indicating septal, anterior, and lateral wall subendocardial ischemia or infarction. (The T axis is −90°, if you're plotting these out or thinking in three dimensions.) There is no atrial or ventricular hypertrophy.

The most common cause of this EKG is ischemic heart disease. Is the patient symptomatic? Are there other signs and symptoms to confirm the presence of ischemia or infarction? Is there an old EKG for comparison? Are the cardiac enzymes (biochemical markers) abnormal?

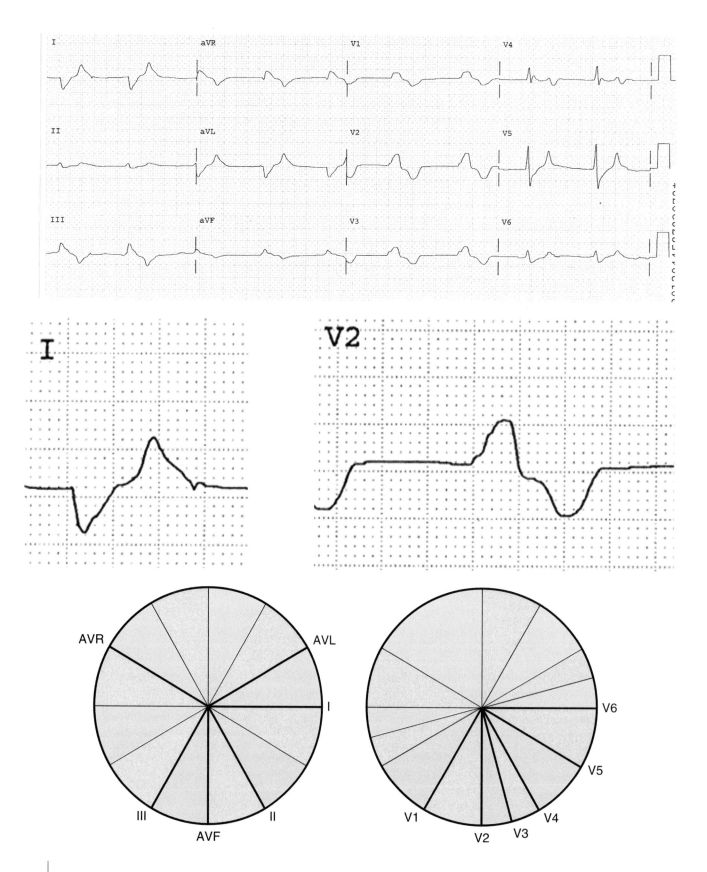

Heart Rate:

Rhythm:

Intervals (measured in the limb leads)

PR: short (< .12)
         normal (.12 to .20)
         long (>0.20 seconds); this is 1st degree AV
         block

QRS: normal (≤0.09 seconds)
         prolonged (.10 or .11); this is intraventricular
         conduction delay (IVCD)
         Bundle Branch Block (.12 seconds or greater)

QT:

P axis: normal
             rightward
             arm-lead reversal or dextrocardia
             junctional rhythm

QRS axis: normal
             left anterior hemiblock
             left posterior hemiblock
             indeterminate

T wave inversion (ischemia or infarction):

II,III,AVF	inferior
I, AVL	lateral
V1, without V2	nonspecific septal
V1 and V2	septal
V3 and V4	anterior
V5 and V6	lateral
V6, without V5	nonspecific lateral

ST Elevation (acute infarction):

II,III,AVF	inferior
I, AVL	lateral
V1, without V2	nonspecific septal
V1 and V2	septal
V3 and V4	anterior
V5 and V6	lateral
V6, without V5.	nonspecific lateral

ST Depression (ischemia or infarction):

| I,II,III,AVL,AVF | diffuse subendocardial ischemia or infarction |
| V2,V3,V4,V5 | diffuse subendocardial ischemia or infarction |

Q waves (infarction):

II,III,AVF	inferior
I, AVL	lateral
V1, without V2	nonspecific septal
V1 and V2	septal
V3 and V4	anterior
V5 and V6	lateral
V6, without V5	nonspecific lateral

Hypertrophy:

Right atrial: Tall P wave 2.5 mm in II, III, or AVF

Left atrial: Deep negative part of P wave in V1

LVH: R wave in 1 + S wave in III ≥ 25mV
     S wave in V1 + R wave in V5 ≥ 35mV

RVH: Mean QRS either anterior, or rightward

Bizarre wide QRS in a sine wave pattern. Rule out severe hyperkalemia immediately.

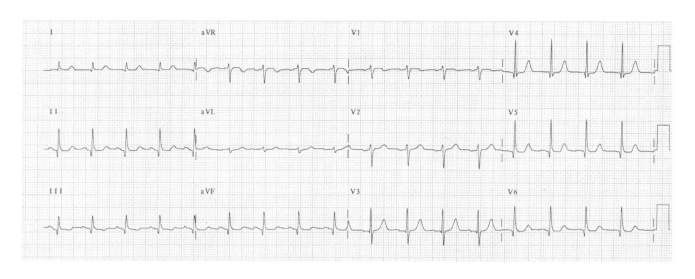

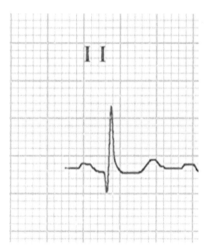

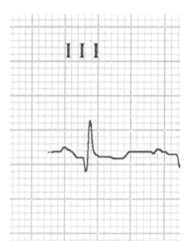

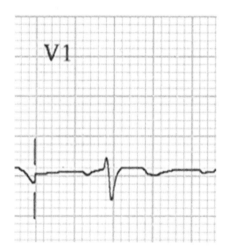

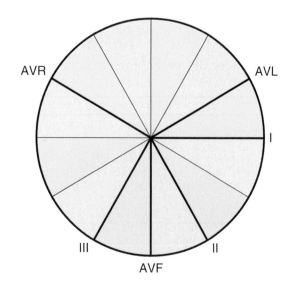

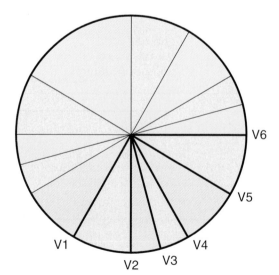

Heart Rate:

Rhythm:

ST Elevation (acute infarction):

II,III,AVF	inferior
I, AVL	lateral
V1, without V2	nonspecific septal
V1 and V2	septal
V3 and V4	anterior
V5 and V6	lateral
V6, without V5.	nonspecific lateral

Intervals (measured in the limb leads)

PR: short (< .12)
normal (.12 to .20)
long (>0.20 seconds); this is 1st degree AV block

QRS: normal (≤0.09 seconds)
prolonged (.10 or .11); this is intraventricular conduction delay (IVCD)
Bundle Branch Block (.12 seconds or greater)

QT:

ST Depression (ischemia or infarction):

I,II,III,AVL,AVF	diffuse subendocardial ischemia or infarction
V2,V3,V4,V5	diffuse subendocardial ischemia or infarction

P axis: normal
rightward
arm-lead reversal or dextrocardia
junctional rhythm

QRS axis: normal
left anterior hemiblock
left posterior hemiblock
indeterminate

Q waves (infarction):

II,III,AVF	inferior
I, AVL	lateral
V1, without V2	nonspecific septal
V1 and V2	septal
V3 and V4	anterior
V5 and V6	lateral
V6, without V5	nonspecific lateral

T wave inversion (ischemia or infarction):

II,III,AVF	inferior
I, AVL	lateral
V1, without V2	nonspecific septal
V1 and V2	septal
V3 and V4	anterior
V5 and V6	lateral
V6, without V5	nonspecific lateral

Hypertrophy:

Right atrial: Tall P wave 2.5 mm in II, III, or AVF

Left atrial: Deep negative part of P wave in V1

LVH: R wave in 1 + S wave in III ≥ 25mV
S wave in V1 + R wave in V5 ≥ 35mV

RVH: Mean QRS either anterior, or rightward

The heart rate is 107 beats per minute. The rhythm is sinus tachycardia. The PR interval measures 0.16 seconds. The QRS interval measures 0.09 seconds. The QT interval measures 0.32 seconds. The P axis is +90°. The mean QRS axis in the frontal plane is +60° and in the horizontal plane is −7.5°. The axis for the initial part of the QRS is abnormal (the initial 0.04 seconds points at −60° in the frontal plane) and points away from the inferior wall (q waves in II, III, and AVF). This indicates transmural infarction of the inferior wall. The ST segments are not perfectly normal, so the infarction is "possibly acute." It is possible to nitpick the timing of the infarction (ST elevation would be "acute," ST depression or T wave inversion would be "recent," and normal T and ST would be "old" or "age indeterminate." There are critical exceptions to this clinical classification of the timing of infarction, and we think this is to no avail and can be misleading. The ST segments are abnormal and can be read as nonspecific inferior ST changes, because they are not 1 mm deep. In the horizontal plane, the initial QRS is abnormal and points away from the lateral walls in V5 and V6. This is consistent with transmural infarction of the lateral wall.

The most likely cause of this EKG is a ruptured atherosclerotic plaque in the right coronary artery that produced a 100% occlusion with complete obstruction to flow to the inferior wall. The lateral infarction may have been due to occlusion of either the circumflex or even the LAD depending on the underlying coronary anatomy. In a patient with a "dominant circumflex," occlusion of the circumflex artery could cause a lateral and inferior wall infarction.

There was likely ST elevation earlier. The formation of Q waves indicates that attempts to open the artery with thrombolytic or surgical therapy were unsuccessful.

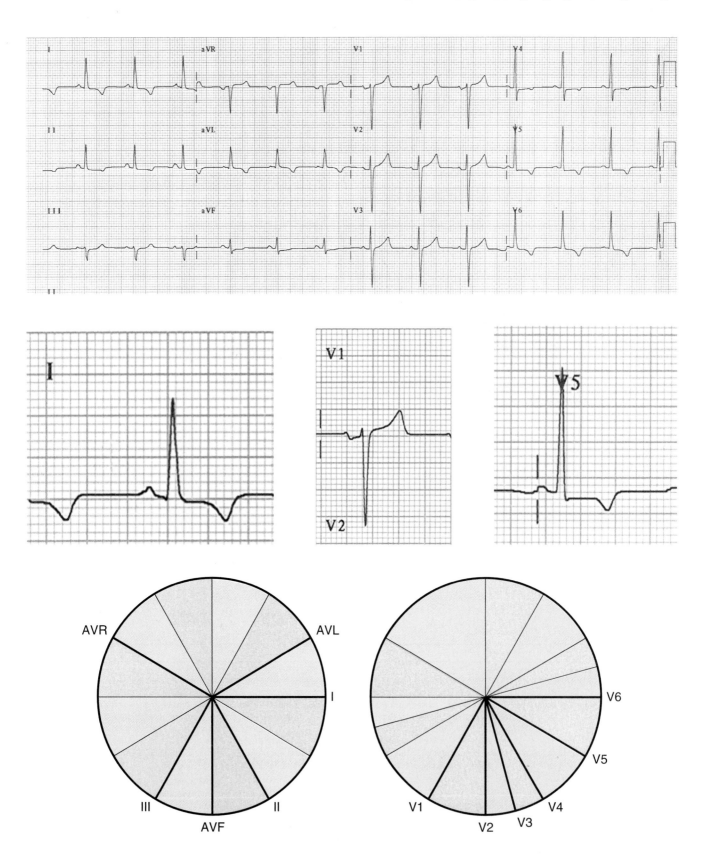

Heart Rate:

Rhythm:

ST Elevation (acute infarction):

II,III,AVF	inferior
I, AVL	lateral
V1, without V2	nonspecific septal
V1 and V2	septal
V3 and V4	anterior
V5 and V6	lateral
V6, without V5.	nonspecific lateral

Intervals (measured in the limb leads)

PR: short (< .12)
 normal (.12 to .20)
 long (>0.20 seconds); this is 1st degree AV block

QRS: normal (≤0.09 seconds)
 prolonged (.10 or .11); this is intraventricular conduction delay (IVCD)
 Bundle Branch Block (.12 seconds or greater)

QT:

ST Depression (ischemia or infarction):

I,II,III,AVL,AVF	diffuse subendocardial ischemia or infarction
V2,V3,V4,V5	diffuse subendocardial ischemia or infarction

P axis: normal
 rightward
 arm-lead reversal or dextrocardia
 junctional rhythm

QRS axis: normal
 left anterior hemiblock
 left posterior hemiblock
 indeterminate

Q waves (infarction):

II,III,AVF	inferior
I, AVL	lateral
V1, without V2	nonspecific septal
V1 and V2	septal
V3 and V4	anterior
V5 and V6	lateral
V6, without V5	nonspecific lateral

T wave inversion (ischemia or infarction):

II,III,AVF	inferior
I, AVL	lateral
V1, without V2	nonspecific septal
V1 and V2	septal
V3 and V4	anterior
V5 and V6	lateral
V6, without V5	nonspecific lateral

Hypertrophy:

Right atrial: Tall P wave 2.5 mm in II, III, or AVF

Left atrial: Deep negative part of P wave in V1

LVH: R wave in 1 + S wave in III ≥ 25mV
 S wave in V1 + R wave in V5 ≥ 35mV

RVH: Mean QRS either anterior, or rightward

The heart rate is 75 beats per minute. The PR interval measures 0.12 seconds. The QRS measures 0.09 seconds. The QT interval measures 0.36 seconds. The P axis is normal at +45°. The mean QRS axis in the frontal plane is +15°, and in the horizontal plane is −22.5°. A left atrial abnormality is present. The S wave in lead V1 (17 mm) and the R wave in lead V5 (17 mm) total 34 mm. Voltage criteria for LVH require 35 mm. There are borderline criteria for LVH present. The presence of the LAA makes the presence of LVH more likely. *The sensitivity (ability to detect disease) of an echocardiogram (90%) is higher than that of an EKG (only 60%) for the diagnosis of LVH. Therefore, an echocardiogram would be helpful to rule in or our LVH.* The ST segments point away from the lateral wall, which could be secondary to LVH or could indicate lateral subendocardial ischemia or infarction.

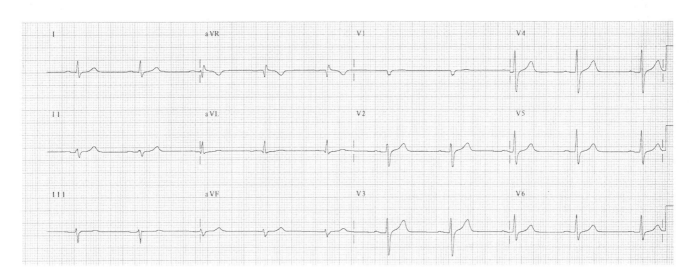

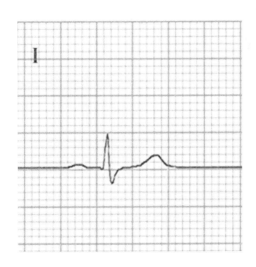

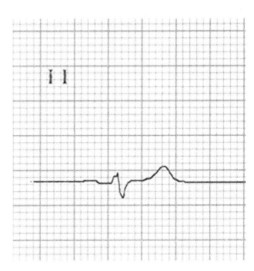

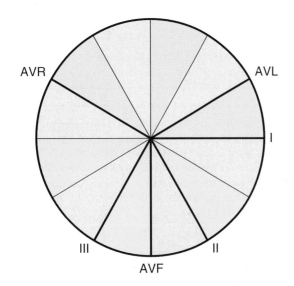

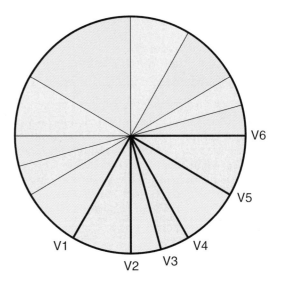

Heart Rate:

Rhythm:

Intervals (measured in the limb leads)

PR: short (< .12)
normal (.12 to .20)
long (>0.20 seconds); this is 1st degree AV block

QRS: normal (≤0.09 seconds)
prolonged (.10 or .11); this is intraventricular conduction delay (IVCD)
Bundle Branch Block (.12 seconds or greater)

QT:

P axis: normal
rightward
arm-lead reversal or dextrocardia
junctional rhythm

QRS axis: normal
left anterior hemiblock
left posterior hemiblock
indeterminate

T wave inversion (ischemia or infarction):

II,III,AVF	inferior
I, AVL	lateral
V1, without V2	nonspecific septal
V1 and V2	septal
V3 and V4	anterior
V5 and V6	lateral
V6, without V5	nonspecific lateral

ST Elevation (acute infarction):

II,III,AVF	inferior
I, AVL	lateral
V1, without V2	nonspecific septal
V1 and V2	septal
V3 and V4	anterior
V5 and V6	lateral
V6, without V5.	nonspecific lateral

ST Depression (ischemia or infarction):

I,II,III,AVL,AVF	diffuse subendocardial ischemia or infarction
V2,V3,V4,V5	diffuse subendocardial ischemia or infarction

Q waves (infarction):

II,III,AVF	inferior
I, AVL	lateral
V1, without V2	nonspecific septal
V1 and V2	septal
V3 and V4	anterior
V5 and V6	lateral
V6, without V5	nonspecific lateral

Hypertrophy:

Right atrial: Tall P wave 2.5 mm in II, III, or AVF

Left atrial: Deep negative part of P wave in V1

LVH: R wave in 1 + S wave in III ≥ 25mV
S wave in V1 + R wave in V5 ≥ 35mV

RVH: Mean QRS either anterior, or rightward

The heart rate is 58 beats per minute. The PR interval measures 0.18 seconds. The QRS interval measures 0.10 seconds (IVCD). The QT interval measures 0.36 seconds. This is short and suggests a drug or electrolyte problem. Hypercalcemia should be considered. The P axis is +90°. The mean QRS axis is −60° and indicates LAHB. The mean QRS axis in the horizontal plane is −22.5°. There is no atrial or ventricular hypertrophy. The ST and T segments are normal.

The most common cause of a long or short QT interval is drug effect/toxicity or electrolyte imbalance.

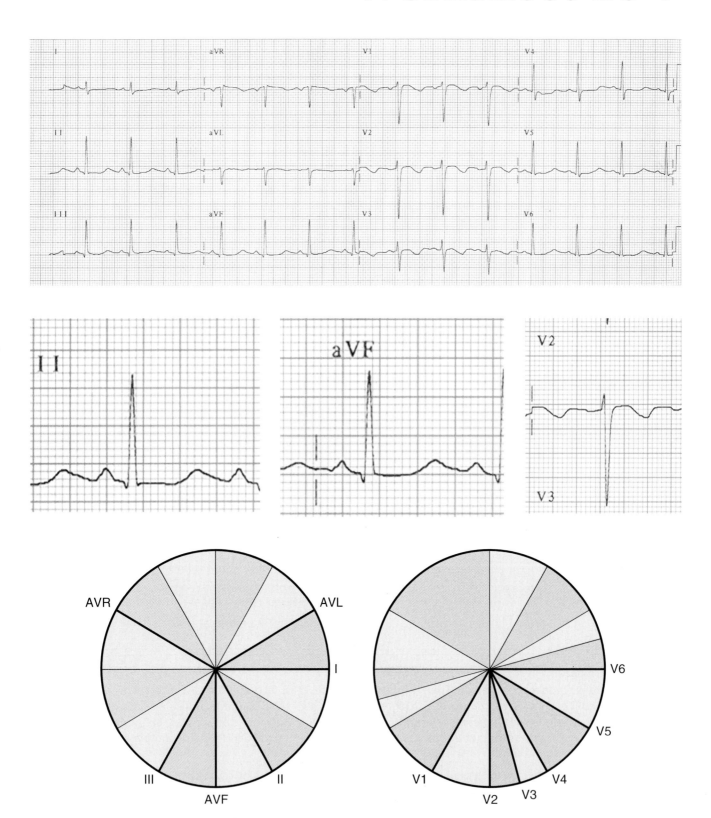

Heart Rate:

Rhythm:

Intervals (measured in the limb leads)

PR: short (< .12)
normal (.12 to .20)
long (>0.20 seconds); this is 1st degree AV block

QRS: normal ($\leq$0.09 seconds)
prolonged (.10 or .11); this is intraventricular conduction delay (IVCD)
Bundle Branch Block (.12 seconds or greater)

QT:

P axis: normal
rightward
arm-lead reversal or dextrocardia
junctional rhythm

QRS axis: normal
left anterior hemiblock
left posterior hemiblock
indeterminate

T wave inversion (ischemia or infarction):

II,III,AVF	inferior
I, AVL	lateral
V1, without V2	nonspecific septal
V1 and V2	septal
V3 and V4	anterior
V5 and V6	lateral
V6, without V5	nonspecific lateral

ST Elevation (acute infarction):

II,III,AVF	inferior
I, AVL	lateral
V1, without V2	nonspecific septal
V1 and V2	septal
V3 and V4	anterior
V5 and V6	lateral
V6, without V5.	nonspecific lateral

ST Depression (ischemia or infarction):

I,II,III,AVL,AVF	diffuse subendocardial ischemia or infarction
V2,V3,V4,V5	diffuse subendocardial ischemia or infarction

Q waves (infarction):

II,III,AVF	inferior
I, AVL	lateral
V1, without V2	nonspecific septal
V1 and V2	septal
V3 and V4	anterior
V5 and V6	lateral
V6, without V5	nonspecific lateral

Hypertrophy:

Right atrial: Tall P wave 2.5 mm in II, III, or AVF

Left atrial: Deep negative part of P wave in V1

LVH: R wave in 1 + S wave in III $\geq$ 25mV
      S wave in V1 + R wave in V5 $\geq$ 35mV

RVH: Mean QRS either anterior, or rightward

The heart rate is 83 beats per minute. The PR interval measures 0.16 seconds. The QRS interval measures 0.09 seconds. The QT interval measures 0.50 seconds. At this heart rate, the corrected QT (QTc) is greater than 500 ms. This is dangerously long. The T wave amplitude is low. This indicates hypokalemia. The P axis is normal (+60°). The mean QRS axis is +75° in the frontal plane and −22.5° in the horizontal plane. The diffuse ST and T wave changes throughout the EKG may represent subendocardial ischemia or be due to hypokalemia or both.

Long or short QT intervals suggest drug effect/toxicity or electrolyte imbalance. The combination of low-amplitude T waves, a long QT interval, and diffuse ST segment changes all suggest severe hypokalemia.

The most common cause of this EKG is hypokalemia. The most common cause of hypokalemia is renal loss due to diuretics or GI loss.

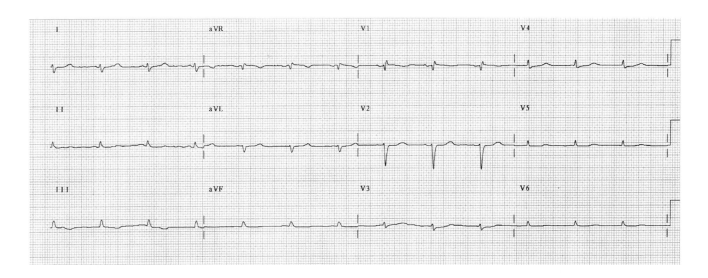

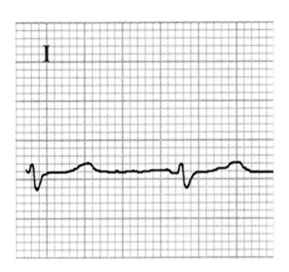

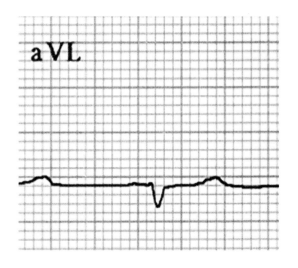

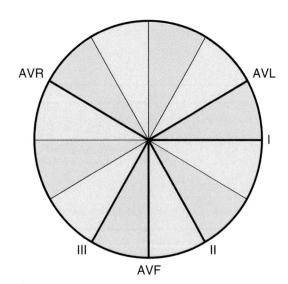

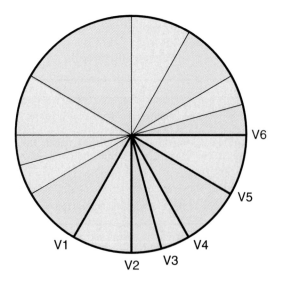

Heart Rate:

Rhythm:

Intervals (measured in the limb leads)

PR: short (< .12)
        normal (.12 to .20)
        long (>0.20 seconds); this is 1st degree AV block

QRS: normal (≤0.09 seconds)
        prolonged (.10 or .11); this is intraventricular conduction delay (IVCD)
        Bundle Branch Block (.12 seconds or greater)

QT:

P axis: normal
           rightward
           arm-lead reversal or dextrocardia
           junctional rhythm

QRS axis: normal
             left anterior hemiblock
             left posterior hemiblock
             indeterminate

T wave inversion (ischemia or infarction):

II,III,AVF	inferior
I, AVL	lateral
V1, without V2	nonspecific septal
V1 and V2	septal
V3 and V4	anterior
V5 and V6	lateral
V6, without V5	nonspecific lateral

ST Elevation (acute infarction):

II,III,AVF	inferior
I, AVL	lateral
V1, without V2	nonspecific septal
V1 and V2	septal
V3 and V4	anterior
V5 and V6	lateral
V6, without V5.	nonspecific lateral

ST Depression (ischemia or infarction):

I,II,III,AVL,AVF	diffuse subendocardial ischemia or infarction
V2,V3,V4,V5	diffuse subendocardial ischemia or infarction

Q waves (infarction):

II,III,AVF	inferior
I, AVL	lateral
V1, without V2	nonspecific septal
V1 and V2	septal
V3 and V4	anterior
V5 and V6	lateral
V6, without V5	nonspecific lateral

Hypertrophy:

Right atrial: Tall P wave 2.5 mm in II, III, or AVF

Left atrial: Deep negative part of P wave in V1

LVH: R wave in 1 + S wave in III ≥ 25mV
        S wave in V1 + R wave in V5 ≥ 35mV

RVH: Mean QRS either anterior, or rightward

The heart rate is 75 beats per minute. The PR interval measures 0.12 to 0.14 seconds. Although the P wave is present in lead I, it is of very low voltage and difficult to read with confidence. The QRS complexes also have low voltage. The QRS interval is 0.09 seconds. The QT interval measures 0.36 seconds. The P axis cannot be determined. The mean QRS axis in the frontal plane is +105°. This indicates RVH or possibly LPHB. The T waves are of low voltage, as are all the waves and complexes on the EKG. They are diffusely but nonspecifically abnormal at most.

The most common cause of low voltage and a rightward QRS axis (RVH) is COPD. A large pericardial effusion could give low voltage, but unless there was hypothyroidism, the heart rate would typically be faster. Pulmonary embolism does not produce low voltage.

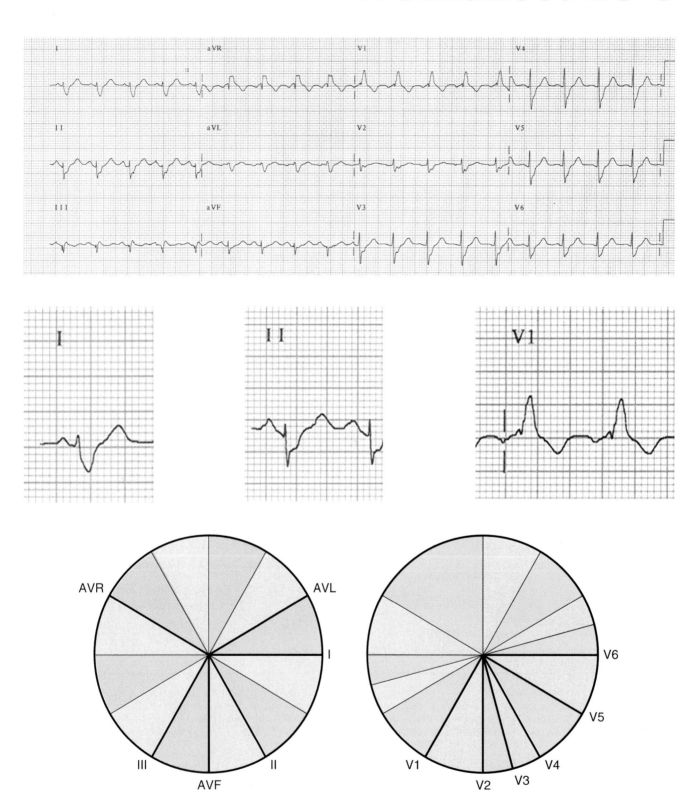

Heart Rate:

Rhythm:

Intervals (measured in the limb leads)

PR: short (< .12)
     normal (.12 to .20)
     long (>0.20 seconds); this is 1st degree AV
     block

QRS: normal (≤0.09 seconds)
     prolonged (.10 or .11); this is intraventricular
     conduction delay (IVCD)
     Bundle Branch Block (.12 seconds or greater)

QT:

P axis: normal
           rightward
           arm-lead reversal or dextrocardia
           junctional rhythm

QRS axis: normal
           left anterior hemiblock
           left posterior hemiblock
           indeterminate

T wave inversion (ischemia or infarction):

II,III,AVF	inferior
I, AVL	lateral
V1, without V2	nonspecific septal
V1 and V2	septal
V3 and V4	anterior
V5 and V6	lateral
V6, without V5	nonspecific lateral

ST Elevation (acute infarction):

II,III,AVF	inferior
I, AVL	lateral
V1, without V2	nonspecific septal
V1 and V2	septal
V3 and V4	anterior
V5 and V6	lateral
V6, without V5.	nonspecific lateral

ST Depression (ischemia or infarction):

| I,II,III,AVL,AVF | diffuse subendocardial ischemia or infarction |
| V2,V3,V4,V5 | diffuse subendocardial ischemia or infarction |

Q waves (infarction):

II,III,AVF	inferior
I, AVL	lateral
V1, without V2	nonspecific septal
V1 and V2	septal
V3 and V4	anterior
V5 and V6	lateral
V6, without V5	nonspecific lateral

Hypertrophy:

Right atrial: Tall P wave 2.5 mm in II, III, or AVF

Left atrial: Deep negative part of P wave in V1

LVH: R wave in 1 + S wave in III ≥ 25mV
      S wave in V1 + R wave in V5 ≥ 35mV

RVH: Mean QRS either anterior, or rightward

The heart rate is 107 beats per minute. The rhythm is sinus tachycardia. The PR interval measures 0.16 seconds. The QRS interval measures 0.14 seconds. This is BBB. The last part of the QRS points toward the right ventricle. This indicates RBBB. The mean QRS axis in the frontal plane is 180°. This is an unusual axis, but probably represents LPHB. The ST segment in V1 points away from the last part of the QRS, and this is the expected result in RBBB. A left atrial abnormality is present.

The most likely cause of this EKG is conduction disease. By itself, RBBB, even with LPHB or LAHB, does not indicate that ischemic disease is present.

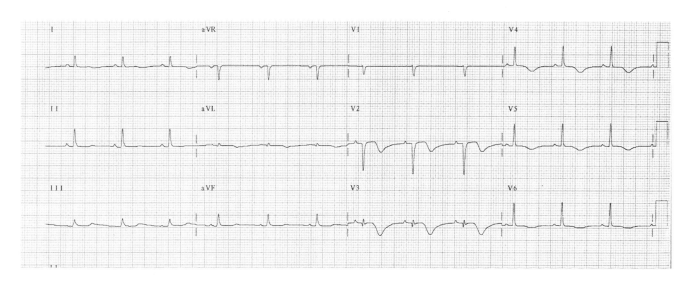

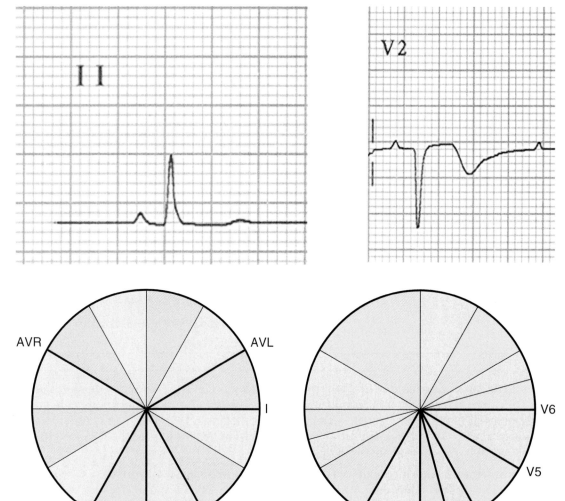

Heart Rate:

Rhythm:

Intervals (measured in the limb leads)

PR: short (< .12)
     normal (.12 to .20)
     long (>0.20 seconds); this is 1st degree AV
     block

QRS: normal (≤0.09 seconds)
     prolonged (.10 or .11); this is intraventricular
     conduction delay (IVCD)
     Bundle Branch Block (.12 seconds or greater)

QT:

P axis: normal
          rightward
          arm-lead reversal or dextrocardia
          junctional rhythm

QRS axis: normal
          left anterior hemiblock
          left posterior hemiblock
          indeterminate

T wave inversion (ischemia or infarction):

II,III,AVF	inferior
I, AVL	lateral
V1, without V2	nonspecific septal
V1 and V2	septal
V3 and V4	anterior
V5 and V6	lateral
V6, without V5	nonspecific lateral

ST Elevation (acute infarction):

II,III,AVF	inferior
I, AVL	lateral
V1, without V2	nonspecific septal
V1 and V2	septal
V3 and V4	anterior
V5 and V6	lateral
V6, without V5.	nonspecific lateral

ST Depression (ischemia or infarction):

I,II,III,AVL,AVF	diffuse subendocardial ischemia or infarction
V2,V3,V4,V5	diffuse subendocardial ischemia or infarction

Q waves (infarction):

II,III,AVF	inferior
I, AVL	lateral
V1, without V2	nonspecific septal
V1 and V2	septal
V3 and V4	anterior
V5 and V6	lateral
V6, without V5	nonspecific lateral

Hypertrophy:

Right atrial: Tall P wave 2.5 mm in II, III, or AVF

Left atrial: Deep negative part of P wave in V1

LVH: R wave in 1 + S wave in III ≥ 25mV
     S wave in V1 + R wave in V5 ≥ 35mV

RVH: Mean QRS either anterior, or rightward

The heart rate is 74 beats per minute. The PR interval measures 0.14 seconds. The QRS interval measures 0.08 seconds. The QT interval measures 0.40 seconds (which is long) but is difficult to measure, suggesting hypokalemia. The P axis is normal. The mean QRS axis is +60° in the frontal plane and −15° in the horizontal plane. The frontal plane T axis is nonspecific. In the horizontal plane, the initial QRS axis is abnormal and points away from the septum and anterior wall, indicating transmural infarction. Because the ST and T axes are abnormal, the infarction is possibly acute.

The most common cause of this EKG is a ruptured atherosclerotic plaque in the LAD. A superimposed thrombus formed a 100% obstruction to flow that led to ST elevation and a subsequent transmural infarction. Hypokalemia or a QT prolonging drug may be present.

Answers to EKGs

CHAPTER 4: Some additional diagnoses.

Question 1: The PR is 0.16. The QRS is 0.08. The QT is 0.34, normal. The P axis (+45°) is normal. The mean QRS axis is −15° in the frontal plane and −45° in the horizontal plane. The ST axis in the frontal plane is +150°, and in the horizontal plane +150°. There is a voltage criterion for LVH in the frontal plane (R in I plus the S in III measure >25 mm). There is a left atrial abnormality. The initial QRS is abnormal in leads II and III (Q waves are present). This can be due to inferior wall infarction or possibly by a false-positive finding due to LVH. Remember, the most common cause of LVH is hypertension, which is a major risk factor for CAD. The ST segment abnormality may be secondary to LVH to ischemia.

Question 2: The PR is 0.12, the QRS 0.09, and the QT 0.38 sec. The QTc is long. The P axis is normal (+75°). The mean QRS is +75° (FP) and −7.5° (HP). The T axis is +60° (FP) and +60 (HP). The voltage present does not meet our criteria for LVH, but because it appears larger than normal, it can be documented by calling it "high QRS voltage."

Question 3: The PR is 0.12, the QRS 0.08, and the QT 0.44, all of which are normal. The P axis (+30°) is normal. The mean QRS axis is +45° (FP) and −7.5° (HP). The T axis is +30° (FP) and +15° (HP). The horizontal T axis is nonspecific.

Question 4: The PR interval is 0.12, the QRS 0.09, and the QT 0.28; all are normal. The P axis (+30°) is normal. The mean QRS axis is +75° (FP) and −7.5° (HP) and is normal. The T axis is +30° (FP) and +30° (HP), which is normal. The initial QRS is borderline abnormal in II, III, and AVF. This is nonspecific inferior Q waves. There is high QRS voltage.

Question 5: The PR interval is 0.14, the QRS 0.08, and the QT 0.30; all are normal. The P axis (+60°) is normal. The mean QRS is +45° (FP) and −7.5° (HP), which is normal. **ST depression is present in V5 and V6, but it doesn't reach 1 mm in depth, so it is less specific (nonspecific lateral ST changes).**

CHAPTER 5

Question 1: The P axis (+75°) is normal. The mean QRS is +15° (FP) and −22.5° (HP). There are nonspecific inferior Q waves. There is borderline criteria in the V leads for LVH. The initial QRS is negative in V1 and borderline in V2. **This may represent QRS changes due to LVH or represent the possibility of septal infarction.**

Question 2: The P axis is normal. The mean QRS is +15° (FP) and +15° (HP). The QRS axis is anterior in the horizontal plane but not enough to confidently call it RVH. The T axis in the frontal plane is indeterminate due to its low amplitude and is normal in the horizontal plane. **There are diffuse nonspecific ST and T wave abnormalities, which are likely due to hypokalemia.**

Question 3: The P axis is normal. The mean QRS axis is +60° (FP) and −22.5° (HP). The T axis is +60° (FP) and +60° (HP). There are diffuse ST segment abnormalities, likely due to electrolyte or drug effect.

Question 4: The P axis is normal. The mean QRS is +45° (FP) and −7.5° (HP). The T waves and ST segments are diffusely but nonspecifically abnormal and are likely due to the underlying electrolyte disturbance. **The initial QRS axis is negative in V1 and V2. Causes of this include septal infarction, large breasts, COPD, and thyroid disease.** Obviously, this should be correlated with the clinical history.

Question 5: The P axis is difficult to see, but is probably in the normal range; call it normal or indeterminate. **The mean QRS axis is isoelectric in every lead in the frontal plane. This is called "indeterminate QRS axis."** The initial QRS is abnormal in the V leads and is negative in V1, V2, and V3, consistent with septal and anterior wall infarction. **The conduction disease may have been caused by the septal infarction.** The inferior leads demonstrate Q waves as well and suggest inferior infarction.

CHAPTER 6: Additional diagnoses

Question 1: There is LVH, LAA, and borderline RAA.

Question 2: **The initial QRS is negative in V1 and borderline in V2. Septal infarction, large breasts, COPD, can all cause this.**

Question 3: None.

Question 4: Nonspecific inferior Q waves.

Question 5: LVH. The ST segments are diffusely abnormal, secondary to LVH or electrolyte abnormalities.

Question 6: LBBB. The ST segments are abnormal and consistent with LBBB. Do not diagnose hemiblock in the setting of LBBB. **Do not diagnose septal and anterior MI, and do not read Q waves in the face of LBBB.**

Question 7: The QT interval is long for this rate. The Q waves in I and AVL are nonspecifically abnormal, and should be correlated with other clinical data.

CHAPTER 7: Additional diagnoses

Question 1: Don't read any further when the limb leads are reversed. Repeat the EKG.

Question 2: None.

Question 3: Don't read any further. Repeat the EKG with all the leads (limb and precordial) done in a mirror image reversal about the patient's midline.

Question 4: Borderline LVH. (Call that "high QRS voltage"). There are ST segment changes in the lateral leads, which may be due to LVH.

Question 5: T wave changes in leads V1 and V2 suggest septal ischemia or infarction. However, digitalis causes ST and T changes. Worry about both.

CHAPTER 8: Additional diagnoses

Question 1: None.

Question 2: None.

Question 3: Because LPHB is present, the diagnosis of LVH is less reliable in the frontal plane. Nonspecific inferior T changes.

Question 4: RBBB. The ST segment axis does not point away from the last part of the QRS. Therefore, ischemia must be included in the suggested diagnoses. (Anterior subendocardial ischemia or infarction.)

Question 5: Nonspecific inferior Q waves are present. Inferior MI should be ruled out clinically or by other means.

CHAPTER 9: Additional diagnoses

Question 1: None (don't **diagnose RVH in the presence of RBBB**).

Question 2: None.

Question 3: None.

Question 4: The initial QRS is abnormal and points away from the septal consistent with septal infarction. (Q waves are present in V1 and V2.) RBBB does not alter the initial forces of the QRS.

Question 5: The initial QRS in V1, V2, and V3 is borderline negative. Again, this may be due to infarction, COPD, large breasts, thyroid disease, or pericardial effusion.

CHAPTER 10: Additional diagnoses

Questions 1, 2, 3: None.

Questions 4, 5: LAA.

CHAPTER 11: Additional diagnoses

Question 1: None.

Question 2: LVH.

Question 3: Initial QRS is abnormal and points away from the septum, consistent with septal infarction.

Question 4: LAA.

Question 5: RAA. The Q in III is nonspecific.

Question 6: Borderline low voltage.

Question 7: High QRS voltage. Voltage appears increased but doesn't meet criteria for LVH.

Question 8: RAA, high QRS voltage.

CHAPTER 12: Additional diagnoses

Questions 1, 2: None.

Question 3: Low voltage. Initial QRS is abnormal in V1 through V4. This is due to septal and anterior infarction or to whatever is causing the low voltage. **COPD could cause both low voltage and abnormal initial QRS complexes in the septal and anterior leads.**

Question 4: The initial QRS in the inferior leads (II, III, and AVF) is abnormal. This suggests inferior wall infarction. The initial QRS is abnormal in V1 and V2 and suggests the possibility of posterior infarction as well.

Question 5: LAA, nonspecific septal Q wave.

Question 6: None.

CHAPTER 13: Additional diagnoses

Question 1: The initial QRS points away from the septum and anterior wall (V1, V2, and V3), consistent with septal and anterior transmural infarction, possibly acute. These ST segment elevations may be 6 hours old with an acute 100% occlusion, or 1 year old in the presence of a left ventricular aneurysm. Clinical information is critical. LAA.

Question 2: The initial QRS points away from the septum and anterior wall (V1, V2, and V3), consistent with septal and anterior transmural infarction, possibly acute.

Question 3: Nonspecific inferior Q waves.

Question 4: Borderline LVH (or "high QRS voltage"). Initial QRS is abnormal in I and AVL and suggests lateral infarction.

Question 5: None.

CHAPTER 14: Additional diagnoses

Questions 1, 2: None.

Question 3: LAA, LVH.

Question 4: LVH.

Question 5: Low voltage.

CHAPTER 15: Additional diagnoses

Question 1: Low voltage. The initial QRS in V1 and V2 is abnormal. This suggests infarction. However, because low voltage is present, the cause of the low voltage (COPD, large breasts, thyroid disease) may also reduce the voltage in V1 and V2, giving the (false-positive) appearance of a septal infarction. Clinical determination should be made by other means.

Question 2: None.

Question 3: Low voltage. This reduces the specificity of the septal and anterior Q waves, as in question 1 of this chapter.

Questions 4, 5: None.

CHAPTER 16: Additional diagnoses

Question 1, 2, 4, 5: None.

Question 3: High QRS voltage.

CHAPTERS 17, 18, 19, 20: Additional diagnoses
None.

Index

A

Amplitude of waves, 18
Anatomy of heart, 1–4
Anterior descending artery, left, 7, 9, 10
   complete occlusion of, transmural infarction resulting from, 298–304
Aortic regurgitation, left ventricular hypertrophy and, 336
Aortic stenosis, left ventricular hypertrophy and, 337
Aortic valve, 6
Artifacts, with change in EKG leads, 15
ASD (atrial septal defect), right ventricular hypertrophy with, 355
Atherosclerosis
   coronary artery occlusion in, 211, 282
      transmural ischemia due to, 259–260
   in end arteries, 12
Atria, 4
   abnormalities of, 316–323
      in dilated cardiomyopathy, 379
      in mitral valve disease, 321–323
   depolarization of
      in dextrocardia, 140
      with junctional rhythm, 139
      P wave axis with, 140
   electrical activation of. *See* Atria, depolarization of; P waves
   left, 4, 6
      abnormalities of, 316, 319–320, 323, 379
      dilation of, mitral stenosis and, 322
   right, 4, 6
      abnormalities of, 316, 317–318
      enlargement of, 138, 316, 317, 318
      hypertrophy of, 138, 316, 317, 322
      P wave axis with abnormalities of, 138
      sinoatrial node, 22
Atrial appendage, left, 319
Atrial fibrillation, heart rate in, 34
Atrial septal defect (ASD), right ventricular hypertrophy with, 355
Atrioventricular (AV) block, first degree, 52, 53
Atrioventricular (AV) bypass tract, 52, 54
Atrioventricular (AV) node, 21, 24
Axis, 74–120
   calculation in frontal plane, 79–85
      combination of leads and, 88, 91, 95, 98, 105
      frontal plane leads as observers and, 79
      lead AVF and, 83–85, 87, 91, 95, 97, 98, 100, 102, 103, 105, 107
      lead AVL and, 92–95, 103–104
      lead AVR and, 105–106, 107
      lead I and, 80–82, 86, 91, 95, 96, 98, 100, 101, 103, 105, 107
      lead II and, 103–104, 105, 107
      lead III and, 89–91, 95, 99–100
   calculation in horizontal plane, 108–120
      combination of leads and, 116, 118, 120
      horizontal plane leads as observers and, 109
      lead V2 and, 112–113, 115, 116, 118, 120
      lead V3 and, 118–119, 120
      lead V4 and, 116–117, 118, 120
      lead V6 and, 110–111, 114, 116, 118, 120
   frontal plane axis diagram and, 77–78
   as means of understanding and interpreting EKG, 74–76
   P wave, 136–141
      in dextrocardia, 140, 375
      with junctional rhythm, 139
      normal, 137
      with right atrial abnormality, 138
   QRS. *See* QRS axis
   T wave. *See* T axis

B

Baseline, 17
   waves above and below, 18
Bradycardia
   hypoxia and, 387
   sinus, 32
      in hypothyroidism, 380
Bundle branch block, 152
   left, 192–198
      in dilated cardiomyopathy, 379
      frontal plane concept of, 196
      horizontal plane concept of, 197
      initial forces and, 193
      late (terminal) forces and, 195
      middle force and, 194

Bundle branch block (*continued*)
    right, 174–181
        frontal plane concept of, 179
        horizontal plane concept of, 179
        late or terminal forces and, 178
        normal QRS interval and, 175–177
        QRS interval in, 174
    ST segment depression due to, 238
Bundle branches, 24
    disease of, long QRS intervals due to, 58
    hemiblock and, 152–162
        left anterior, 154–157
        left posterior, 158–161
    left, 21, 24, 152
        in right bundle branch block, 178
    right, 21, 24, 152
Bundle of His, 21, 24

C

Calcium
    high levels of, 383
        with cancer, 389
    low levels of, 384
Cancer, 389
Cardiomyopathy, dilated, 379
CFX (circumflex) artery, 7, 9, 11
Chemotherapy, 389
Chronic obstructive pulmonary disease (COPD)
    hypoxia in, 387
    low voltage in, 386
    right ventricular hypertrophy in, 355, 359
Circulation, collateral, 12
Circumflex (CFX) artery, 7, 9, 11
Collateral circulation, 12
Conduction disturbances. *See also* Bundle branch
        block; Hemiblock
    in hypothyroidism, 380
COPD (chronic obstructive pulmonary disease)
    hypoxia in, 387
    low voltage in, 386
    right ventricular hypertrophy in, 355, 359
Coronary arteries, 7–12. *See also* Left anterior de-
        scending (LAD) artery
    complete occlusion of
        by ruptured plaque and superimposed throm-
            bus. *See* Transmural infarction
        ST segment elevation with. *See* ST segment el-
            evation (STE)
    as end arteries, 12
    left, 7, 9
    plaque in, 211, 282
    right, 7, 8
Corrected QT (cQT), 62

cQT (corrected QT), 62
Cuspid valves, 6

D

Deflections, first, 22
Degenerative diseases, PR interval in, 53
Depolarization, 22
    atrial
        in dextrocardia, 140
        with junctional rhythm, 139
        P wave axis with, 139, 140
    ventricular. *See also* QRS complex
        electrical force from, 75–76
        factors affecting, 59
        QRS complex and, 176, 177
Dextrocardia, 375
    P wave axis with, 140
Diastole, 4
    ventricular, 4
Digitalis, 385
Dilated cardiomyopathy, 379
Drug effects
    on PR interval, 53
    on QT interval, 59, 61, 385
    on ST segment, 385
    on U waves, 385

E

Einthoven, William, 14
EKG development, 14
EKG leads, 15
    artifact with change in, 15
    limb, 15, 393
        axis measurement and. *See* Axis
        intervals measured in, 48, 50
    precordial, 15, 48, 393
        axis measurement and. *See* Axis
EKG measurements, 18
EKG paper, 16
Electrical axis. *See* Axis
Electrical force, axis and, 74–76
Electrical system of heart, 20–31
    components of, 21
Electrolyte disturbances, 381–384
    QT interval and, 61, 62, 63
Embolism, pulmonary, 388
    right ventricular hypertrophy with, 355, 360
Endocardium, 2, 3
Epicardial arteries. *See* Coronary arteries; Left ante-
        rior descending (LAD) artery
Epicardium, 2, 3
Exercise, ST segment depression induced by, 239

F

Fibrillation, atrial, heart rate in, 34
Frontal plane
    axis measurement in. *See* Axis, calculation in
        frontal plane
    QRS axis in, in right ventricular hypertrophy, 356
    QRS complex in, normal, 177
    Q wave in, inferior, 286–287
    ST segment depression in, 240, 242
    T axis in, 219
    ventricular depolarization in, QRS complex and,
        177
    ventricular hypertrophy in
      left, EKG criteria for, 339
      right, EKG criteria for, 356
Frontal plane axis diagram, 77–78
Frontal plane concept
    of left bundle branch block, 196
    of right bundle branch block, 179

H

Heart
    anatomy of, 1–4
    chambers of, 4. *See also* Atria; Ventricles
    electrical system of, 20–31
      structures of, 21
    layers of, 3
    left side of, 4
    position in dextrocardia, 375
    right side of, 4
Heart rate, 32–36
    abnormal, 32
    in atrial fibrillation, 34
    calculating, 36
    importance of, 33
    measurement of, 33
    normal, 32
    QT interval correction for, 62
    table of, 35
Heart valves, 6. *See also* Valvular heart disease
Hemiblock, 152–162
    left anterior, 154–157
      example of, 155
      lead pattern with, 157
    left bundle branch and, 153
    left posterior, 158–161
      example of, 159
      lead pattern with, 182
His, bundle of, 21, 24
Horizontal plane
    axis measurement in. *See* Axis, calculation in
        horizontal plane

left ventricular hypertrophy in, EKG criteria for, 340
    QRS complex in, normal, 176
    Q waves in, anterior, 303–304
    right ventricular hypertrophy in
      EKG criteria for, 357
      QRS axis in, 357
    ST segment depression in, 241, 243
    T axis in, 220
    ventricular depolarization in, QRS complex and,
      176
Horizontal plane concept
    of left bundle branch block, 197
    of right bundle branch block, 179
Hypercalcemia, 383
    with cancer, 389
Hyperkalemia, 381
    with cancer, 389
Hypocalcemia, 384
Hypokalemia, QT interval and, 63, 382
Hypothyroidism, 380
Hypovolemia, 388
    with cancer, 389
Hypoxia, in chronic obstructive pulmonary disease,
    387

I

Infarction
    myocardial, 260
    transmural. *See* Transmural infarction
Inferior vena cava, 4
Intervals, 48–63
    measurement of, 48
    PR, 48, 49–54
      examples of, 50–52
      long, 52, 53
      normal, 49
      short, 52, 54
    QRS. *See* QRS interval
    QT. *See* QT interval
    R-R, 33
Intraventricular conduction delay (IVCD), 58
    left, QRS interval slowing in, 192
    right, QRS interval slowing in, 174
Ischemia
    myocardial, 213
    PR interval and, 53
    ST segment elevation due to, 258
    subendocardial. *See* Subendocardial ischemia
    transmural. *See* Transmural ischemia
Isoelectric complexes, 82
IVCD (intraventricular conduction delay), 58
    left, QRS interval slowing in, 192
    right, QRS interval slowing in, 174

J

Junctional rhythm, P wave axis with, 139

K

Kidney failure, with cancer, 389

L

LAD (left anterior descending) artery, 7, 9, 10
  complete occlusion of, transmural infarction resulting from, 298–304
LBBB. *See* Bundle branch block, left
Leads, 15
  axis measurement and. *See* Axis
  in frontal plane axis diagram, 77–78
  in hemiblock
    left anterior, 157
    left posterior, 182
  limb, 15
    intervals measured in, 48, 50
  precordial, 15, 48
Left anterior descending (LAD) artery, 7, 9, 10
  complete occlusion of, transmural infarction resulting from, 298–304
Left ventricular hypertrophy (LVH), 334–342
  aortic regurgitation and, 336
    aortic stenosis and, 337
  EKG criteria for, 338
    in frontal plane, 339
    in horizontal plane, 340
  mechanism of, 335
  mitral regurgitation and, 323
  mitral stenosis and, 322
  simulating anterior wall infarction, 342
  ST segment changes in, 238, 341
Limb leads, 15, 393
  axis measurement and. *See* Axis
  intervals measured in, 48, 50
Love, 390
Lung disease, chronic obstructive
  hypoxia in, 387
  low voltage in, 386
  right ventricular hypertrophy in, 355, 359
LVH. *See* Left ventricular hypertrophy (LVH)

M

Malignancies, 389
Metastatic disease, 389
Mitral regurgitation, 323
  left atrial abnormalities in, 319
Mitral stenosis, 322

Mitral valve, 6
Myocardial infarction, 260
Myocardial ischemia, 213
Myocardium, 2, 3
  blood supply to, 13
  loss of, with coronary artery occlusion, 259

N

Natural pacemaker, 21, 22
Negative complexes, 83
Negative waves, 18

P

Pacemaker, natural, 21, 22
Pain, sinus tachycardia and, 388
Paper, EKG, 16
Parietal pericardium, 2
P axis, in dextrocardia, 375
Pericardial effusion, 378
  with cancer, 389
Pericardial space, 2
Pericarditis, 376–377
Pericardium
  anatomy of, 2
  parietal, 2
  visceral, 2, 3
Plaque, in coronary arteries, 211, 282
Pleural effusion, 374
Pneumothorax, 373, 388
Positive complexes, 83
Positive waves, 18
Postoperative patients, sinus tachycardia in, 388
Potassium
  high levels of, 381
    with cancer, 389
  low levels of, QT interval and, 63, 382
Precordial leads, 15, 48, 393
  axis measurement and. *See* Axis
PR intervals, 48, 49–54
  examples of, 50–52
  long, 52, 53
  normal, 49
  short, 52, 54
PT segment depression, in pericarditis, 377
Pulmonary artery, 6
Pulmonary disease, chronic obstructive
  hypoxia in, 387
  low voltage in, 386
  right ventricular hypertrophy in, 355, 359
Pulmonary embolism, 388
  right ventricular hypertrophy with, 355, 360
Pulmonary veins, 4

Pulmonic valve, 6
Purkinje fibers, 21, 24
P wave axis, 136–141
    in dextrocardia, 140
    with junctional rhythm, 139
    normal, 137
    with right atrial abnormality, 138
P waves, 22, 23
    absence of, 23
    amplitude of, 23
    baseline and, 17
    in hyperkalemia, 381
    positive and negative, 23
    in right atrial abnormalities, 316–318

Q

QRS axis, 75–76
    hemiblock and
        left anterior, 154–156
        left posterior, 158–160, 162
    in left ventricular hypertrophy, 338–340
    in right ventricular hypertrophy
        in frontal plane, 356
        in horizontal plane, 357
QRS complex
    heart rate calculation using, 33, 34
    in hyperkalemia, 381
    initial part of. *See* Q waves
    as isoelectric complex, 82
    normal, 175–177
        in frontal plane, 177
        in horizontal plane, 176
        initial forces and, 176
        main forces and, 177
    parts of, 26–30
        examples of, 29–30
    in pneumothorax, 373
    in right ventricular hypertrophy, 354
QRS interval, 48, 55–58
    examples of, 56–57
    in left bundle branch block, 192–197
    in left intraventricular conduction delay, 192
    long, 58
    normal, 55, 175, 177
    in right bundle branch block, 174, 178–180
    in right intraventricular conduction delay, 174
QR waves, 29
Qr waves, 29
qR waves, 29
QS waves, 28, 29
QT interval, 48, 59–63
    corrected, 62
    digitalis and, 385

    examples of, 60–61
    in hypercalcemia, 383
    in hypocalcemia, 384
    in hypokalemia, 63, 382
    in hypothyroidism, 380
    indeterminate, 63
Q waves, 26, 27
    anterior, 298–304
        in horizontal plane, 303–304
        in transmural infarction, 299–304
    inferior, 280–287
        in frontal plane, 286–287
        normal, 281, 286
        in transmural infarction, 282–287
q waves, 281

R

Radiation therapy, 389
RBBB. *See* Bundle branch block, right
Regurgitation, valvular, 321, 323
    aortic, left ventricular hypertrophy and, 336
    mitral, 319, 323
    tricuspid, right ventricular hypertrophy with, 355
Renal failure, with cancer, 389
Repolarization, ventricular. *See* T axis; T waves
Right ventricular hypertrophy (RVH), 354–360
    in chronic obstructive pulmonary disease, 359
    EKG criteria for
        in frontal plane, 356
        in horizontal plane, 357
    with pulmonary embolism, 360
    ST segment changes in, 238, 358
R-R interval, 33
RR′ waves, 337
RSr′ waves, 29
rSR′ waves, 29
RS waves, 29
Rs waves, 29, 337
rS waves, 29, 337
RVH. *See* Right ventricular hypertrophy (RVH)
R waves, 26, 27, 29, 337
    heart rate calculation using, 33
R′ (R prime) waves, 29

S

SA (sinoatrial) node, 21, 22
Semilunar valves, 6
Septum, 4
Sinoatrial (SA) node, 21, 22
Sinus bradycardia, 32
    in hypothyroidism, 380
Sinus rhythm, 32

Sinus tachycardia, 32
    with cancer, 389
    in pericardial effusion, 378
    in pericarditis, 376
    in postoperative patients, 388
Standardized voltage, 19
STE. *See* ST segment elevation (STE)
Stenosis, valvular, 321, 323
    left ventricular hypertrophy and, 337
    mitral, 322
ST segment
    depression of, 238–244
        exercise induction of, 239
        frontal plane, 240, 242
        horizontal plane, 241, 243
        summary chart of, 244
    digitalis and, 385
    in hypokalemia, 382
    in left ventricular hypertrophy, 341
    in pericarditis, 377
ST segment elevation (STE), 258–268
    bulging upward, 258
    sway back, 258
    transmural ischemia and, 259–268, 282
        anterior wall, 265
        apical wall, 264
        inferior wall, 261–263
        lateral wall, 264
        pathophysiology of, 259–260
        septal, 265
ST waves, in right ventricular hypertrophy, 358
Subendocardial ischemia, 211–213, 266, 268
    anatomy of, 211–212
    anterior wall, 218, 219, 220, 221
    apical wall, 217, 219, 220, 221
    inferior wall, 215, 219, 220, 221
    lateral wall, 215, 219, 220, 221
    septal, 218, 221
    ST segment depression in, 239
Subendocardial tissue, blood supply to, 13
Superior vena cava, 4
S waves, 27, 179, 180
s waves, 27
Systole
    left ventricle in, 20
    ventricular, 25

T

Tachycardia, sinus, 32
    with cancer, 389
    in pericardial effusion, 378
    in pericarditis, 376

    in postoperative patients, 388
T axis, 210–221
    calculating, 84
    frontal plane, 219
    horizontal plane, 220
    inversions of, chart of, 221
    normal, 214
    subendocardial ischemia and, 211–213
        anatomy of ischemia and, 211–212
        of anterior wall, 218
        of apical wall, 217
        of inferior wall, 215
        of lateral wall, 216
        septal, 218
Thromboembolism, venous, 360
Thrombus
    complete occlusion of coronary arteries by rup-
        tured plaque and. *See* Transmural infarction
    in left atrial appendage, 319
Time lines, 32
Transmural infarction, 282–287, 298–304
    anterior wall, 299, 302, 303, 304
    apical, 284, 286, 287
    inferior wall, 283, 286, 287
        left ventricular hypertrophy simulating, 342
    lateral wall, 284, 286, 287, 302, 303, 304
    nonspecific inferior Q waves and, 285, 286
    posterior wall, 303, 304
    septal, 299, 300–301, 303, 304
        left bundle branch block complicating, 301
        left ventricular hypertrophy simulating, 342
        right bundle branch block and left arterial
            hemiblock complicating, 300
Transmural ischemia
    anterior wall, 265, 267, 268
    apical, 264, 266, 268
    inferior wall, 261–262, 266, 268
        posterior extension of, 263
        reciprocal changes in, 262
    lateral wall, 264, 266, 267, 268
    posterior wall, 267
    septal, 265, 267, 268
    ST segment elevation due to. *See* ST segment ele-
        vation (STE)
Tricuspid regurgitation, right ventricular hypertro-
        phy with, 355
Tricuspid valve, 6
T waves, 31
    baseline and, 17
    factors affecting, 59
    in hyperkalemia, 381
    in hypokalemia, 382
    in right ventricular hypertrophy, 358

U

U waves
  digitalis and, 385
  in hypokalemia, 382

V

Valves. *See* Heart valves
Valvular heart disease
  aortic, 336–337
  atrial abnormalities in, 321–323
  mitral, 319, 322–323
  regurgitation as, 319, 321, 323, 336, 337, 355
    aortic, left ventricular hypertrophy and, 336
    mitral, 319, 323
    tricuspid, right ventricular hypertrophy with, 355
  stenotic, 321, 322, 323, 337
    left ventricular hypertrophy and, 337
    mitral, 322
  tricuspid, 355
Vena cavae, 4
Venous thromboembolism (VTE), 360
Ventricles, 4
  hypertrophy of. *See* Left ventricular hypertrophy (LVH); Right ventricular hypertrophy (RVH)
  left, 4, 6, 25
    in systole, 20
  right, 4, 6, 25

Ventricular depolarization, 25. *See also* QRS complex
  electrical force from, 75–76
  factors affecting, 59
  QRS complex and
    in frontal plane, 177
    in horizontal plane, 176
Ventricular diastole, 4
Ventricular repolarization. *See* T axis; T waves
Visceral pericardium, 2, 3
V leads, 15, 48
  axis measurement and. *See* Axis
Voltage
  low
    with cancer, 389
    in chronic obstructive pulmonary disease, 386
    with chronic obstructive pulmonary disease, 359
    in dextrocardia, 375
    in hypothyroidism, 380
    with pleural effusion, 374
    with pneumothorax, 373
  standardized, 19
VTE (venous thromboembolism), 360

W

Wolff-Parkinson-White (WPW) syndrome, 52, 54